The Pap Smear: Controversies in Practice

Edited by

Barbara S Ducatman MD
Department of Pathology
Robert C Byrd Health Sciences Center of West Virginia
University
Morgantown, WV, USA

Helen H Wang MD DRPH
Department of Pathology
Beth Israel Deaconess Medical Center
Harvard Medical School
Boston, MA, USA

A member of the Hodder Headline Group
LONDON • NEW YORK • NEW DELHI

First published in Great Britain in 2002 by
Arnold, a member of the Hodder Headline Group,
338 Euston Road, London NW1 3BH

http://www.arnoldpublishers.com

Distributed in the United States of America by
Oxford University Press Inc.,
198 Madison Avenue, New York, NY10016
Oxford is a registered trademark of Oxford University Press

Whilst the advice and information in this book are believed to be true and
accurate at the date of going to press, neither the authors nor the publisher
can accept any legal responsibility or liability for any errors or omissions
that may be made. In particular (but without limiting the generality of the
preceding disclaimer) every effort has been made to check drug dosages;
however it is still possible that errors have been missed. Furthermore,
dosage schedules are constantly being revised and new side-effects
recognized. For these reasons the reader is strongly urged to consult the
drug companies' printed instructions before administering any of the drugs
recommended in this book.

British Library Cataloguing in Publication Data
A catalogue record for this book is available from the British Library

Library of Congress Cataloging-in-Publication Data
A catalog record for this book is available from the Library of Congress

ISBN 0 340 75928 3 (hb)

1 2 3 4 5 6 7 8 9 10

Publisher: Georgina Bentliff
Development Editor: Michael Lax
Production Editor: Anke Ueberberg
Production Controller: Bryan Eccleshall

Typeset in 10/12 Minion by Charon Tec Pvt. Ltd, India
Printed and bound in Malta by Gutenberg Press

This book is dedicated to our mothers: Rosina Steinmetz and to the memory of Tien-yuan Wang (1924–1996), to whom we owe our existence, who we are and what we are; and to mothers everywhere.

Contents

Contributors

Catherine S Abendroth MD
Chief, Anatomic Pathology and Medical Director of Cytopathology, The Penn State Milton S Hershey Medical Center, Associate Professor of Pathology, Pennsylvania State University College of Medicine, Hershey, PA

Graziella Abu-Jawdeh MD
Assistant Professor of Pathology, Beth Israel Deaconess Medical Center, Harvard Medical School, Boston, MA

Linda L Cook MD
Assistant Professor of Pathology, Robert C Byrd Health Sciences Center of West Virginia University, Morgantown, WV

Barbara S Ducatman MD
Professor and Chair, Department of Pathology, Robert C Byrd Health Sciences Center of West Virginia University, Morgantown, WV

Linnea W Garcia MD
Department of Pathology, North Shore Medical Center Salem – Hospital, Salem, MA

David R Genest MD
Associate Professor of Pathology, Brigham and Women's Hospital, Harvard Medical School, Boston, MA

Jorge L Gonzalez MD
Director of Cytopathology, Dartmouth-Hitchcock Medical Center, Assistant Professor of Pathology, Dartmouth Medical School, Lebanon, NH

Robert A Goulart MD
Department of Pathology, Baystate Medical Center, Assistant Professor of Pathology, Tufts University School of Medicine, Springfield, MA

Shirley E Greening, MS JD CFIAC
Professor and Chairman, Department of Laboratory Sciences, Program Director, Cytotechnology, Health Policy Liaison, College of Health Professions, Thomas Jefferson University, Philadelphia, PA

Christina Isacson MD
Assistant Professor of Pathology, New York Presbyterian Hospital – Cornell Medical Center, Joan and Sanford I. Weill Medical College of Cornell University, New York, NY

R Gerald Pretorius MD
Department of Obstetrics and Gynecology, Southern California Permanente Medical Center – Fontana, Fontana, CA

Mark E Sherman MD
Associate Professor of Pathology and Oncology, The Johns Hopkins University, School of Medicine, Baltimore, MD

Jeffrey A Stead MD
Associate Professor of Pathology, Robert C Byrd Health Sciences Center of West Virginia University, Morgantown, WV

R Shawn Underwood CT (ASCP)
Department of Pathology, Dartmouth-Hitchcock Medical Center, Lebanon, NH

Helen H Wang MD DRPH
Director of Cytopathology, Beth Israel Deaconess Medical Center, Associate Professor of Pathology, Harvard Medical School, Boston, MA

Preface

Few medical laboratory tests have altered so little for so long and then generated so much controversy as the Pap smear. For approximately 40 years collection, preparation and diagnosis remained virtually unchanged. Recently, a series of regulatory, scientific and technologic shocks transformed this humble test. Its future is exciting and unpredictable.

This book is designed to provide a comprehensive overview of cervical neoplasia screening at the start of the new millennium to pathologists, cytotechnologists, gynecologists, nurse practitioners and public health personnel. We have chosen to emphasize the introduction and discussion of new technologies and approaches to problematic areas rather than to concentrate on a more traditional morphological approach. In doing so, we have striven to provide the most up to date information available at the time and hope that it will help the reader to understand future developments.

We hope that this book aids in the diagnosis and management of women with abnormal Pap smears. However, we caution that we must remember to treat our patients rather than their test results. Furthermore, we acknowledge sadly that the most common reason for cervical cancer death is still lack of access to any Pap smear testing. We hope we have succeeded in conveying the rewards, challenges and frustrations of dealing with a population-based screening test that, nonetheless, carries important implications for each individual woman.

Acknowledgments

The authors wish to acknowledge several individuals for their help with this book. For help with many of the pictures we thank Linda Tomago. For preparation of bibliographies for most of the chapters we thank Edith Hurney.

In addition, we thank our long-suffering chapter authors for their patience with this long and sometimes painful process. Our editor, Georgina Bentliff, has been unflagging in her support and advice. Finally, we acknowledge each other. This book has been a collaboration via email and telephone. Without our long-standing and deep friendship, we would never have completed it.

Introduction

HELEN H WANG, BARBARA S DUCATMAN

HISTORICAL PERSPECTIVE

Background

The least understood important concept of the Pap smear for patients, pathologists, gynecologists and nurses is perhaps its actual purpose. Contrary to popular belief, the purpose of the Pap smear is to screen for cervical cancer and its precursor lesions, not to diagnose them. This distinction is crucial for understanding the use, misuse and limitations of the procedure. This first and most crucial misunderstanding is just one of many myths that have arisen over time.

George Papanicolaou, the 'father' of the Pap smear, was actually neither a pathologist nor a gynecologist. He was an anatomist; the original Papanicolaou smear was designed to assess the hormonal status of mice. This was not a cervical smear, rather, it used vaginal pool material initially in mice and later in women.[1,2] Papanicolaou was not the first to propose cellular sampling as a means of cervical cancer diagnosis. A Romanian pathologist, Aurelia Babes, initially described a direct cervical smear a year earlier than Papanicolaou's earliest reports.[3,4] J. Ernest Ayre, a Canadian gynecologist, designed the spatula, named in his honor, which was used for many years thereafter to directly sample the cervix.[5]

Although the American Cancer Society endorsed the Pap smear in 1945, the reception was not overwhelmingly enthusiastic. In particular, the more senior pathology community expressed reservations, a situation not unfamiliar to those who witnessed the development of fine needle aspiration cytology in the USA some 30 years later. Despite these initial doubts, the popularity of the test among the medical and lay community increased until it became standard practice for a woman to undergo an annual Pap test.

In the celebration of the triumph of the Pap smear, an unjustified expectation of Pap smears was established. The dramatic decrease in incidence and mortality rates of cervical cancer since the introduction of the screening program with Pap smear reached a plateau in the 1980s.[6] At the same time, those that contributed to this triumph – cytology laboratories with cytotechnologists and cytopathologists – did not receive comparable credit or compensation for the work they performed. It was as though the Pap smears became the hero at the expense of those who made them possible. Routine Pap smears themselves became an unjustified assurance of freedom from cervical cancer without enforcement of proper reading of the Pap smears.

Unfortunately, the Pap smear is by no means a panacea for cervical carcinoma, and problems, exacerbated by poor laboratory practices, led to an article on Pap smears in 1987 by Walt Bogdanich in the *Wall Street Journal*.[7] It is truly unfortunate that the gynecology and particularly the pathology communities had previously turned a blind eye to the abuses of screening described. These problems were made worse by the increasing commercialization of reference laboratories, but are by no means unique to commercial laboratories. Owing to the large volume of Pap smears, cervical screening had become a significant industry. The lack of regulation made it readily exploitable by a few profit-oriented commercial laboratories. In such laboratories, cytotechnologists were under pressure to read large volumes of material quickly – up to 100 cases in a 3.5-hour period. At this rate, a cytotechnologist would be screening a Pap smear every 2.1 min. In order to encourage their employees, such high-volume, low-cost laboratories often paid by piecework (as little as 50 cents per slide), thus resembling the 'sweatshops' of the turn of the century and, in fact, were often called 'Pap factories' or 'Pap mills'. Supervision was lax and, with a low prevalence of dysplasia, random rescreening of 10 per cent of cases failed to disclose significant errors. These laboratories succeeded because '… their bargain rates also appeal to budget-conscious administrators of group health plans and government-funded clinics. Thus, at a time when pressures are great to restrain medical expenses, problems with Pap-testing accuracy exemplify the possible trade-off in quality of care'.[7] On the other hand, the lack of effective cytopathology training in many pathology residency programs often led to pathologists poorly qualified to supervise cytologists or, as is the case in many smaller community hospitals, to screen Pap smears.

Whenever a story of an unfortunate fatal cervical cancer as a result of repeated false-negative Pap smears was made known, the issue of Pap smears became an easy target of sensation-seeking media. This attention helped the public to realize the importance of quality control and assurance of cytology laboratories and cytotechnologists. The historically poor compensation and the new work load limitation created a serious shortage of cytotechnologists. Consequently, the compensation of cytotechnologists increased dramatically within a short period of time. The *Wall Street Journal* brought forth some positive results in the field of cytology. However, the reimbursement for Pap smears has not been adjusted in proportion to the increased cost of Pap smears, and cytology has become a loss leader in pathology laboratories.

The initial report and follow-up and concomitant furor in the medical and lay communities undoubtedly led directly to many provisions of the Clinical Laboratory Improvement Amendments of 1988 (CLIA'88) and strict federal guidelines, making the Pap smear perhaps the most regulated of all laboratory tests. Along with federal guidelines, increasing numbers of women with cervical cancer took their physicians and laboratories to court for missed diagnoses. As a result, Pap smears have also attained the unfortunate distinction of being the most litigated laboratory procedure. Although there are benefits to the spotlight the Pap smear has been held in (remembering the abuses that led to the 1987 article), the crucial distinction that Pap smear is a screening test seems to have been lost by all but the public health community. An overreaction to the *Wall Street Journal* article is endangering the practice of cytology since it is virtually impossible to achieve 100 per cent sensitivity. The Pap smear has succeeded, for the most part admirably, in its role as a screening test and has reduced the incidence of cervical cancer, but cannot diagnose every case of cancer or pre-neoplastic lesions. It is vitally important that all who are connected with this test understand the epidemiological basis for the test and communicate its successes and limitations to the women it serves.

What is a screening test?

GOALS AND PRINCIPLES OF SCREENING

Screening was defined by the US Commission on Chronic Illness as 'the presumptive identification of unrecognized disease or defect by the application of tests, examinations, or other procedures which can be applied rapidly. Screening tests sort out apparently well persons who probably have a disease from those who probably do not'.[8] According to this definition, a screening test is applied to those who are apparently well, i.e. either asymptomatic subjects or subjects with unrecognized symptoms of the disease. The definition also emphasizes that screening is not designed to generate a definitive diagnosis; a diagnostic work-up is required for those with positive results for a screening test in order to establish the diagnosis.

On the basis of this definition, a World Health Organization monograph[9] provided a set of principles for determining when screening is appropriate on a population basis, consisting in essence of the following requirements:

1 The condition to be screened is an important cause of morbidity, disability, or mortality and is so recognized by the target population.
2 The natural history of the disease is sufficiently well known with a detectable preclinical stage identified, and treatments for the preclinical stage of the disease are more effective than those for a later stage.
3 The test has a high level of sensitivity and specificity (sensitivity is defined as the proportion of the subjects who have the disease will have a positive test result, and specificity is defined as the proportion of subjects who do not have the disease will have a negative test result).
4 The test has low risk and is acceptable to the target population and their physicians.
5 Diagnostic work up is available to those with positive test results.
6 Efficacy in reducing morbidity, disability or mortality is high enough to conclude that detection of the disease through screening will lead to a net benefit to the target population and that the resources required to administer the test under screening conditions are justified in terms of the net benefits.

It should be noted that no absolute figure or weight is attached to any of the conditions. Therefore, value judgment plays a large role in assessing the cost, risk and benefit of a screening program and in the balancing of all these costs, risks and benefits to determine the overall efficacy.

EPIDEMIOLOGICAL AND PUBLIC HEALTH CONCEPTS OF SCREENING WITH PAP SMEARS

Although Pap smears were introduced with the interest of individual women in mind, it eventually became one of the most successful public health tools to reduce the incidence and mortality of one of the most common cancer killers of women worldwide, cervical cancer. It is considered by most that what is best for the individual in a society is also the best for the society. However, this concept is not always correct. From the perspective of an individual woman, the goal of Pap smears as a screening test is to detect the disease as early as possible, not only to prevent mortality secondary to the disease but also to prevent any significant morbidity either associated with the disease itself or with the appropriate treatment for the stage of the disease. From the perspective of society, the goal of early detection also involves financial considerations, i.e. not only to minimize the morbidity and mortality (and therefore productive person-years lost) associated with the disease but also to minimize the cost incurred in the diagnosis and treatment of the disease. A highly sensitive test would satisfy the requirement of a good screening test for an individual, but for a test to be considered beneficial to society it also needs to be specific as well as low in cost. High specificity reduces the expenses incurred in the diagnostic work-up of subjects with false-positive results from the screening test.

Unfortunately, the result of a screening test is often not simply dichotomized into normal versus abnormal, and this is particularly true with Pap smears. Not only is the result of Pap smears a continuum, it is also quite subjective, especially in the borderline abnormal zone. The results of Pap smears are not only categorized as normal versus abnormal but also involve varying degrees of abnormality, if any is identified. A cytotechnologist/cytopathologist needs to determine the point at which a morphological aberration deserves to be flagged as abnormal and to what degree this abnormality should be categorized. Sensitivity can be increased at the expense of specificity and vice versa. Sensitivity and specificity cannot easily be increased simultaneously without significantly increasing the cost of the test, i.e. either having one cytotechnologist and/or cytopathologist scrutinize and ponder over a smear for a long time or having multiple technologists/pathologists review each smear. After an abnormal result is issued for a Pap smear, the clinician then needs to decide when (i.e. at which point on the diagnostic spectrum) further evaluation is indicated. If the threshold for such a work-up is low, significant lesions are less likely to be missed and more individuals have their lesions detected at an early stage. However, at the same time, more women are likely to have unnecessary diagnostic tests for either false-positive results or very early lesions that do not require treatment. The attempts to increase the sensitivity of Pap smears with better technology, such as computer-assisted rescreening, are likely to do so with much reduced cost-effectiveness. The attempts to increase both sensitivity and specificity with improved slide preparation appear to be a more rational approach, although it is still unclear whether the higher sensitivity and specificity will pay for the much increased cost of preparing optimal Pap smears.

Impact on cervical cancer incidence rate worldwide

It has been well established that Pap smears have significantly reduced the incidence rate of squamous cell carcinomas of the uterine cervix in the developed countries.[10–12] However, cervical cancer is still the most common cancer among women worldwide and the leading cancer cause of death in many developing and third-world countries.[13,14] Obviously, the availability and the acceptability of Pap smears are not as widespread in these countries as in the developed countries. The majority of cervical cancer mortality worldwide is now from these countries.

At present, the screening program with Pap smears would be most cost effective in those countries where the incidence rate of cervical cancer is still high. By the same token, in the developed countries the screening program would be most cost effective in the high-risk populations where Pap smears have not been widely used. In those populations that have Pap smears on a regular basis, the cost per case of high-grade squamous intraepithelial lesion or invasive carcinoma identified is already considerable, and much higher than that in the high-risk populations that do not have routine Pap smears. Any attempts to improve Pap smears in the former population are going to further increase such cost and decrease the cost-effectiveness of Pap smears significantly.

A trend of increasing incidence of invasive cervical carcinoma and cervical intraepithelial neoplasia has been noted among young women in many countries,[10–12,15–19] particularly for adenocarcinoma.[13,20–22] It is worth noting that the mass screening programs for cervical cancer has not made an impact on the incidence or mortality rate of cervical adenocarcinoma.[23] This increasing trend for cervical cancer may be due to the increasing prevalence of human papilloma virus (HPV) infection, a cause of cervical neoplasms, increasing prevalence of cofactors of cervical neoplasms, or a change in disease definition and reporting and screening pattern, or a combination of these.[24] While the increase in cervical intraepithelial lesions may be due to disease criteria and/or reporting, the increase in invasive carcinoma incidence is more likely caused by an increase in the prevalence of risk factors of cervical cancer and/or a change in screening pattern. At present, the reason for the increasing trend of cervical cancer is unclear and the potential increase may have been partly prevented by the screening program and we now are observing a tempered increase.

OVERVIEW OF CURRENT PROBLEMS

The reasons why Pap smears have not eradicated cervical cancer in the developed countries are many and include: failure of women to be screened at optimal intervals, or at all; failure of physicians to obtain an adequate smear, smears not being prepared adequately, failure of cytotechnologists to identify abnormal cells; failure of pathologists to classify correctly the abnormal cells; failure of physicians to recommend or provide proper follow-up and management; and failure of women to adhere to the recommended follow-up and management.[25] A discussion of each of these points and other current problems follows.

Participation/coverage of women in screening with Pap smears

Raising the participation/coverage of women in screening is the most effective measure to reduce the incidence of invasive carcinoma – much more so than changing the screening interval or increasing the specificity or sensitivity of the test.[26] According to the 1987 National Health Interview Survey in the USA, over 70 per cent of women interviewed had a Pap smear within the previous three years.[27] The proportion of women having never heard of a Pap smear was comparable for whites (2.6 per cent) and blacks (5.1 per cent), but was much higher for Hispanic women (19.7 per cent). The unfortunate paradox is that those who need to be screened the most are most likely to have no or infrequent Pap smears. This is not only true in terms of developed versus developing countries but also true on an individual basis. Based on computerized records of a large health maintenance organization in the USA with prepayment,[28] 22 per cent of women with a cancer diagnosis had no record of screening within the past 5 years compared with 8.5 per cent of the total group. It thus shows that women at highest risk for cervical cancer seemed less likely to obtain Pap smear screening, even when cost is not a barrier to care. Overall, the most frequently reported reason for not having a recent Pap smear was procrastination or not believing it was necessary.[27] Access to health care appears not to be the only barrier for women to attend Pap smear screening. However, an in-depth discussion on health education, which is clearly needed in this regard, is beyond the scope of this book.

Sampling and preparation of Pap smears

The sampling device for Pap smear has come a long way since the introduction of Ayre's spatula.[5] The various devices currently available on the market appear to be comparable in effectiveness and share a common goal of adequate sampling of the transformation zone and endocervical canal. It would be interesting to see if this will have an impact on the efficacy of detecting precursors of adenocarcinoma by Pap smears. Traditionally, the physicians or nurses who take the materials for Pap smears also prepare the smears. The cytotechnologists and cytopathologists are at the mercy of these health-care providers to prepare a proper smear for proper screening and interpretation. With the advent of thin-layer preparation techniques the cytology laboratories have the option of taking over the preparation of Pap smears to ensure quality. Another advantage of thin-layer preparation is to have material for ancillary study, such as HPV testing, if necessary. It is controversial whether the improved quality of the smear and the consequent higher detection rate of abnormal cells justify the added cost. The costs and benefits of thin-layer preparation are discussed in Chapter 3.

Accuracy of Pap smear

False-negative results are inherent in screening with Pap smears. Although efforts should be made to minimize the false-negative rate, they should not be made at the expense of accessibility to Pap smears. It has been well documented that most of the patients with invasive cervical cancer either never had a Pap smear or had not had a Pap smear in the 3–5 years before the diagnosis.[29] Less than perfectly accurate reading of Pap smears is a minor contributor to the failure of Pap smear when compared with the low participation rate among high-risk women.[29] As devastating as the impact false-negative results may be on individuals involved, an increased false-negative rate does not significantly compromise the effectiveness of reducing cervical cancer incidence rate by Pap smear screening. For example, compared with an 89 per cent reduction in the incidence rate of invasive cervical cancer for women who are at an average risk and undergo Pap smear screening annually, a 15 per cent increase in the false-negative rate for Pap smears can still cause an 88 per cent reduction in the incidence rate of invasive cervical cancer in these women.[30] Given the same 15 per cent higher false-negative rate, the reduction in the incidence rate of invasive cervical cancer is 80 per cent for those who have a Pap smear every 3 years.[30] Similarly, a recent study of the cost-effectiveness of three methods (ThinPrep, AutoPap-assisted rescreen and PAPNET-assisted rescreen) to enhance the sensitivity of Papanicolaou testing also showed that they did not decrease the mortality rate of cervical cancer and only barely reduced the incidence rate compared with a conventional Pap smear with routine 10 per cent random rescreen when women undergo annual Pap smear.[31] The impact of the increased sensitivity of new technologies on mortality and incidence rates of cervical cancer is more apparent when the interval between Pap smears increases.[31] It appears that the most effective approach is to ensure that women have frequent, regular Pap smears instead of working on the reduction of false-negative rate.

Furthermore, the false-negative rate or sensitivity is closely related to the threshold for abnormal smears (see discussion on sensitivity and specificity of Pap smears). In a study on the relationship between detection of carcinoma *in situ* of the cervix and the subsequent reduction in invasive cancer, Bergstrom et al.[32] found that detection of 100 extra cases of cancer *in situ* per 100 000 women per year in 1975 resulted in a reduction of 1.0 cases of invasive cancer 10 years later. This indicates that relaxed morphologic criteria for neoplasia/carcinoma, or lower sensitivity (thus higher false-negative rate), do not significantly increase the subsequent incidence of invasive carcinoma in a stable population undergoing regular screening. This may be due to spontaneous regression or the fact that the lesion will be identified at a later date, but still before it becomes invasive. However, relaxed criteria for neoplasia or any abnormality would significantly reduce extensive, unnecessary work-up and treatment.

Another issue associated with a reduced false-negative rate is the associated increase in cost. CLIA'88 is aimed at decreasing the false-negative rate. Consequently, the cost of Pap smears is increased in order to comply with the regulations. According to a recent mathematical model to examine the health consequences of diminished access to Pap testing,[33] the regulatory effect of CLIA'88 is very sensitive to the degree of improvement in the false-negative rate and the increase in price that the regulations cause. The proposed regulations could greatly reduce or greatly increase the incidence of invasive cancer, especially among high-risk and uninsured women, depending on how much the false-negative rate is reduced and how much the cost is increased. Therefore, the overall impact of CLIA'88 is still unclear. The full implementation of these regulations deserves further consideration. This issue is also discussed in Chapter 4.

Frequency of routine Pap smears

Regular repeats of Pap smears serve two purposes: to identify new lesions that occur after the last test and to identify old lesions that have been missed owing to either sampling error or screening/interpretation error on the previous tests. If our understanding of the natural history of cervical cancer is correct in that it takes years for an intraepithelial neoplastic lesion to progress to invasive cancer, there is no biological reason to repeat Pap smears more frequently than every 3–5 years in order to detect it just before it becomes invasive. However, because of the irreducible false negative rate of Pap smears and the possible existence of a rapidly progressing type of cervical neoplasia, it is necessary to repeat Pap smears more frequently than every 3–5 years.

The optimal interval for Pap smears is ultimately determined by resources and value judgment.[34] Theoretically, the false-negative rate should enter into the equation of calculating the optimal interval. However, it is difficult to estimate this rate, which varies according to the clinician and cytology laboratory. Both mathematical modeling and empirical data indicate that screening every 2, 3, 5, and 10 years retains 99 per cent, 97 per cent, 89 per cent and 69 per cent, respectively, of the effectiveness of annual screening, measured as a reduction in frequency of invasive cancer.[30,35] However, the reduction in cost is 50 per cent, 67 per cent, 80 per cent and 90 per cent, respectively, for screening every 2, 3, 5, and 10 years when compared with annual screening.[35] A collaborative study of screening programs in eight countries demonstrated that there was little difference in the protection afforded by screening every year compared with every 3 years, but screening only once every 5 or 10 years offered appreciably less protection.[36]

Three case-control studies that investigated the issue of frequency of Pap smears independently concluded that screenings at intervals of 2 years are virtually as effective as annual screening in preventing invasive carcinoma of cervix.[37–39] Two of the studies[38,39] also showed that screening at intervals of 3 or 5 years is associated with a much increased risk of invasive carcinoma. From another perspective, the incidence of invasive cervical carcinoma increases with the length of time since the last negative smear and reaches the level of unscreened women within 5–10 years.[40,41] Therefore, the risk associated with screening at intervals of 5 years is perhaps too great to tolerate. It is probably safe to say that screening every 2 years is almost as effective as annual screening in terms of prevention of cervical cancer but is much more cost-effective. Screening every two or more years seems desirable from the perspective of proper allocation of resources for public health.[34] However, compared with annual screening, there will be a small but definite increase in patients that develop invasive cervical cancer. When they are identified, who will be responsible for the compensation of such individuals? It is therefore doubtful that anyone who is directly responsible for the care of individual patients would recommend screening at an interval longer than 1 year.

A rational approach to this issue may be individualization of frequency of Pap smears. The American Cancer Society has used previous Pap smear results to triage patients and has recommended that women with three consecutive annual negative Pap smears can be screened less frequently. Perhaps, a better variable for triaging patients would be factors independent of Pap smears, such as social history and/or HPV test results. This issue is also discussed in Chapter 2.

Increasing rate of abnormal results, particularly ASCUS

One way to decrease the false-negative rate is to decrease the threshold of designating Pap smears as abnormal, as discussed above. PAPNET has been shown to detect abnormal cells that are missed by primary manual screening.[42] However, most of the abnormal cells thus identified are categorized as atypical squamous cells of undetermined significance (ASCUS).[42] In fact, ASCUS has already become prevalent without the assistance of PAPNET. It is common to find non-specific poorly preserved cells retrospectively when the smear is known to be from a woman with a diagnosis of high-grade squamous intraepithelial lesions (HSIL) or invasive cervical cancer. These cells have been dubbed as litigation cells, since they are difficult to interpret prospectively and can be called ASCUS if the cytopathologist is concerned about the potential of litigation.[43] The result of an increasing rate of abnormal Pap smears is the increased use of colposcopy and biopsy and consequently increased (probably unnecessary) cost involved in the prevention of cervical cancer. This issue is discussed in detail in Chapter 8.

It should be noted that the possibility of a real increase in the rate of preinvasive cervical neoplasia exists, as discussed above. However, this should not be a selective increase of ASCUS only. Therefore, ASCUS to squamous intraepithelial lesions (SIL) ratio is a good indicator of whether the ASCUS category has been abused.

Increasing liability

Pathology has been transformed from a low-risk specialty, as far as malpractice suits are concerned, to a high-risk specialty primarily because of false-negative Pap smears. As mentioned above, the public expects a zero false-negative rate from Pap smears when in fact no medical tests can reach such a goal. In many of the well-publicized unfortunate cases resulting from false-negative Pap smears, the Pap smear was incorrectly used as a diagnostic test instead of a screening test. For patients who present with symptoms, such as bleeding, colposcopy and biopsy instead of, or in addition to, Pap smears are indicated. Pap smears may be used as an adjunct test in such a case but should never be used as the sole diagnostic test. However, the cytology laboratory and its personnel unfortunately often get all the blame for improperly used and improperly interpreted Pap smears.

False-negative Pap smears are inevitable even in cytology laboratories with the best quality control program. The difference is in the degree and extent. Although it is inevitable, the responsible cytology laboratory is still liable when it occurs. This issue is covered in Chapter 5.

Decreasing reimbursement

Despite the increasing cost of Pap smears owing to work-load limitations, increased compensation for the cytotechnologists, increased liability and increased requirement for quality assurance/improvement, the reimbursement of Pap smears has not increased proportionally. Such a combination has made the practice of Pap smears increasingly difficult. A new charge code has been introduced for ThinPrep processing of cervical/vaginal cytological materials. Many insurance companies have announced consent to abide by the higher charge code for ThinPrep Pap smears. This is an opportunity to adjust appropriately the reimbursement for Pap smears. However, a blow to this move was the issue of a press release in August 1998 of a Committee Opinion by the Committee on Gynecologic Practice of the American College of Obstetricians and Gynecologists, which stated that new Pap smear technologies '... do not represent the current standard of care in cervical cancer screening ...'. The new technologies include ThinPrep, AutoPap and PAPNET. PAPNET has since been removed from the market because of its lack of cost-effectiveness, as discussed above and in Chapter 3.

FUTURE DIRECTIONS

Standard of care

Although the standard of care for Pap smears could conceivably be established for cytology laboratories in terms of quality control/assurance programs and fulfillment of CLIA'88 requirements, it is difficult, if not impossible, to establish the standard on an individual basis, except perhaps the application of 'new technologies'. Therefore, it is unlikely that a standard of care can be used to defend cytology laboratories in a malpractice suit. However, educating clinicians and women to realize the limits of Pap smears may decrease their unrealistic expectation of this test and help to put Pap smear results in the appropriate context. This issue is discussed in detail in Chapter 5.

Automated primary screening

In contrast to automated rescreening, automated primary screening has the potential to reduce the cost of Pap smears. For example, AutoPap eliminates a certain percentage of smears from manual screening without compromising the sensitivity of Pap smears. Please see Chapter 3 for details.

Ancillary studies, such as HPV and/or other antibody testing

With ThinPrep for Pap smears, the remaining materials can be used for ancillary studies, if indicated. This can improve the specificity of the test without increasing the cost of routine smears. Please see Chapters 6 and 9 for details.

Adenocarcinoma and its precursors

Although one study showed that the mass screening program has reduced the mortality rate of adenocarcinoma,[44] perhaps owing to detection at an earlier stage, screening for cervical cancer has been shown in most studies to have had no effect on the incidence rate of adenocarcinoma of the cervix.[44–46] Most recently, the incidence rate of adenocarcinoma of the uterine cervix has been shown to be increasing in both black and white women in the USA.[22] Therefore, adenocarcinoma has become relatively frequent and more important as a target for screening. The sensitivity of Pap smears to detect cervical adenocarcinoma is poor, and has been estimated to be 42 per cent.[46] However, with improved sampling device for endocervical canal, ThinPrep preparation of the material,[47,48] and greater awareness of the glandular lesions, Pap smears may become more useful in detecting glandular precursor lesions and thus make an impact on the mortality as well as morbidity of adenocarcinoma.

REFERENCES

1 Koss LG. Cervical (Pap) smear. New directions. *Cancer* 1993; **71**: 1406–12.
2 Papanicolaou GN. New cancer diagnosis. *Proc of the 3rd Race Betterment Conference*. Battle Creek, MI: RBF, 1928: 528–34.
3 Daniel C, Babes A. Diagnosticul cancerului colului uterin prin frotiu. *Proc Bucharest Gynecology Society, Bucharest*, April 5, 1927: 23.

4 Naylor B. The century for cytopathology. *Acta Cytol* 2000; **44**: 709–25.

5 Ayre JE. Selective cytology smear for diagnosis of cancer. *Am J Obstet Gynecol* 1947; **53**: 609–17.

6 Parker SL, Tong T, Bolden S, Wingo PA. Cancer statistics, 1966. *CA Cancer J Clin* 1996; **46**: 5–27.

7 Bogdanich W. Lax Laboratories: the Pap test misses much cervical cancer through lab's errors. *Wall Street J*, Nov 2, 1987: 1.

8 United States Commission on Chronic Illness. *Chronic illness in the United States 1.* Cambridge, MA: Harvard University Press, 1957: 267.

9 Wilson J, Jungner G. *Principles and practices of screening for disease: public health paper 34.* Geneva: World Health Organization, 1968: 26–39.

10 Free K, Roberts S, Bourne R, et al. Cancer of the cervix – old and young, now and then. *Gynecol Oncol* 1991; **43**: 129–36.

11 Macgregor JE, Campbell MK, Mann EM, Swanson KY. Screening for cervical intraepithelial neoplasia in northeast Scotland shows fall in incidence and mortality from invasive cancer with concomitant rise in preinvasive disease. *BMJ* 1994; **308**: 1407–11.

12 Parkin DM, Nguyen-Dinh X, Day NE. The impact of screening on the incidence of cervical cancer in England and Wales. *Br J Obstet Gynaecol* 1985; **92**: 150–7.

13 Herrero R. Epidemiology of cervical cancer. *J Natl Cancer Inst Monogr* 1996: 1–6.

14 Tkeshelashvili VT, Bokhman JV, Kuznetzov VV, Maximov SJ, Chkuaseli GT. Geographic peculiarities of endometrial and cervical cancer incidence in five continents (review). *Eur J Gynaecol Oncol* 1993; **14**: 89–94.

15 Bonett A, Davy M, Roder D. Cervical cancer in South Australia: trends in incidence, mortality and case survival. *Aust NZ J Obstet Gynaecol* 1989; **29**: 193–6.

16 Cook GA, Draper GJ. Trends in cervical cancer and carcinoma *in situ* in Great Britain. *Br J Cancer* 1984; **50**: 367–75.

17 Kainz C, Gitsch G, Heinzl H, Breitenecker G. Incidence of cervical smears indicating dysplasia among Austrian women during the 1980s. *Br J Obstet Gynaecol* 1995; **102**: 541–4.

18 Seow A, Chia KS, Lee HP. Cervical cancer: trends in incidence and mortality in Singapore 1968–1987. *Ann Acad Med Singapore* 1992; **21**: 328–33.

19 Weiss LK, Kau TY, Sparks BT, Swanson GM. Trends in cervical cancer incidence among young black and white women in metropolitan Detroit. *Cancer* 1994; **73**: 1849–54.

20 Schwartz SM, Weiss NS. Increased incidence of adenocarcinoma of the cervix in young women in the United States. *Am J Epidemiol* 1986; **124**: 1045–7.

21 Stockton D, Cooper P, Lonsdale RN. Changing incidence of invasive adenocarcinoma of the uterine cervix in East Anglia. *J Med Screen* 1997; **4**: 40–3.

22 Zheng T, Holford TR, Ma Z, et al. The continuing increase in adenocarcinoma of the uterine cervix: a birth cohort phenomenon. *Int J Epidemiol* 1996; **25**: 252–8.

23 Kjaer S, Brunton LA. Adenocarcinomas of the uterine cervix: the epidemiology of an increasing problem. *Epidemiol Rev* 1993; **15**: 486–98.

24 Noller KL. Incidence and demographic trends in cervical neoplasia. *Am J Obstet Gynecol* 1996; **175**: 1088–90.

25 Miller AB. Editorial: failures of cervical cancer screening. *Am J Public Health* 1995; **85**: 761–2.

26 Sherlaw-Johnson C, Gallivan S, Jenkins D, Jones MH. Cytological screening and management of abnormalities in prevention of cervical cancer: an overview with stochastic modelling. *J Clin Pathol* 1994; **47**: 430–5.

27 Harlan LC, Bernstein AB, Kessler LG. Cervical cancer screening: who is not screened and why? *Am J Public Health* 1991; **81**: 885–91.

28 Rolnick S, LaFerla JJ, Wehrle D, Trygstad E, Okagaki T. Pap smear screening in a health maintenance organization: 1986–1990. *Prev Med* 1996; **25**: 156–61.

29 Janerich DT, Hadjimichael O, Schwartz PE, et al. The screening histories of women with invasive cervical cancer, Connecticut. *Am J Public Health* 1995; **85**: 791–4.

30 Eddy DM. Screening for cervical cancer. *Ann Intern Med* 1990; **113**. 214–26.

31 Brown AD, Garber AM. Cost-effectiveness of 3 methods to enhance the sensitivity of Papanicolaou testing. *JAMA* 1999; **281**: 347–53.

32 Bergstrom R, Adami HO, Gustafsson L, Ponten J, Sparen P. Detection of preinvasive cancer of the cervix and the subsequent reduction in invasive cancer. *J Natl Cancer Inst* 1993; **85**: 1050–7.

33 Helfand M, O'Connor GT, Zimmer-Gembeck M, Beck JR. Effect of the Clinical Laboratory Improvement Amendments of 1988 (CLIA'88) on the incidence of invasive cervical cancer. *Med Care* 1992; **30**: 1067–82.

34 Waugh N, Robertson A. Costs and benefits of cervical screening. II. Is it worthwhile reducing the screening interval from 5 to 3 years? *Cytopathology* 1996; **7**: 241–8.

35 Eddy DM. The frequency of cervical cancer screening. Comparison of a mathematical model with empirical data. *Cancer* 1987; **60**: 1117–22.

36 IARC Working Group on Evaluation of Cervical Cancer Screening Programmes. Screening for squamous cervical cancer: duration of low risk after negative results of cervical cytology and its implication for screening policies. *BMJ* 1986; **293**: 659–64.

37 Clarke EA, Hilditch S, Anderson TW. Optimal frequency of screening for cervical cancer: a Toronto case-control study. *IARC Sci Publ* 1986; **76**: 125–31.

38 Herbert A, Stein K, Bryant TN, Breen C, Old P. Relation between the incidence of invasive cervical cancer and the screening interval: is a five year interval too long? *J Med Screen* 1996; **3**: 140–5.

39 Shy K, Chu J, Mandelson M, Greer B, Figge D. Papanicolaou smear screening interval and risk of cervical cancer. *Obstet Gynecol* 1989; **74**: 838–43.

40 Lynge E, Poll P. Incidence of cervical cancer following negative smear. A cohort study from Maribo County, Denmark. *Am J Epidemiol* 1986; **124**: 345–52.

41 van Oortmarssen GJ, Habbema JD. Duration of preclinical cervical cancer and reduction in incidence of invasive cancer following negative pap smear. *Int J Epidemiol* 1995; **24**: 300–7.

42 O'Leary T, Tellado M, Buckner S-B, Ali I, Stevens S, Ollayos C. PAPNET-assisted rescreening of cervical smears. Cost and accuracy compared with a 100 per cent manual rescreening strategy. *JAMA* 1998; **279**: 235–7.

43 Frable W. Litigation cells: definition and observations on a cell type in cervical vaginal smears not addressed by the Bethesda System [editorial]. *Diagn Cytopathol* 1994; **11**: 213–15.

44 Nieminen P, Kallio M, Hakama M. The effect of mass screening on incidence and mortality of squamous and adenocarcinoma of cervix uteri. *Obstet Gynecol* 1995; **85**: 1017–21.

45 Herbert A, Breen C, Bryant TN, et al. Invasive cervical cancer in Southampton and South West Hampshire: effect of introducing a comprehensive screening programme. *J Med Screen* 1996; **3**: 23–8.

46 Sigurdsson K. Quality assurance in cervical cancer screening: the Icelandic experience 1964–1993. *Eur J Cancer* 1995; **31A**: 728–34.

47 Ashfaq R, Gibbons D, Vela C, Saboorian MH, Iliya F. ThinPrep Pap test. Accuracy for glandular disease. *Acta Cytol* 1999; **43**: 81–5.

48 Bai H, Sung CJ, Steinhoff MM. ThinPrep Pap Test promotes detection of glandular lesions of the endocervix. *Diagn Cytopathol* 2000; **23**: 19–22.

2

Clinical decision-making

R GERALD PRETORIUS

INTRODUCTION

Clinicians use Papanicolaou (Pap) smears to screen women for cervical or vaginal neoplasia, based on the assumption that the risks and cost of cytological screening are outweighed by the benefits of lower morbidity and mortality as a result of screening. Despite virtual universal acceptance of Pap smears, it seems that few truly understand the effectiveness of Pap smears in preventing cervical cancer and the magnitude of the risks and cost of cytological screening. It remains controversial which women should be screened, how often they should be screened, and how women with 'abnormal' smears should be managed. The confusion concerning the appropriate use of Pap smears has recently been further compounded by the introduction of a new reporting system of Pap smears (the Bethesda system),[1] an increasing rate of 'abnormal' smears and an increase in malpractice suits against alleged false-negative Pap smears.[2]

The purpose of this chapter is to propose an optimal way to use the Pap smear and to suggest a way for clinicians to improve outcomes based on Pap smear screening. These goals will be achieved through six sections of this chapter.

OBTAINING A SATISFACTORY PAP SMEAR

Obtaining a Pap smear requires visualizing the cervix, scraping it with one or more instruments, and transferring the cells from the instrument to a glass slide. Recently, the instruments used to scrape the cervix and the methods by which the cells are transferred to the glass slide have changed. Initially, Pap smears were obtained by aspiration of fluid from the vaginal fornix.[3] As noted by Ayre,[4] vaginal aspiration specimens consisted of cells that had already been exfoliated. Ayre advised using a small spatula to gently scrape the surface of the tissues at the squamocolumnar junction. Pund et al.[5] obtained specimens for cytological evaluation by inserting a cotton-tipped swab into the cervical canal, twirling it a few times in one direction, and then rolling the swab on the slide. Johansen et al.[6] concluded that the combination of an endocervical swab and a cervical scraping was superior to either technique alone. By the 1970s, the standard method of obtaining Pap smears was a combination of an ectocervical scrape with a wooden or plastic spatula and an endocervical sample with a cotton-tipped swab or aspiration with a plastic tube and a rubber bulb.[7] However, some still advocated an additional vaginal pool specimen be obtained in perimenopausal and postmenopausal women.[8] Although both endocervical and ectocervical specimens were important, according to a study by Shingleton et al.[7] on a colposcopy clinic experience the ectocervical specimen was more effective in detecting cervical neoplasia than was the endocervical specimen obtained with cotton-tipped swab or aspiration. In that study, separate endocervical and ectocervical smears were obtained from 300 women. Of the 78 women with marked dysplasia or cancer 65 had abnormal endocervical and ectocervical smears, 10 had abnormal ectocervical but negative endocervical smears, none had normal ectocervical and abnormal endocervical smears, and three had normal ectocervical and endocervical smears.[7]

In 1983, Elias et al.[9] reported that cytological smears obtained with Ayre spatula that contained endocervical cells had 4.4 times more chance of detecting severe dysplasia or carcinoma *in situ* when compared with smears that did not contain endocervical cells. Vooijs et al.[10] corroborated Elias et al.'s study in 1985 and found that smears with endocervical cells were 1.7 times more likely to have slight to moderate dysplasia than were smears without these. These two reports fueled a search for methods of obtaining Pap smears that increased the yield of endocervical cells, on the assumption that there would be a concomitant increase in the detection of neoplastic lesions. Cytobrush was thus introduced.[11] Ectocervical smears were collected in the same fashion with an Ayre spatula but the endocervical specimen was collected by rotating the cytobrush within the external cervical os. When compared with the spatula alone or spatula plus cotton-tipped swab combination, smears obtained with the cytobrush were more likely to contain endocervical cells.[12] Unfortunately, smears obtained with the cytobrush were not more likely to be of optimum quality,[13,14] and only one[15] of six randomized trials comparing spatula plus cytobrush with spatula plus cotton-tipped swab showed the cytobrush smears to have a higher detection rate of dysplastic cells.[12–17] These results are not entirely surprising given the less important role of the endocervical specimen in the detection of cervical dysplasia as concluded by Shingleton et al.[7] A major advantage of obtaining endocervical smears with the cytobrush is that endocervical cells are an indicator for the adequacy of the smear obtained with the swab while they are not an indicator for adequacy of smear obtained with the cytobrush.[12] If a cytobrush is used to sample the endocervix, it is not necessary to repeat smears lacking endocervical cells. Two exceptions to this rule are women in whom glandular neoplastic lesions are suspected and women who have been treated for cervical intraepithelial neoplasia (CIN) and have cervical stenosis.[12] Although the efficacy of the use of the cytobrush during pregnancy has been confirmed by two studies,[14,18] the manufacturer does not recommend its use in pregnancy.

Other improvements on the Ayre spatula, such as extending the tip to improve sampling of the endocervix,[19] the Eisenstein Ecto–Endo Cervical Scraper,[20] the Bayne brush,[12] and the Cervex brush,[14,16] have also been introduced. The last two methods are associated with an increased yield of endocervical cells but, as with the cytobrush, neither has been conclusively shown to increase either the proportion of smears of optimum quality or the proportion of smears with dysplastic cells.[12,14,16] The conventional method of transferring cells to the slide is to smear the sampling device onto the glass slide. It is not important whether both endocervical and ectocervical specimens are smeared onto one slide or onto separate slides. What is important is to roll the cotton-tipped swab or endocervical brush onto the slide rather than sweeping the slide with only one side of the swab or brush. While smearing the specimen onto a slide appears to be an easy and inexpensive way of preparing the specimen, it often results in smears of varying quality with potential obscuring and loss of neoplastic squamous and endocervical cells. New, fluid-based, thin-layer systems have recently been developed. In these systems, the instruments used to obtain the endocervical and ectocervical specimens are rinsed in a transport medium. The cells in the transport medium are dispersed, collected on a filter, and then transferred as a thin layer to a glass slide.[21] This subject is discussed in detail in Chapter 3. From the clinicians' viewpoint, the fluid-based cytology preparation has the advantage of providing a sample for high-risk human papillomavirus (HPV) typing from the same specimen without requiring a second visit of the patient for a second specimen.[22]

COMPARISON OF STATISTICS FROM TWO CYTOLOGICAL SCREENING POPULATIONS – 1989 VERSUS 1996

Many changes have recently taken place in the cytological screening system. The introduction of the Bethesda system for reporting cervical/vaginal cytological smears and the increased proportion of abnormal smears between 1989 and 1996 are among the most important. In order to examine these changes in more detail, this section compares two large databases from 1989 and 1996. The database from 1989 antedates the Bethesda system and comes from a prospective trial involving 11 061 women in Southern California Kaiser Permanente.[12] The objective of this trial was to determine which of three methods of obtaining Pap smears had the highest detection rate of cervical neoplasia. The trial showed no significant differences in the detection rates of cervical neoplasia with these three methods. The original data from this trial were reanalyzed to determine the rate of abnormal smears and the yield of significant neoplastic lesions per 1000 smears as a function of patient age. In 1989, the Southern California Permanente Cytopathology Laboratory reported smears as cancer, dysplasia, condyloma, inconclusive, inappropriate appearance of endometrial cells, inflammation or negative. For the purposes of this analysis, an 'abnormal' smear was defined as a smear reported as other than negative or inflammation. As shown in Table 2.1, the most common method of determining a final diagnosis was histological examination of colposcopically directed biopsy.

The data from 1996 was obtained by reviewing the cancer prevention program within the Fontana Southern California Permanente Medical Group. In 1996, 44 989 cervical or vaginal

Table 2.1 *Comparison of methods of obtaining a histological diagnosis in women with abnormal Pap smears in 1989 and 1996 in the Southern California Kaiser Permanente system*

Method of diagnosis	1989 (*n* = 296)	1996 (*n* = 1818)
LETZ,[a] cervical conization, or hysterectomy	33 (11%)	191 (11%)
Colposcopic directed biopsy	242 (82%)	1068 (59%)
Colposcopic impression	21 (7.1%)	552[b] (30%)
Endometrial or vulvar biopsy	0	7 (0.4%)

[a]LETZ, loop excision of the transformation zone.
[b]Virtually all of the women in whom the diagnosis was based solely on colposcopic impression (543 out of 552) had no cervical lesion.

cytological smears on women aged 10 years or older were obtained at the Fontana facility. The Southern California Permanente Cytopathology Laboratory had adopted the Bethesda system of reporting cytological smears by 1996. Smears were reported as cancer, high-grade squamous intraepithelial lesions (HSIL), low-grade squamous intraepithelial lesions (LSIL), atypical squamous cells of uncertain significance (ASCUS), atypical glandular cells of uncertain significance (AGUS), and negative. At the Fontana facility, abnormal smears were defined as any diagnosis other than negative. Although all 2790 women with abnormal smears at the Fontana facility in 1996 were referred for colposcopy, the statistics in this review were based on a subset of 1818 women with abnormal smears evaluated between March 1996 and January 1997. This was due to the introduction of a computer-based data collection system into the cancer prevention center in March of 1996. The predictive value of each cytological diagnosis was calculated for each 5-year age group (the predictive value of a cytological diagnosis is the proportion of women with that cytological diagnosis who actually have cervical, vaginal, uterine, or ovarian neoplasia or HPV). These values were then extrapolated to estimate the predictive values of each cytological diagnosis for each age group for the entire year of 1996. As shown in Table 2.1, and similar to the data set from 1989, the majority of women had their final diagnosis based on colposcopic-directed biopsy. Almost all of the women in whom the diagnosis was based solely on colposcopic impression in the 1996 data (543 of 552 cases) had no cervical lesion.

The comparison of the rates of abnormal smears in 1989 and 1996 is presented in Fig. 2.1. In 1989, 2.8% of all Pap smears were abnormal. Women under the age of 25 years had more than twice the abnormal rate (6.0%) of women aged 25 years or older (2.3%). By 1996, the total abnormal rate had more than doubled (6.2%) and the curve had shifted to an older age, such that the abnormal rate for women under the age of 25 years (8.2%) was only slightly higher than that for women aged 25 years and older (5.7%). Furthermore, as seen in Table 2.2, this increase is secondary to the increase in the proportion of ASCUS, AGUS and LSIL smears; the proportion of smears reported as HSIL or cancer remained constant.

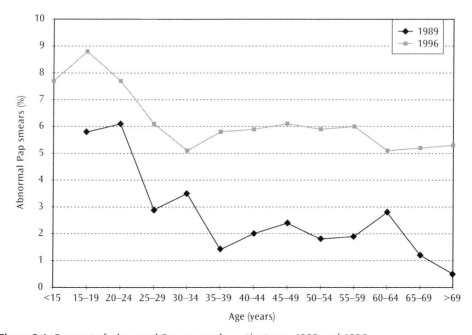

Figure 2.1 *Per cent of abnormal Pap smears by patient age, 1989 and 1996.*

Table 2.2 *Per cent of ASCUS/AGUS/LGSIL and HGSIL/cancer diagnoses on Papanicolaou smears from Southern California Permanente Medical Group, 1990–95[a]*

Year	ASCUS/AGUS/LSIL (%)	HSIL/cancer (%)
1990	2.5	0.4
1991	3.0	0.2
1992	5.1	0.3
1993	4.7	0.3
1994	6.0	0.3
1995	5.9	0.2

[a]ASCUS, atypical squamous cells of undetermined significance; AGUS, atypical glandular cells of undetermined significance; LSIL, low-grade squamous intraepithelial lesions; HSIL, high-grade squamous intraepithelial lesions.

The age distribution of the yield of CIN II, CIN III, vaginal intraepithelial neoplasia II (VAIN III), vaginal intraepithelial neoplasia III (VAIN III), endometrial hyperplasia or cancer (significant neoplastic lesions) on histology per 1000 Pap smears in 1989 and 1996 is compared in Fig. 2.2. Three conclusions can be drawn. First, the yield of significant neoplastic lesions in 1989 (the area under the 1989 curve) is lower (4.0 per 1000 smears) than in 1996 (5.7 per 1000 smears). Second, the age at which the yield is highest (i.e. the age at which the screening system is most efficient) has shifted from age 30–34 years in 1989 to age 20–24 years in 1996. Third, in 1996 there is an increase in the yield of significant neoplastic lesions in women over age 60 years (6.0 per 1000 smears) from that in 1989 (1.6 per 1000 smears). Conclusions about the differences between these two databases must be tempered by the limitations of this analysis. The two data sets, while similar, are not from identical populations. The data from the randomized trial from 1989 were obtained from Kaiser Permanente members at San Diego, Fontana, and Los Angeles, while the data from 1996 were obtained only from members in Fontana. The evaluation of the patients is not entirely equivalent as the final diagnosis was based on colposcopic impression alone in 30% of the women in the 1996 series, while it was in only 7.1% of the women in the 1989 series. It is also possible that there was a shift in the threshold of histological CIN II in 1996 as opposed to 1989 (some have suggested that lesions interpreted as CIN I in 1989 may now be interpreted as CIN II).

Each of the conclusions noted above requires some elaboration. The 40% increase in yield of significant neoplastic lesions from 1989 to 1996 is, in part, secondary to the evaluation with colposcopy and biopsy in 1996 of the increased number of women with marginally 'abnormal' smears. This increase in yield is not as great as the increase in the rate of abnormal smears (2.8% to 6.2% or 121%). It is questionable whether the increased yield is worth the increased cost incurred in evaluating the additional women with abnormal smears. The question of cost effectiveness of screening and the optimum rate of abnormal smears is discussed later in this chapter (see section What is an 'abnormal' Pap smear and what should the optimum rate of abnormal smears be?, and Fig. 2.4).

Of greater interest than the overall increased yield of Pap smears is the finding that the age of the peak yield of significant neoplastic lesions decreased by 10 years. While it is possible that part of this shift to a younger age is secondary to interpreting HPV and CIN I as CIN II, it is doubtful that this explanation can account for the entire shift. This decrease in the peak age at which CIN II and CIN III is diagnosed suggests that screening of younger women is important and should be encouraged. The question of when to initiate screening is discussed in detail in the next section of this chapter.

The increase in yield of significant lesions in women over 60 years of age is of concern. Boyes reported in 1981 that the incidence of CIN III in women over 60 years of age attending

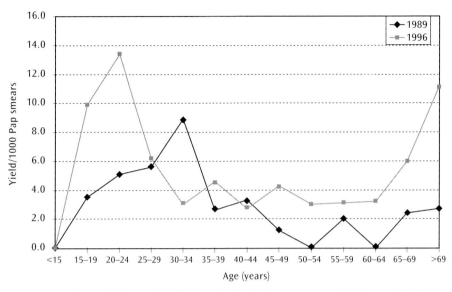

Figure 2.2 *Yield of cervical intraepithelial neoplasia (CIN) II, CIN III, vaginal intraepithelial neoplasia (VAIN) II, VAIN III or cancer per 1000 Pap smears by patient age, 1989 and 1996.*

a screening clinic in Canada was 0.017% and thus concluded that this figure was small enough to recommend no screening for women in this age group.[23] Our 1989 data could be interpreted in a similar fashion as the yield of significant neoplastic lesions in women over 60 years of age was very low. In 1993, van Wijngaarden and Duncan in the UK reported an age distribution of yield of significant neoplastic lesions and found a considerable yield of significant neoplastic lesions in women age 60 years or older (7.8 per 1000 smears); their yield curve was quite similar to our 1996 curve.[24] These authors reviewed the screening history of women age 50 years or older who had significant neoplastic lesions and found that essentially none of them had engaged in periodic screening. They thus concluded that if a woman had participated in periodic screening and had not had an abnormal smear, the yield of significant lesions was small enough to discontinue screening after age 50 years.[24]

To determine whether women in Fontana in 1996 were similar to women in the UK in 1993, the 16 women in Fontana age 60 years or older who had significant neoplastic lesions in 1996 were reviewed. Three had endometrial cancer, and had postmenopausal bleeding and a concurrent positive diagnosis on biopsy. Two of the remaining 13 women had never had a prior Pap smear, two had only one prior Pap smear, two had multiple prior smears, with the last one more than 5 years before, and seven had multiple prior smears, with the last one within the last 3 years. In contrast to the 1993 data from the UK, more than half of the women 60 years of age or older in Fontana with significant lesions in 1996 had prior history of screening. The yield of significant lesions in this age group (6.0 per 1000 smears) is high enough to justify continued screening after age 60 years.

THE TARGET POPULATION OF SCREENING WITH PAP SMEARS

Screening with Pap smears should be performed on women who are at risk for cervical cancer. Ideally, women who are at increased risk should be screened more often. Risk indicators of cervical cancer include country of residence, socioeconomic status, race, number of sexual partners, age at first intercourse, sexual behavior of male partner, HPV infection, Herpes infection, smoking, use of birth-control pills, patient age and previous removal of the cervix.[25] Most of these are in fact related to risk of HPV infection, the etiologic factor in most cases of cervical neoplasia. Although any or all of these factors could be used to define subsets of women at high, medium or low risk of cervical cancer, in most organized screening programs only patient age, history of abnormal Pap smear and previous removal of the cervix are employed. The reason is that it is difficult to obtain accurate information on the other risk indicators. There are special situations in which these other risk indicators may determine frequency of screening (e.g. the patient is a prostitute or has documented HPV infection); judgment is required for this decision.

Four pertinent issues need to be considered in determining a strategy for routine cytological screening. They are: (1) screening for women without a cervix; (2) the ages for initiating and stopping screening; (3) the appropriate frequency of screening; and (4) whether or not it is necessary to have a number of consecutive, annual, negative smears prior to obtaining smears less frequently. Ideally, these questions should have been answered by data obtained from a series of prospective randomized trials. However, such data are not available as too many patients would have been required in order to achieve reasonable statistical power for these trials to be feasible or practical. For example, a 10-year trial to detect a 25% decrease in mortality of cervical cancer in which both arms of the trial involve screening with Pap smears (e.g. 3/10 000 versus 2.25/10 000) would require 725 000 women in each arm. Although no randomized trials have been done to address the above questions, considerable epidemiological data are available.

Should women without a cervix be screened with Pap smears?

The combined incidence of CIN III plus cervical cancer is 44 times higher than the combined incidence of VAIN III plus vaginal cancer.[26] The yield of significant vaginal lesions is not high enough to justify Pap smear screening of women who have had a total hysterectomy for any-thing other than cervical neoplasia.[27,28] Women whose cervix has been removed in the course of treatment for CIN or cervical cancer are at increased risk for VAIN and vaginal cancer and require continued screening.

At what age should screening begin?

In 1986, the International Agency for Research on Cancer (IARC) concluded that screening women under the age of 25 years was not particularly effective because young women had a very low rate of cervical cancer despite their relatively high prevalence of abnormal cytology.[29] Although women under 25 years old are very unlikely to be diagnosed with invasive cervical cancer,[30] the goal of screening with Pap smears is also to prevent the development of cervical cancer by detecting and eliminating CIN II and CIN III. According to our 1996 data from Fontana, the peak incidence of CIN II and CIN III is now in women aged 20–24 years. It no longer seems appropriate to limit screening of women under 25 years old. The enthusiasm for screening women under the age of 25 years must be tempered by the fact that many, if not most, of the women with CIN III do not develop invasive cervical cancer.[31] It should also be noted that the progression rates for CIN III in young women are lower than those in older women.[32] While screening women under the age of 25 years may detect more CIN II and CIN III, it may also lead to unnecessary treatment of young women whose CIN is destined to regress without intervention. As cervical cancer is essentially nonexistent prior to onset of coitus,[33] screening prior to sexual activity is not indicated. The American Cancer Society (ACS), the National Cancer Institute (NCI), the American College of Obstetrics and Gynecology (ACOG)[34] and the US Preventive Task Force[35] have concluded that screening with Pap smears should begin at age 18 years or onset of sexual activity. The US Preventive Task Force also advised to begin screening adolescents whose sexual history is thought to be unreliable at the age of 18 years regardless of the history of coitus.[35]

At what age should screening stop?

As noted above, our Fontana Kaiser data suggest that there is still a yield of significant neoplastic lesions by Pap smears in women aged 60 years or older, even when these women had participated in periodic screening and had not had abnormal smears. This finding suggests that routine screening should continue beyond the age of 60 years. Since it takes time for CIN to progress to clinically significant invasive cancer and women may die of competing causes in the mean time, there should be an upper age limit for cytological screening. No available data permit us to determine with certainty this upper age limit. At present, screening with cytological smears should be continued at least every 3 years until the age of 74 years. Women aged 75 years and over should be screened if they have not participated in periodic screening previously.

What frequency of screening is appropriate?

To date, the strongest data concerning frequency of Pap smears come from the IARC.[29] The IARC concluded that the cumulative reduction in the incidence of squamous cervical cancer in women aged 35–64 years with at least one prior negative smear and with annual Pap smears would be 93.5%; with smears every 2 years, the reduction would be 92.5%; with smears every 3 years, the reduction would be 90.8%; and with smears every 5 years, the reduction would be 83.6%. A frequency of every 3 years is reasonable if the population is compliant, there is an organized recall system, and if the 'tickler' or reminder file for other screening procedures can easily be integrated into 3-year intervals.

The female population in the USA is not particularly compliant. Harlan et al. found that 27% of women aged 18 years or older had not had a Pap smear in the past 3 years.[36] When these women were asked why they had not had a smear, almost half said that they simply 'put it off'. The study of Kottke et al. gave further insight concerning women's attitudes toward screening.[37] Approximately half of the women surveyed in the study would accept screening and wanted their physician to contact them when the screening is due. Seven to 10% of women surveyed would refuse screening even if told it was necessary, and 40–50% would submit to screening if advised, although they preferred not to receive this advice.[37] Organized screening programs in which members of a population are advised of the need for screening and pursued if they fail to obtain screening are superior to opportunistic programs in which women are offered cytological screening when they are seen by a health-care provider for an unrelated condition.[38,39] Unfortunately, most screening done in the USA is done on an opportunistic basis rather than as part of an organized health maintenance program. In addition to the problems of a non-compliant population and our current opportunistic strategy, there is the problem that the guidelines for mammograms are at least every 2 years between the age of 50 and 69 years.[35] If an organized program were to be developed, it would probably be less expensive and more effective to adopt guidelines in which screenings with cytological smears and mammograms are synchronized rather than run a tickler file in which cytological smears are obtained at 3-year intervals and mammograms are obtained at 2-year intervals.

Is it necessary to have a number of consecutive annual negative smears prior to obtaining smears less frequently?

Clearly, the answer to the question above is yes; the question is how many? At least one prior negative smear is required because the IARC data quoted earlier concerning the reduction of cumulative incidence of squamous cervical cancer is based on women who have at least one prior negative smear.[29] It is noteworthy that IARC found that the relative risk of cervical cancer for all lengths of time since the last Pap smear was lower if there were two prior negative smears as opposed to a single negative smear. Furthermore, the variation in the relative risk of invasive cervical cancer from one laboratory to another was less if there were two or more prior negative smears as opposed to a single negative smear. It would appear reasonable that two consecutive annual negative smears are required before a woman can have smears every 2–3 years. The above recommendations differ only somewhat from those adopted by the ACS, ACOG and the NCI in 1988,[34] and are quite similar to those of the US Preventative Task Force.[35]

It is not crucial which exact set of guidelines for cytological screening to prevent cervical cancer is adopted. The important facts are: (1) the entire at-risk population should be screened,[38] and (2) there is still an unscreened population.[36,37,40] Annual screening of women with multiple prior negative smears will not save significantly more lives than screening every 2–3 years.[29] Unfortunately, the unscreened population tends to be the poor and the elderly, exactly the women who are at highest risk for cervical cancer.[40] Redirecting resources by decreasing the frequency of screening in women with multiple negative smears and by developing methodologies for reaching the unscreened population should be a priority for health-care providers.

WHAT IS AN 'ABNORMAL' PAP SMEAR AND WHAT SHOULD THE OPTIMUM RATE OF ABNORMAL SMEARS BE?

An abnormal Pap smear is one that contains neoplastic cells. Unfortunately, to determine which smears are normal and which are 'abnormal' based on the Pap smear reports is not as easy as one might hope. Some examples of Pap smear reports which are not clearly normal or abnormal include inflammatory smears with or without atypia, 'atypical squamous meta-plasia', 'rule-out dysplasia', 'rule-out condyloma', 'smears with endometrial cells', 'ASCUS, favor reactive', and 'AGUS favor reactive'. Assuming that one did understand which reports were 'abnormal' and which were normal, it would still be unclear whether the cytological system would function more efficiently if a different definition of normal were adopted. In addition, there is the confusion concerning the adequacy of a smear. An example is a smear that is reported as 'satisfactory but limited by ...' . Should such a smear be treated as negative?

An abnormal cytological smear should have a higher predictive value than does a negative smear. Unfortunately, the predictive value of Pap smears is not readily available or obtained. The classification system for abnormal smears has changed four times since the mid 1970s. Many clinicians were aware that in the classification system just prior to the Bethesda system, roughly 6% of the women with smears interpreted as atypical squamous cells had CIN II or CIN III.[41–43] When the Bethesda system was introduced, there were no immediate studies defining the predictive value of the various categories. Was the category of ASCUS equivalent to the old report of atypical squamous cells? How then does the qualifier of the ASCUS category change the predictive value? The fact that the rate of abnormal smears in many laboratories more than doubled between 1989 and 1996, yet the total yield of significant neoplastic

Table 2.3 *Predictive value of Papanicolaou smears*

Pap smear result[b]	Histological diagnosis[a]		
	HPV +CIN I	CIN II +	Cancer
Negative (See Table 2.4)	–	0.4%	–
ASCUS, Reactive	80/429 (19%)	14/429 (3.3%)	1/429 (0.2%)
ASCUS, NOS	188/828 (23%)	39/828 (4.7%)	0/828 (0%)
ASCUS, Premalignant	46/164 (28%)	25/164 (15%)	0/164 (0%)
LSIL	127/318 (40%)	54/318 (17%)	1/318 (0.3%)
HSIL	9/48 (19%)	31/48 (65%)	4/48 (8.3%)
AGUS	6/25 (24%)	2/25 (8.0%)	1/25 (4.0%)
Adenocarcinoma[50]	2/46 (4.3%)	12/46 (26%)	29/46 (63%)
Squamous carcinoma	0/2 (0%)	0/2 (0%)	2/2 (100%)

[a]Abbreviations: ASCUS, AGUS, LSIL, HSIL: see Table 2.2. HPV, human papillomavirus; CIN, cervical intraepithelial neoplasia.
[b]Data for ASCUS Reactive, ASCUS, ASCUS Premalignant, LGSIL, HGSIL, AGUS, and Squamous cancer are from a review of 1818 women with abnormal smears in Fontana Kaiser Hospital in 1996. Please see test for the diagnosis of Endometrial Cells Out of Phase.

lesions increased only 40% implies that the predictive value of the abnormal Pap smears in general must have decreased. Furthermore, the predictive value of abnormal smears differs from one laboratory to another.

A summary of the predictive value of Pap smears in the Southern California Permanente Cytopathology Laboratory is presented in Table 2.3. The data for the predictive value of ASCUS Reactive, ASCUS NOS, ASCUS Premalignant, LSIL, HSIL, AGUS and Squamous Cancer came from the colposcopy experience between March 1996 and January 1997 at the Fontana Kaiser Hospital, as described previously. The rate of CIN II or worse in women with negative conventional Pap smears was not measured in the 1996 Fontana review and has not been directly measured by others. The data for the positive predictive value of a negative Papanicolaou smear presented in Table 2.3 was inferred from a review of five studies in which women were screened with Pap smears plus cervicography, HPV tests and/or visual inspection.[44–48] In these five studies, women with any abnormal screening test were referred for colposcopy and biopsy. A summary of these five studies is presented in Table 2.4. As shown in the 6th column of the table, the risk of CIN II or worse in women with negative conventional Pap smears was between 0.74% and 1.78% with a mean of 1.06%. The five studies reviewed in Table 2.4 differ from the Fontana 1996 experience in a number of ways. Three of the studies from Table 2.4 (Reid et al.,[46] Cuzick et al.,[45] and Clavel et al.[44]) enrolled subjects from sexually transmitted disease or family planning clinics, and Wright et al.'s study was specifically designed to screen a known high-risk population. It is not surprising that the rate of abnormal Pap smears (6.5–17%) and the rate of CIN II or worse detected (2.2–4.1%) in these four series are much higher than that found in the fifth study reviewed (Tawa et al.[47]) (1.2% and 0.95%) or that found in the Fontana data from 1996 (6.2% and 0.6%).

Although the differences in populations studied make direct comparison of rates of CIN II or worse difficult, the data in Table 2.4 can be used to estimate the risk of CIN II or worse in women with negative Pap smears. Based on the combined data from the five studies from Table 2.4, the sensitivity of Pap smears for CIN II or worse was 60% (see the last column in Table 2.4). If one assumes the same sensitivity for CIN II or worse by Pap smears in the Fontana 1996 series, the number of women with CIN II or worse that had negative Pap smears can be calculated. In the 1996 Fontana review there were 44 898 women screened, 2790 women

Table 2.4 *Review of five studies on Pap smears and a second screening test to determine the risk of cervical intraepithelial neoplasia (CIN) II or worse in women with negative Pap smears and the sensitivity for CIN II or worse by Pap smears*

Author	Screening test	% Colposcopy	% Abnormal Pap	% CIN II or worse	CIN II or worse per negative Pap	Proportion of CIN II or worse detected by Pap (sensitivity)
Tawa[47]	Pap cervigram	385/3271 (12%)	39/3271 (1.2%)	31/3271 (0.95%)	24/3232 (0.74%)	7/31 (23%)
Reid[46]	Pap cervigram HPV	230/1012 (23%)	167/1012 (17%)	23/1012 (2.3%)	10/845 (1.2%)	13/23 (57%)
Cuzick[45]	Pap HPV	231/1985 (12%)	128/1985 (6.5%)	81/1985 (4.1%)	33/1851 (1.8%)	48/81 (59%)
Clavel[44]	Pap HPV	165/1518 (11%)	104/1518 (6.9%)	34/1518 (2.2%)	5/1414 (0.35%)	29/34 (85%)
Wright[48]	Pap HPV cervigram Visual inspection	500/1415 (35%)	216/1415 (15%)	56/1415 (4.0%)	18/1174 (1.5%)	38/56 (68%)
Total					90/8516 (1.1%)	135/225 (60%)

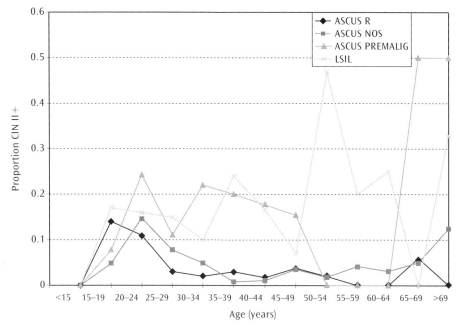

Figure 2.3 *Proportion of women with cervical intraepithelial neoplasia (CIN) II, CIN III, vaginal intraepithelial neoplasia (VAIN) II, VAIN III or cancer with atypical squamous cells of undetermined significance (ASCUS) reactive, ASCUS NOS, ASCUS premalignant and low-grade squamous intraepithelial lesions (LGSIL) smears by patient age (SCPMG Fontana, 1996).*

with abnormal Pap smears, and 254 cases of CIN II or worse detected. If these 254 women represent 60% of the total number of women with CIN II or worse, there must be about 169 women with CIN II or worse who had negative Pap smears. The rate of CIN II or worse in women with negative Pap smears is thus about 169 out of 42 108 or 0.4%.

In the Southern California Permanente Medical Group (SCPMG) cytopathology laboratory, the predictive value of cytological smears reported as ASCUS Reactive and ASCUS NOS are almost identical while the predictive value of smears reported as ASCUS Premalignant is similar to that of LSIL. These similarities are even more striking when the predictive value is plotted as a function of patient age (see Fig. 2.3). For all practical purposes, in the SCPMG laboratory, ASCUS Reactive and ASCUS NOS are the same cytological diagnosis while ASCUS Premalignant and LSIL are the same cytological diagnosis. However, this may not be the experience of all laboratories. In the Northern California Permanente Medical Group study conducted by Manos et al., 65 out of 973 (6.7%) women with ASCUS smears had CIN II or worse.[49] This positive predictive value is quite similar to that of the 1996 Fontana series in which 79 out of 1421 or 5.6% of women with ASCUS smears had CIN II or worse. Although the overall proportion of women with ASCUS smears that had diagnoses of CIN II or worse on biopsy is similar in the two regions, the positive predictive value of the subcategories of ASCUS differs significantly. In Manos et al.'s series, 2.3% of women with ASCUS Reactive smears had CIN II or worse, 9.4% of women with ASCUS NOS smears had CIN II or worse and 11.2% of women with ASCUS Premalignant Preferred smears had CIN II or worse.[49] In the same series, ASCUS NOS and ASCUS Premalignant Preferred have similar, relatively high positive predictive values while ASCUS Reactive smears have very low positive predictive values. Extrapolation of the statistics from Table 2.3 to a global population should be done with caution.

The predictive value of smears reported as adenocarcinoma in Table 2.3 comes from a review of 46 women with smears reported as 'adenocarcinoma', 'rule-out adenocarcinoma', and 'adenocarcinoma *in situ*' by the SCPMG cytopathology laboratory between July 1989 and March 1992 (the number of patients with smears reported as adenocarcinoma in 1996 in Fontana ($n = 1$) is too small for meaningful statistical analysis).[50] Only three of the Fontana series of 1818 had cytological smears reported as having endometrial cells out of phase; none of these three had a significant neoplastic lesion. The predictive value of cytological smears in which normal or atypical endometrial cells are detected depends on the age of the patient and how atypical the endometrial cells are.[51–53] The significance of endometrial cells in Pap smears is discussed in detail in Chapter 11.

The predictive value of cytological smears may also be dependent upon the quality of the smear. The three categories of adequacy, i.e. 'satisfactory for evaluation', 'satisfactory but limited by' and 'unsatisfactory' are defined in the Bethesda system in the following way.[54] 'Satisfactory for evaluation' smears have adequate numbers of well-preserved and well-visualized squamous epithelial cells and at least two clusters of endocervical glandular or squamous metaplastic cells; smears from women with atrophy are not required to have endocervical glandular or squamous metaplastic cells to be considered satisfactory. 'Satisfactory but limited by' smears are those with part of the slide obscured by blood, inflammation, thick areas, poor fixation, air drying or those in which no endocervical glandular or squamous metaplastic cells are seen. 'Unsatisfactory' smears have squamous cells covering less than 10% of the slide or those in which the cells are completely obscured by blood, inflammation, thick areas, poor fixation, air-drying artifact or contaminants. Although the predictive value of smears that are obtained with spatula and endocervical brush and reported as 'satisfactory for evaluation' is probably higher than that of smears reported as 'satisfactory but limited by', there are no data to prove this conclusively. Unless the cytological report is 'unsatisfactory', if the cervix has been sampled by an endocervical brush, the qualification of 'satisfactory but limited by lack of endocervical glandular or squamous metaplastic cells' can probably be ignored. However, this limiting factor cannot be ignored when the patient has had a cervical excision or ablation for cervical neoplasia – e.g. loop excision of the transformation zone (LETZ), conization, cryotherapy, etc. – and now has cervical stenosis, and when the patients has a history of cervical smears or biopsies suggesting glandular lesions. In either situation, the smear should be repeated.

The rate of abnormal Pap smears is of great interest to the clinician, the patient and the administrator. Everyone wishes that Pap smears were analogous to the serum human chorionic gonadotrophin (HCG) levels in the detection of pregnancy. Serum HCG levels are either less than 5 IU/mL (i.e. negative) or they are greater than 5 IU/mL (i.e. positive); there are no atypical pregnancy tests of uncertain significance. In addition, if the serum HCG is less than 5 IU/mL it is highly unlikely that the woman is pregnant, while if the HCG is greater than 5 IU/mL, it is almost certain. While there are false negative pregnancy tests (in the first few days following conception) and there are false positive pregnancy tests (e.g. due to a germ cell tumor of the ovary or other malignancies), they are uncommon. Unfortunately, unlike pregnancy tests, Pap smears are not either normal or abnormal. There are normal smears and then there are eight types of 'abnormal' smears, which can be ranked from minimally abnormal (e.g. ASCUS Reactive) to markedly abnormal (e.g. squamous carcinoma or adenocarcinoma). In addition, the positive predictive value of the abnormal smears is dependent upon the definition of a positive diagnosis. For example, if abnormal is defined as any smear other than negative, and a positive diagnosis includes HPV and CIN I, then the positive predictive value of an abnormal smear in our series is 35%. If only CIN II or worse is defined as positive, then the positive predictive value of an abnormal smear is 9.2%.

Table 2.5 *Proportion of significant neoplastic lesions [vaginal intraepithelial neoplasia (VAIN) II, VAIN III, vaginal cancer, cervical intraepithelial neoplasia (CIN) II, CIN III, cervical cancer, endometrial hyperplasia, endometrial cancer and ovarian cancer] on histology*

Abnormal Pap smear diagnosis[a]	Proportion of significant lesions (from Table 2.3) (%)[b]	Number of smears in 1996[b]	Calculated number of significant lesions in 1996[c]
Endometrial cells out of phase	0/3 (0%)	5	0
ASCUS Reactive	15/429 (3.5%)	664	(664) × (0.035) = 23
ASCUS NOS	39/828 (4.7%)	1279	(1279) × (0.0471) = 60
AGUS	3/25 (12%)	34	(34) × (0.12) = 4.0
ASCUS Premalignant	25/164 (15%)	286	(286) × (0.152) = 43
LSIL	55/318 (17%)	462	(462) × (0.173) = 80
HSIL	35/48 (73%)	57	(57) × (0.714) = 41
Cancer (squamous and glandular)	3/3 (100%)	3	(3) × (1.00) = 3.0
TOTAL	175/1818 (9.6%)	2790	254

[a]See Table 2.2 for abbreviations.
[b]From the subset of 1818 women with available data in Fontana Kaiser Hospital in 1996.
[c]Calculated number for all 2790 women with abnormal smears in Fontana Kaiser Hospital in 1996.

If the minimally abnormal smears (i.e. ASCUS Reactive and endometrial cells out of phase) were considered negative rather than abnormal, then there would have been 669 fewer abnormal smears from the 1996 data, and 23 women with significant neoplastic lesions would have been missed (see Table 2.5). If smears with ASCUS Reactive and endometrial cells out of phase were considered negative, the abnormal smear rate would decline from 6.2% to 4.7%, the positive predictive value of an abnormal Pap smear would increase from 9.7% to 11% and the yield of significant neoplastic lesions would decrease from 5.7 per 1000 to 5.1 per 1000. If the next abnormal smears (i.e. ASCUS NOS) were also considered negative, these changes would be even more pronounced. This calculation has been repeated for each category of the abnormal smears and is presented in Table 2.6 and Fig. 2.4. The yield of significant neoplastic lesions rises quickly as the rate of abnormal smears increases from zero to about 2 per cent and rises much more slowly thereafter. I would interpret the data in Fig. 2.4 as suggesting that the optimum rate of abnormal smears in our population is probably between 2 and 3 per cent rather than its current level of 6.2%.

The reason that the rate of abnormal smears is 6.2% instead of 2–3% is linked to the definition of ASCUS smears and the malpractice liability associated with calling a positive smear negative. There is no absolute line between ASCUS smears and negative smears. When the Bethesda system was first proposed, an attempt was made to limit the number of smears that would be reported as ASCUS by stating that the proportion of ASCUS smears should not exceed two to three times the proportion of other abnormal smears.[54] Using this guideline instead of one in which the absolute rate of ASCUS smears is set to be less than a certain number avoids the problem of varying populations that may have different absolute rates of abnormal smears. The reason why the authors of the Bethesda system recommended that the appropriate ASCUS to squamous intraepithelial lesion (SIL) ratio should be no greater than 3 is unclear. Based on the data presented in Fig. 2.4 and the IARC data[29] (that showed Pap smears to prevent about 90% of cervical cancers with an abnormal smear rate of 3%) the cytological screening system for the prevention of cervical cancer would be more cost-effective if the recommended ASCUS to SIL ratio could be decreased to no greater than 1.

Table 2.6 *Yield of significant neoplastic lesions [vaginal intraepithelial neoplasia (VAIN) II, VAIN III, vaginal cancer, cervical intraepithelial neoplasia (CIN) II, CIN III, cervical cancer, endometrial hyperplasia, endometrial cancer and ovarian cancer] on histology per 1000 smears as a function of rate of abnormal smear*

Smears defined as abnormal[a]	Per cent of abnormal smears	Yield of significant neoplasia
None	0	0
Cancer	3/44 898 = 0.007%	3/44 898 = 0.07 per 1000
Cancer, HSIL	60/44 898 = 0.13%	44/44 898 = 0.98 per 1000
Cancer, HSIL, LSIL	522/44 898 = 1.2%	124/44 898 = 2.8 per 1000
Cancer, HSIL, LSIL, ASCUS Premalignant	808/44 898 = 1.8%	167/44 898 = 3.7 per 1000
Cancer, HSIL, LSIL, ASCUS Premalignant, AGUS	842/44 898 = 1.9%	171/44 898 = 3.8 per 1000
Cancer, HSIL, LSIL, ASCUS Premalignant, AGUS, ASCUS NOS	2121/44 898 = 4.7%	231/44 898 = 5.1 per 1000
Cancer, HSIL, LSIL, ASCUS Premalignant, AGUS, ASCUS NOS, ASCUS Reactive, Endometrial cells out of phase	2790/44 898 = 6.2%	254/44 898 = 5.7 per 1000

[a]See Table 2.2 for abbreviations.

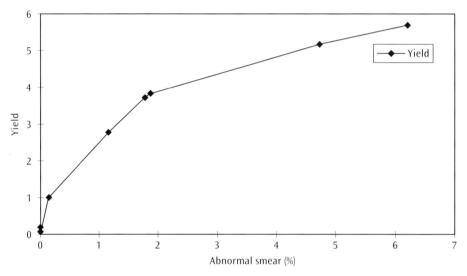

Figure 2.4 *Yield of significant neoplastic lesions per 1000 Pap smears as a function of rate of abnormal smear.*

The rate of 'abnormal' smears may change in the near future. When liquid-based cytology systems are introduced, the rate of 'abnormal' smears is likely to increase. As discussed in other chapters of this book, liquid-based cytology smears detect more CIN II or worse and have a higher rate of 'abnormal' smears. In Vassilakos et al.'s[55] series the rate of smears reported as ASCUS or worse was 4.7% for conventional smears and 5.3% for liquid-based smears, while in Hutchinson et al.'s[56] series the rates were 7% for conventional smears and 13% for liquid-based smears. The inclusion of a test for high-risk HPV as part of the cytological screening

Table 2.7 *Proportion of women with atypical squamous cells of undetermined significance (ASCUS) smears who have cervical intraepithelial neoplasia (CIN) II or worse on histology as a function of the HC II test for high-risk human papillomavirus (HPV) types*

Author	HC II Pos/ Total ASCUS	CIN II+/ HC II Negative	CIN II+/ HC II Positive	CIN II+/ Total ASCUS
Manos[49]	384/973 (39%)	7/589 (1.2%)	57/384 (15%)	64/973 (6.6%)
Pretorius (unpublished data)	306/949 (32%)	7/643 (1.1%)	56/306 (18%)	63/949 (6.6%)
Total	690/1922 (36%)	14/1232 (1.1%)	113/690 (16%)	127/1922 (6.6%)

would decrease the rate of 'abnormal' smears. If the 64% of women with ASCUS smears and negative tests for high-risk HPV (see Table 2.7) were reported as negative rather than ASCUS, the rate of 'abnormal' smears in our population would decrease from 6.2% to 3.2%.

EVALUATION OF WOMEN WITH ABNORMAL PAP SMEARS

Many older clinicians remember the Papanicolaou classification scheme (Class I–V) of the 1960s and 1970s with some fondness. With the old Class I–V reports, most clinicians ignored smears reported as Class I or II, repeated Class IIR, and evaluated women with Classes III –V smears with colposcopy and directed biopsy with or without endocervical curettage (ECC). For the colposcopically directed biopsy result to be considered the definitive diagnosis the following conditions have to be fulfilled: colposcopy needs to be adequate; the cervical lesions must be adequately sampled; the colposcopic impression should be consistent with that of the Pap smear and histology; the endocervical curettage (if performed) has to be negative; and neither the biopsy nor the colposcopic impression suggests an invasive cancer or glandular lesions of the cervix.[57] Women with inadequate colposcopy and negative ECC could be considered adequately evaluated if they met the other criteria listed above and the initial presentation is not strongly suggestive of CIN II, CIN III or cancer (i.e. the Pap smear is not HSIL and the patient has no abnormal vaginal bleeding and no prior history of CIN II or III). Women who could not be adequately evaluated with colposcopically directed biopsy were usually subjected to LETZ or cervical conization.

The current flow diagrams for evaluation of women with abnormal cytological smears are more complex. In large part, the added complexity is secondary to the low risk of CIN II or worse in women with ASCUS smears. Although most clinicians would agree that a risk of CIN II or worse of 12 or 16% seen in women with AGUS, ASCUS Premalignant, and LSIL smears (see Table 2.3) is high enough to justify colposcopy and directed biopsy, many do not believe that the 4% risk seen in women with ASCUS React or ASCUS NOS could justify colposcopy. Many clinicians have thus advocated secondary tests that could be used to triage women with ASCUS React and ASCUS NOS smears. Women with a positive second test would be referred for colposcopy while women with a negative secondary test would have repeat Pap smears in 1 year; if that repeat smear was negative, they would be returned to routine screening. For the secondary test to be effective in triaging women with ASCUS smears, it needs to have a low proportion of abnormal results and the residual prevalence of CIN II or worse in women with ASCUS smears and negative secondary tests needs to be similar to that of women with negative smears (about 0.4%, as seen in Table 2.3 and discussed above). Methods that have been proposed to triage women with ASCUS smears are a repeat cytological smear, HPV test, cervicography or using the patient's age.

A repeat cytological smear in 3–6 months is the oldest of the triage methods for women with low-grade abnormalities on their Pap smears. In Manos et al.'s study of the effectiveness of repeat smear for triage, 596 out of 973 women with ASCUS smears had negative repeat smears while 377 (39%) had abnormal repeat smears.[49] Fifteen of the 596 women (2.5%) with negative repeat smears had CIN II or worse. Triage of women with ASCUS smears on the basis of repeat Pap smear avoids colposcopy in two-thirds of the women. However, the prevalence of CIN II or worse in women who have negative repeat Pap smears (2.5%) is probably still higher than the risk of CIN II or worse in women with negative smears. Given the risk of CIN II or worse of 2.5% in women with ASCUS smears and negative repeat Pap smears, it is prudent not to return such women to routine screening.

HPV DNA has been detected in virtually all cases of primary invasive cervical cancer.[58] Certain types of HPV are not usually associated with invasive cancer (types 6, 11, 42, 43 and 44), while the 'high-risk' types are associated with the development of CIN II, CIN III or invasive cancer (types 16, 18, 31, 33, 35, 39, 45, 51, 52, 56, 58, 59 and 60).[59,60] Given the strong association of high-risk HPV types and cervical neoplasia, one might expect that triage of ASCUS smears based on the presence or absence of high-risk HPV would be useful. Recently, two large studies on triaging women with ASCUS smears on the basis of detection of high-risk HPV with the second-generation hybrid capture test (HC II developed by Digene, Inc., Gaithersburg, MD, USA) have been completed. The one by Manos et al.[49] was published in 1999; the other is a recently completed and yet unpublished study of the efficacy of HPV testing at the time of colposcopy that we did in 1999. These two studies are summarized in Table 2.7. In the combined data, 36% of women with ASCUS smears tested positive for high-risk HPV. The risk of CIN II or worse in women with ASCUS smears and negative HC II tests was 14 out of 1232 (1.1%). This figure is probably still higher than the risk of CIN II or worse in women with negative smears, but is lower than the risk found in women with ASCUS smears and negative repeat Pap smears. Given the uncertainty of the calculation of the risk of CIN II or worse in women with negative Pap smears and the inaccuracy of single measurements in determining HPV status,[61] we would advise follow-up of women with ASCUS smears and negative HPV tests with a repeat Pap smear and HPV test in 12 months and to return them to routine screening only if the second repeat test is negative.

Although the data cited above supports the concept of triaging women with ASCUS smears on the basis of HC II tests for high-risk HPV, a recently completed but unpublished study raises some question about the category of ASCUS Premalignant smears. Since approximately 90% of the ASCUS smears are ASCUS React or ASCUS NOS, the importance of ASCUS Premalignant smears tends to be overshadowed. Based on the unpublished data of our most recent study, the risk of CIN II or worse in women with ASCUS Premalignant smears was 13%, and 65% of the women with ASCUS Premalignant smears tested positive with second-generation hybrid capture test (HC II). Only one of the 36 women (2.8%) with ASCUS Premalignant smears and a negative HC II had CIN II or worse. These numbers are similar to those for LSIL smears in which 21% of such women had CIN II or worse, 76% had positive HC II and the risk of CIN II or worse in women with negative HC II was 4.5%. For this reason, we have chosen to treat women with ASCUS Premalignant the same way as we do to those with LSIL and not to triage them on the basis of HC II tests. We advise that women with ASCUS Premalignant smears undergo colposcopy with directed biopsy.

Cervicography provides a permanent, objective documentation of normal and abnormal cervical patterns.[62] Cervigrams are obtained by cleaning the cervix with 4% acetic acid and then taking a picture of the cervix with a 35 mm camera to which a 100 mm macro lens and ring strobe light have been adapted. At present, there are no studies on triage of women with ASCUS smears with cervigrams. ASCUS smears are similar to the atypical squamous smears that antedate the Bethesda system. Table 2.8 summarizes three studies of cervicography in women

Table 2.8 *Cervicography in women with atypical Papanicolaou smears*

Author	Defective	Suspicious	Negative	False-negative
Spitzer[43]	15/97	64/97	18/97	1/18
August[41]	41/586	246/586	299/586	11/299
Jones[42]	35/236	106/236	95/236	5/95
Total	91/919 (9.9%)	416/919 (45%)	412/919 (45%)	17/412 (4.1%)

Table 2.9 *Effect of patient age on the rate of cervical intraepithelial neoplasia (CIN) II, CIN III, vaginal intraepithelial neoplasia (VAIN) II, VAIN III or cancer on histology in women with atypical squamous cells of undetermined significance (ASCUS) smears*

	Age <30 years	Age >30 years	Total
ASCUS, Reactive	7/70 (10%)	8/359 (2.2%)	15/429 (3.5%)
ASCUS, NOS	22/237 (9.3%)	17/591 (2.9%)	39/828 (4.7%)
ASCUS, Premalignant	13/82 (16%)	12/82 (15%)	25/164 (15%)

with atypical Pap smears.[41–43] Approximately 10% of cervigrams were defective or unsatisfactory, 45% were suspicious, 45% were negative and 4% were false negative. Cervigrams are neither sensitive nor specific enough to be of great use in the triage of women with ASCUS smears.

A number of authors have noted that the predictive value of atypical smears is dependent upon patient age. Kaminski et al. found that 184 out of 787 (23.4%) women aged 40 years or less with atypical smears had HPV or CIN while only 18 out of 287 (6.3%) women over the age of 40 years with atypical smears had HPV or CIN.[63] He concluded that colposcopy was indicated for women under the age of 40 years and that repeat Pap smear was indicated for women aged over 40 years. Data from the colposcopy study conducted at Kaiser Fontana on the effect of age upon the predictive value of ASCUS smears is presented in the Table 2.9. The predictive value of ASCUS Reactive and ASCUS NOS smears falls significantly in women aged over 30 years, suggesting that it might be reasonable to refer women aged 30 years or less with ASCUS Reactive and ASCUS NOS smears directly to colposcopy and to repeat the smear for triage in women aged 30 years or older. Triage of women with ASCUS Reactive and ASCUS NOS smears on the basis of age alone cannot be advocated because the prevalence of CIN II or worse in the women over aged 30 years is still 2.6%. As with repeat Pap smears, this proportion is probably too high to return the patients to routine screening.

The problem of AGUS smears is heightened by the inability of colposcopically directed biopsy and endocervical curettage to exclude glandular lesions of the cervix;[64–66] the only reliable way to exclude glandular lesions of the cervix is to perform a cervical conization in which virtually all of the endocervical glands are removed.[67] Since large conizations of the cervix are associated with bleeding and cervical stenosis and are probably associated with cervical incompetence,[68] clinicians have been reluctant to employ them in the evaluation of women who have only a 12% chance of having CIN II or worse (see Table 2.3). As with ASCUS NOS and ASCUS Reactive smears, testing for high-risk HPV may be of clinical utility in determining which women with AGUS smears need aggressive evaluation and which deserve follow-up. In the study of Ronnett et al., 14 out of 15 women with AGUS smears and diagnoses of CIN II or worse tested positive with HC II.[69] In a recent unpublished study all five women with AGUS smears and CIN II or worse tested positive with HC II.

Our current strategy for evaluating women with 'abnormal' Pap smears is as follows. Women with ASCUS Reactive or ASCUS NOS smears return to the clinic to have HC II tests.

The HC II test can be done on the remaining cells if a liquid-based cytology is employed, thus avoiding a second visit. If the HC II test is positive for high-risk HPV, women with ASCUS NOS or ASCUS Reactive smears are referred for colposcopy and directed biopsy. If the HC II test is negative, they have a repeat Pap smear and HPV test in 1 year; if both tests are negative, they are returned to routine screening (routine screening in our system is a smear every 2–3 years once two negative smears are documented in our system). Women with all other abnormal smears are referred for colposcopy with directed biopsy and HC II test. The HC II test is performed at the time of colposcopy because it was found that colposcopy with directed biopsy is not particularly effective in diagnosing HPV and CIN I. This conclusion is supported both by the 1996 data on the 1818 women who were evaluated for abnormal Pap smears and by recent experience. Of the 1818 women, 732 had adequate colposcopy, cervical biopsies and negative endocervical curettage. Of these 732 women, 335 had a colposcopic impression of no lesions and in these women, cervical biopsies revealed CIN I or HPV in 91 (27%). An adequate colposcopy with no lesion seen and a negative ECC are clearly inadequate to exclude the diagnosis of HPV or CIN I. The unpublished data of our recent study showed that 217 out of 749 women (29%) who had colposcopy and were assigned a final diagnosis of negative had positive HC II tests. Even among women with smears other than ASCUS Reactive and ASCUS NOS, the addition of HC II at the time of colposcopy added important information; in this group, 94 out of 179 women (53%) who were assigned a negative diagnosis had a positive HC II test. Virtually all of the non-pregnant women referred for colposcopy have ECC. In addition to colposcopy with directed biopsy and ECC, women with AGUS smears have endometrial biopsy to exclude endometrial neoplasia and pelvic examination or sonography to exclude adnexal masses.

Our rules for loop electrocautery excision procedure (LEEP) and conization are similar to those quoted at the beginning of this section.[57] In general, we reserve conization for women who have a significant risk of invasive cancer and those in whom we are trying to exclude glandular lesions of the cervix.

FOLLOW-UP OF WOMEN WITH CERVICAL OR VAGINAL NEOPLASIA OR HPV

The appropriate follow-up of those women with biopsy-proven cervical or vaginal neoplasia or HPV and of those tested positive for high-risk types of HPV during the evaluation for an 'abnormal' Pap smear depends on the diagnosis, the certainty of the diagnosis and the chance that a concurrent or subsequent significant neoplastic process (i.e. CIN II, CIN III or invasive cancer) exists. Appropriate follow-up of such women ranges from repeating the Pap smear in 2–3 years to repeating colposcopy, Pap smear, HPV test and ECC in 6 months. Performing loop excision of the transformation zone (LETZ) or conization is not part of the follow-up of women with cervical neoplasia but should be considered part of the initial evaluation of the abnormal smear. Possible final diagnoses of women with cervical or vaginal neoplasia or HPV run the neoplastic spectrum from invasive squamous carcinoma or adenocarcinoma of the cervix or vagina to HPV or glandular atypia.

Women with biopsies showing CIN II, CIN III, VAIN II or VAIN III are usually treated with either LETZ, conization, cryotherapy, laser vaporization of the transformation zone, partial vaginectomy, laser therapy of the vagina, or 5-day courses of 5-fluorouracil (5-FU). The rate of recurrence of moderate and severe dysplasia of the cervix and vagina depends on the size of the lesion, degree of dysplasia, margin status of the LETZ or conization, and the series that is quoted. It is reasonable to summarize the extensive literature on this subject with the following statement, 'Cryotherapy, laser of the transformation zone, electrocoagulation diathermy, electrocautery and LETZ will prevent recurrence of CIN II and CIN III in about 90% of cases'.[57] Cervical conization with clear margins and hysterectomy are more effective and prevent 95–98% of recurrences.[57] The failure rates for VAIN II and III treated with excision, laser, or 5-FU are somewhat higher than those for CIN II and CIN III and range from 11% to 25%.[70]

Since the failure rate of treatment for CIN II or III is about 10%, and that for VAIN II or VAIN III is about 15%, women who have been treated for these conditions require follow-up. Traditionally, follow-up of women after treatment of CIN II or worse has included repeat Pap smears every 6 months for 2 years.[71] Falcone and Ferenczy[72] followed a series of women who had been treated for CIN with cryotherapy and found that if colposcopy, ECC and Pap smear were performed at 3–4 months after cryotherapy, almost all failures could be diagnosed at the first follow-up visit. Relying on negative colposcopy, ECC and Pap smear to exclude persistence of CIN has been our standard approach until recently. Recent studies by Ho et al.[73] and Nobbenhuis et al.[74] have concluded that virtually all women who develop CIN III persistently test positive for high-risk HPV. Nobbenhuis et al. performed colposcopy on 353 women with dyskaryosis on Pap smear.[74] Instead of being evaluated with biopsy followed by treatment, the women were followed with Pap smears, electro-immunoassay (EIA)–polymerase chain reaction (PCR) based HPV tests, and colposcopy until they either progressed to CIN III covering three or more quadrants of the cervix, had a Pap suggestive of invasive cancer, or reached the end point of the study (at the last visit of the study they all underwent colposcopically directed biopsy or random biopsies if no abnormality was noted). The median follow-up time was 33 months. A total of 122 women had persistent infection with high-risk HPV from baseline to last visit. All 33 women who reached clinical progression had persistent infection with high-risk HPV. End histology of CIN III was present in 103 women, of whom 98 had persistent high-risk HPV. The five women who tested negative for high-risk HPV were retested with type-specific PCR and all five tested positive. No subjects had clinical progression or end histology of CIN III without high-risk HPV infection. In the study by Nobbenhuis et al., an HPV test at the 6-month follow-up had a sensitivity for detecting CIN III of 97% while a Pap smear at 6-month follow-up had a sensitivity for CIN III of only 70%.[74]

Owing to the high prevalence rate of high-risk HPV among women who eventually progress to CIN III and cervical cancer, and the higher sensitivity for CIN III of the HPV test than the repeat Pap smear, it was decided to integrate HPV testing into the follow-up of women that have been treated for CIN II or worse. Currently, we follow women who have been treated for CIN II or worse (usually with LEEP or conization) with colposcopy, ECC, Pap smear and HPV test (HC II) at 6 months. If any of the tests is abnormal, women are further evaluated on a case-by-case basis depending on their risk of having invasive cervical cancer. If all of the tests at 6 months are negative, they have a Pap smear and HPV test 1 year later (at 18 months from the treatment of CIN II or worse). If the Pap smear and HPV at 18 months are normal, they are followed subsequently with annual Pap smears. If the patient has cervical stenosis, it may be necessary to dilate the cervix prior to obtaining follow-up smears and ECC.

Appropriate follow-up of women with CIN I, VAIN I and HPV is unclear. The reasons are many and include the following: significant inter- and intra-observer variation in the histopathological diagnosis of CIN I and HPV, inability to differentiate between high- and low-risk HPV types based on histomorphology and, until recently, the lack of an understanding of the natural history of these lesions. The significant difficulty in the histopathological diagnosis of CIN I and HPV is shown in the series of Ismail et al.,[75] Robertson et al.,[76] and Binder.[77] In Ismail et al.'s and Robertson et al.'s series only 42 out of 77 and 15 out of 37, respectively, cervical biopsies initially interpreted as CIN I were reported as CIN I on a second review.[75,76] In Binder et al.'s series 62 out of 317 colposcopically directed biopsies were initially interpreted as HPV, two were interpreted as HPV plus CIN I, and 27 were interpreted as CIN I; on review,

111 were interpreted as HPV, eight were interpreted as HPV plus CIN I and six were interpreted as CIN I.[77]

It has been known for some time that women with CIN I and high-risk HPV were much more likely to develop CIN III than those without these findings.[59,78–80] Recent data suggest that many women who are exposed to HPV will resolve their infection and that the women who are persistently HPV positive are those at high risk for progression to CIN III and invasive cervical cancer. The median duration of HPV infection (oncogenic and non-oncogenic types) in Ho et al.'s series was 8 months.[73] In Franco et al.'s series it was 8.2 months for the non-oncogenic types of virus and 13.5 months for the oncogenic types.[81] In Nobbenhuis et al.'s series, the median time to clearance of HPV of oncogenic type was 25 months.[74] As noted above, women who are persistently high-risk HPV positive in these studies are at risk for development of CIN III and invasive cervical cancer.[73,74,82] In our clinic, women with a diagnosis of high-risk HPV or CIN I are followed with Pap smear and HPV test annually until both are negative twice. They are then returned to routine screening. We are not willing to return women with a prior diagnosis of high-risk HPV or CIN I to routine follow-up on the basis of one negative Pap and HPV test because Wheeler et al.[61] determined that single-point measurements of cervical HPV have limitations when assessing an individual's HPV status. If the Pap smear is abnormal or the HPV test is persistently positive, they are referred for colposcopy and directed biopsy to exclude progression to CIN II or worse.

Whether progression of HPV or CIN I to CIN III can be prevented by ablation or removal of the cervical transformation zone is unclear. Successful treatment of HPV and/or CIN I with ablation or removal of the transformation zone has been reported by Bekassy et al.,[83] Sesti et al.,[84] Kiviat[85] and Ward et al.[86] Each of these series suffers from relatively short follow-up and none has a suitable control group. Enthusiasm for treatment of women with HPV or CIN I is tempered by the large number of young women who have the disease,[73,81] spontaneous clearance of the virus without intervention in many women,[73,74,81] and recurrent detectable HPV 6–12 months following laser excision or LETZ for CIN and clinical clearance of HPV.[87] The effectiveness of treatment of HPV and CIN I is questionable enough that the follow-up of women with a diagnosis of CIN I or HPV should not depend upon whether they were treated.

What should be the follow-up of women with a diagnosis of cervical atypical glandular epithelium or cervical adenocarcinoma *in situ*? Since it is necessary to perform cervical conization to exclude invasive cancer in women with glandular neoplasia of the cervix, almost all women with cervical glandular lesions will have had cervical conization.[64–66] As shown in Table 2.10, if the cervical conization has negative margins, there is still a 20% chance that there is residual glandular neoplasia on subsequent hysterectomy or second conization; if the margins are positive, there is a 61% chance of residual neoplasia. Unless the patient strongly desires fertility, the high probability of residual neoplasia at the time of subsequent hysterectomy is an indication for hysterectomy. This absolute recommendation for hysterectomy may be tempered somewhat by the study of Ronnett et al.[69] In Ronnett et al.'s series, all five women with cervical adenocarcinoma *in situ* tested positive for high-risk HPV with the newer second-generation hybrid capture test (HC II).[69] Women who have had cervical conization for glandular neoplasia of the cervix and who subsequently test negative for high-risk HPV could possibly be followed with Pap smear, HPV test and ECC every 6 months for 1 year and then annually. It is important to sample the endocervix; if the patient has cervical stenosis following conization, then dilatation of the canal prior to performing the Pap smear, HPV test, or ECC will be needed.

A more germane question concerning follow-up of women with glandular lesions of the cervix is: 'What is the appropriate follow-up of a woman with a Pap smear showing AGUS who has negative colposcopy with directed biopsies, negative ECC, negative endometrial biopsy (EMB) and no adnexal mass?' In our clinic, if the second-generation HPV test is negative,

Table 2.10 *Residual adenocarcinoma* in situ *or invasive adenocarcinoma in hysterectomy or repeat conization specimens in patients with cervical conization showing adenocarcinoma* in situ

Author	Cone margins negative	Cone margins positive
Ostor[66]	0/3	4/6
Bertrand[67]	0/4	0/1
Hopkins[88]	1/7	4/5
Andersen[64]	0/4	2/4
Muntz[89]	1/12	7/10
Poynor[90]	4/10	7/14
Im[91]	4/9	4/6
Total	10/49 (20%)	28/46 (61%)

a Pap smear, HPV test and ECC are obtained on such patients at 6 months. If these tests are negative, the patient has a Pap smear at 1 year. If that is again negative, the patient is returned to routine screening. This follow-up schema is based on the fact that once an endometrial cancer has been excluded, the risk of CIN II or worse among women with AGUS smears and negative second-generation HPV tests is only about 1%.[69] If the patient with an AGUS smear has an initial negative evaluation but has a positive test for high-risk HPV, strong consideration should be given to further evaluation with conization and dilatation and curettage (D&C). The risk of CIN II or worse in women with AGUS smears and positive HPV tests was five out of nine (56%) in our Fontana series and 16 out of 39 (43%) in Ronnett et al.'s series.[69] Combining these two series gives a risk of CIN II or worse in women with AGUS smears and positive HPV tests of 21 out of 48 or 44%. Given this risk of CIN II or worse and the fact that colposcopy with directed biopsy and ECC are poor methods of excluding glandular lesions of the cervix,[64–66] it appears prudent to perform further work-up. As some of the women with AGUS on smears desire future fertility and conizations designed to exclude glandular lesions of the cervix are large,[67] it is difficult to make a general rule that everyone with an AGUS smear, a positive HPV test but a negative evaluation requires cervical conization and D&C. Certainly, if fertility is not an issue, patients with AGUS smears, positive HPV tests and negative evaluations should undergo conization with D&C.

In determining follow-up strategies one must remember a key assumption, i.e. the diagnosis was correct in the first place. If the initial evaluation was inappropriate or if the cervical conization had positive margins, the chance of neoplasia may be much greater than the previous diagnosis would suggest. As an example, 13 out of 21 women who developed invasive cervical cancer following cryotherapy for CIN or HPV clearly had inappropriate evaluation prior to cryotherapy.[71] When performing follow-up of abnormal Pap smears, one must review the colposcopy prior to the diagnosis and/or treatment of HPV or CIN to determine whether the initial evaluation was appropriate.

SUMMARY

Screening with Pap smears will prevent most, but not all, of the deaths from cervical cancer. Most students of the disease agree that cytological screening should begin at the age of 18 years or onset of sexual activity, should be performed at least every 3 years and should be discontinued if the cervix is removed for reasons other than cervical neoplasia. An upper age limit for screening has not been determined, but in women with previous negative screening histories, 75 years may be reasonable. Most also believe that an organized screening system that screens the entire at-risk population is much more effective than an opportunistic system that screens only part of the at-risk population. There is no universal agreement concerning the appropriate ratio of ASCUS to SIL smears; the guidelines from the Bethesda system suggest that this ratio should not exceed 3; however, we have presented data suggesting that the cytological screening system would be better served if the ratio did not exceed 1. Triage of women with ASCUS Reactive and ASCUS NOS smears with HC II is advised. Women with abnormal smears other than ASCUS Reactive and ASCUS NOS should be evaluated with colposcopy and high-risk HPV testing. The indications for cervical conization or loop excision of the transformation zone in the evaluation of women with an abnormal Pap smear include: a colposcopic impression of invasive cancer; a cervical biopsy interpreted as microinvasive squamous cancer; atypical glandular neoplasia or adenocarcinoma *in situ*; a positive (CIN II or worse) endocervical curettage; discordance of the Pap smear; colposcopic impression and biopsy; and a strong suspicion of cervical glandular neoplasia.[57]

Women with a diagnosis of CIN II or CIN III should have ablation or removal of their transformation zone and be followed with colposcopy, ECC, HPV test and Pap smear at 6 months. If this evaluation is negative, they should be followed with Pap smear and HPV test at 18 months; if this again is negative, they should be followed with Pap smears yearly for life. Women with a diagnosis of HPV or CIN I may or may not benefit from ablation or removal of their transformation zones and may be followed with yearly Pap smears and HPV tests. If Pap smear and HPV test are negative for two consecutive years, they may be returned to routine screening. Women with a diagnosis of cervical atypical glandular neoplasia are at a high risk for failure and the lesions are difficult to follow, therefore, most should be advised to have hysterectomy. If the clinician follows the above guidelines, they will make few mistakes in screening women for cervical neoplasia. One must realize, however, that guidelines are only guidelines, they are never a substitute for knowledge of the disease and good clinical judgment. In this regard, it is helpful to remember that any abnormal cytological smear is more significant if the woman is over the age of 35 years, she has abnormal vaginal bleeding, has not been screened at least every 3 years, or has a history of abnormal smears. In addition, no one is absolutely sure of the diagnosis at the time of colposcopy. If the patient is at high risk for cervical neoplasia, more liberal use of repeat evaluation, LETZ or conization should be employed.

REFERENCES

1 Sherman ME, Schiffman MH, Erozan YS, Wacholder S, Kurman RJ. The Bethesda System. A proposal for reporting abnormal cervical smears based on the reproducibility of cytopathologic diagnoses. *Arch Pathol Lab Med* 1992; **116**: 1155–8.

2 Troxel DB, Sabella JD. Problem areas in pathology practice. Uncovered by a review of malpractice claims [see comments]. *Am J Surg Pathol* 1994; **18**: 821–31.

3 Papanicolaou GN, Traut HF. The diagnostic value of vaginal smears in carcinoma of the uterus. *Am J Obstet Gynecol* 1941; **42**: 193–206.

4 Ayre JE. Selective cytology smear for diagnosis of cancer. *Am J Obstet Gynecol* 1947; **53**: 609–17.

5 Pund ER, Nieburgs HE, Nettles JB, Caldwell JD. Preinvasive carcinoma of the uterine cervix. *Arch Pathol* 1947; **44**: 571–7.

6 Johansen P, Arffmann E, Pallesen G. Evaluation of smears obtained by cervical scraping and an endocervical swab in the diagnosis of neoplastic disease of the uterine cervix. *Acta Obstet Gynecol Scand* 1979; **58**: 265–70.

7 Shingleton HM, Gore H, Austin JM, Littleton HJ, Straugin JM. The contribution of endocervical smears to cervical cancer detection. *Acta Cytol* 1975; **19**: 261–4.

 8 Koss LG. The Papanicolaou test for cervical cancer detection. A triumph and a tragedy [see comments]. *JAMA* 1989; **261**: 737–43.

 9 Elias A, Linthorst G, Bekker B, Vooijs PG. The significance of endocervical cells in the diagnosis of cervical epithelial changes. *Acta Cytol* 1983; **27**: 225–9.

10 Vooijs PG, Elias A, van der Graaf Y, Veling S. Relationship between the diagnosis of epithelial abnormalities and the composition of cervical smears. *Acta Cytol* 1985; **29**: 323–8.

11 Trimbos JB, Arentz NP. The efficiency of the Cytobrush versus the cotton swab in the collection of endocervical cells in cervical smears. *Acta Cytol* 1986; **30**: 261–3.

12 Pretorius RG, Sadeghi M, Fotheringham N, Semrad N, Watring WG. A randomized trial of three methods of obtaining Papanicolaou smears. *Obstet Gynecol* 1991; **78**: 831–6.

13 Koonings PP, Dickinson K, d'Ablaing Gd, Schlaerth JB. A randomized clinical trial comparing the Cytobrush and cotton swab for Papanicolaou smears. *Obstet Gynecol* 1992; **80**: 241–5.

14 McCord ML, Stovall TG, Meric JL, Summitt Jr RL, Coleman SA. Cervical cytology: a randomized comparison of four sampling methods. *Am J Obstet Gynecol* 1992; **166**: 1772–7; discussion 7–9.

15 Murata PJ, Johnson RA, McNicoll KE. Controlled evaluation of implementing the Cytobrush technique to improve Papanicolaou smear quality. *Obstet Gynecol* 1990; **75**: 690–5.

16 Boon ME, de Graaff Guilloud JC, Rietveld WJ. Analysis of five sampling methods for the preparation of cervical smears. *Acta Cytol* 1989; **33**: 843–8.

17 Hughes RG, Haddad NG, Smart GE, et al. The cytological detection of persistent cervical intraepithelial neoplasia after local ablative treatment: a comparison of sampling devices [see comments]. *Br J Obstet Gynaecol* 1992; **99**: 498–502.

18 Orr Jr JW, Barrett JM, Orr PF, Holloway RW, Holimon JL. The efficacy and safety of the cytobrush during pregnancy. *Gynecol Oncol* 1992; **44**: 260–2.

19 Colon VF, Linz LE. The extended tip spatula for cervical cytology. *J Fam Pract* 1981; **13**: 37–41.

20 Eisenstein MI. Eisenstein ecto-endo cervical scraper. *NY J Med* 1961; **61**: 591–2.

21 Hutchinson ML, Cassin CM, Ball HGD. The efficacy of an automated preparation device for cervical cytology. *Am J Clin Pathol* 1991; **96**: 300–5.

22 Sherman ME, Schiffman MH, Lorincz AT, et al. Cervical specimens collected in liquid buffer are suitable for both cytologic screening and ancillary human papillomavirus testing. *Cancer* 1997; **81**: 89–97.

23 Boyes DA. The value of a Pap smear program and suggestions for its implementation. *Cancer* 1981; **48**: 613–21.

24 van Wijngaarden WJ, Duncan ID. Rationale for stopping cervical screening in women over 50 [published erratum appears in *BMJ* 1993; **306**: 1373] [see comments]. *BMJ* 1993; **306**: 967–71.

25 Armstrong BK, Munoz N, Bosch FX. Epidemiology of cancer of the cervix. In: Coppleson M, ed. *Gynecologic Oncology*. Edinburgh: Churchill Livingstone, 1992: 11–30.

26 Cusano MM, Young JLJ. *Forty-five years of cancer incidence in Connecticut: 1935–79, National Cancer Institute Monograph 70;NIH Pub. No. 86-2652*. Bethesda, MD: NIH, 1986.

27 Mandelblatt J. Papanicolaou testing following hysterectomy. *JAMA* 1991; **266**: 1289.

28 Pearce KF, Haefner HK, Sarwar SF, Nolan TE. Cytopathological findings on vaginal Papanicolaou smears after hysterectomy for benign gynecologic disease [see comments]. *N Engl J Med* 1996; **335**: 1559–62.

29 Screening for squamous cervical cancer: duration of low risk after negative results of cervical cytology and its implication for screening policies. IARC Working Group on evaluation of cervical cancer screening programs. *Br Med J (Clin Res edn)* 1986; **293**: 659–64.

30 Kavanagh AM, Santow G, Mitchell H. Consequences of current patterns of Pap smear and colposcopy use. *J Med Screen* 1996; **3**: 29–34.

31 Mitchell MF, Schottenfeld D. The natural history of cervical intraepithelial neoplasia and management of the abnormal Papanicolaou smear. In: Rubin SC, Hoskins WJ, eds. *Cervical cancer and preinvasive neoplasia*. Philadelphia: Lippincott-Raven, 1996: 109.

32 Kinlen LJ, Spriggs AI. Women with positive cervical smears but without surgical intervention. A follow-up study. *Lancet* 1978; **ii**: 463–5.

33 Hulka BS. Risk factors for cervical cancer. *J Chronic Dis* 1982; **35**: 3–11.

34 *ACOG Technical Bulletin*; 1993 August. No. 183.

35 US Preventive Services Task Force. *Guide to clinical preventive services*. Baltimore: Williams & Wilkins, 1996.

36 Harlan LC, Bernstein AB, Kessler LG. Cervical cancer screening: who is not screened and why? *Am J Public Health* 1991; **81**: 885–91.

37 Kottke TE, Trapp MA, Fores MM, et al. Cancer screening behaviors and attitudes of women in southeastern Minnesota [see comments]. *JAMA* 1995; **273**: 1099–105.

38 Laara E, Day NE, Hakama M. Trends in mortality from cervical cancer in the Nordic countries: association with organised screening programs. *Lancet* 1987; **i**: 1247–9.

39 Law M. 'Opportunistic' screening [editorial]. *J Med Screen* 1994; **1**: 208.

40 Makuc DM, Freid VM, Kleinman JC. National trends in the use of preventive health care by women. *Am J Public Health* 1989; **79**: 21–6.

41 August N. Cervicography for evaluating the 'atypical' Papanicolaou smear. *J Reprod Med* 1991; **36**: 89–94.

42 Jones DE, Creasman WT, Dombroski RA, Lentz SS, Waeltz JL. Evaluation of the atypical Pap smear. *Am J Obstet Gynecol* 1987; **157**: 544–9.

43 Spitzer M, Krumholz BA, Chernys AE, Seltzer V, Lightman AR. Comparative utility of repeat Papanicolaou smears, cervicography, and colposcopy in the evaluation of atypical Papanicolaou smears. *Obstet Gynecol* 1987; **69**: 731–5.

44 Clavel C, Masure M, Bory JP, et al. Hybrid Capture II-based human papillomavirus detection, a sensitive test to detect in routine high-grade cervical lesions: a preliminary study on 1518 women. *Br J Cancer* 1999; **80**: 1306–11.

45 Cuzick J, Szarewski A, Terry G, et al. Human papillomavirus testing in primary cervical screening [see comments]. *Lancet* 1995; **345**: 1533–6.

46 Reid R, Greenberg MD, Lorincz A, et al. Should cervical cytologic testing be augmented by cervicography or human papillomavirus deoxyribonucleic acid detection? *Am J Obstet Gynecol* 1991; **164**: 1461–9; discussion 9–71.

47 Tawa K, Forsythe A, Cove JK, Saltz A, Peters HW, Watring WG. A comparison of the Papanicolaou smear and the cervigram: sensitivity, specificity, and cost analysis. *Obstet Gynecol* 1988; **71**: 229–35.

48 Wright Jr TC, Denny L, Kuhn L, Pollack A, Lorincz A. HPV DNA testing of self-collected vaginal samples compared with cytologic screening to detect cervical cancer [see comments]. *JAMA* 2000; **283**: 81–6.

49 Manos MM, Kinney WK, Hurley LB, et al. Identifying women with cervical neoplasia: using human papillomavirus DNA testing for equivocal Papanicolaou results [see comments]. *JAMA* 1999; **281**: 1605–10.

50 Pretorius R, Binstock M, Sadeghi M, Hodges W. Cervical and vaginal cytologic smears suggestive of adenocarcinoma. *J Reprod Med* 1996; **41**: 478–82.

51 Cherkis RC, Patten Jr SF, Andrews TJ, Dickinson JC, Patten FW. Significance of normal endometrial cells detected by cervical cytology. *Obstet Gynecol* 1988; **71**: 242–4.

52 Ng AB, Reagan JW, Hawliczek S, Wentz BW. Significance of endometrial cells in the detection of endometrial carcinoma and its precursors. *Acta Cytol* 1974; **18**: 356–61.

53 Yancey M, Magelssen D, Demaurez A, Lee RB. Classification of endometrial cells on cervical cytology. *Obstet Gynecol* 1990; **76**: 1000–5.

54 Kurman RJ, Soloman D. *The Bethesda system for reporting cervical/vaginal cytologic diagnosis: Definitions, criteria and explanatory notes for terminology and specimen adequacy*. New York: Springer-Verlag, 1994.

55 Vassilakos P, Schwartz D, de Marval F, et al. Biopsy-based comparison of liquid-based, thin-layer preparations to conventional Pap smears. *J Reprod Med* 2000; **45**: 11 16.

56 Hutchinson ML, Zahniser DJ, Sherman ME, et al. Utility of liquid-based cytology for cervical carcinoma screening: results of a population-based study conducted in a region of Costa Rica with a high incidence of cervical carcinoma. *Cancer* 1999; **87**: 48–55.

57 Coppleson M, Atkinson KH, Dalrymple C. Cervical squamous and glandular intraepithelial neoplasia: clinical features and review of management. In: Coppleson M, ed. *Gynecologic Oncology*. Edinburgh: Churchill Livingstone, 1992: 571–608.

58 Walboomers JM, Jacobs MV, Manos MM, et al. Human papillomavirus is a necessary cause of invasive cervical cancer worldwide [see comments]. *J Pathol* 1999; **189**: 12–19.

59 Koutsky LA, Holmes KK, Critchlow CW, et al. A cohort study of the risk of cervical intraepithelial neoplasia grade 2 or 3 in relation to papillomavirus infection. *N Engl J Med* 1992; **327**: 1272–8.

60 Lorincz AT, Reid R, Jenson AB, Greenberg MD, Lancaster W, Kurman RJ. Human papillomavirus infection of the cervix: relative risk associations of 15 common anogenital types. *Obstet Gynecol* 1992; **79**: 328–37.

61 Wheeler CM, Greer CE, Becker TM, Hunt WC, Anderson SM, Manos MM. Short-term fluctuations in the detection of cervical human papillomavirus DNA. *Obstet Gynecol* 1996; **88**: 261–8.

62 Stafl A. Cervicography: a new method for cervical cancer detection. *Am J Obstet Gynecol* 1981; **139**: 815–25.

63 Kaminski PF, Stevens Jr CW, Wheelock JB. Squamous atypia on cytology. The influence of age. *J Reprod Med* 1989; **34**: 617–20.

64 Andersen ES, Arffmann E. Adenocarcinoma *in situ* of the uterine cervix: a clinico-pathologic study of 36 cases. *Gynecol Oncol* 1989; **35**: 1–7.

65 Luesley DM, Jordan JA, Woodman CB, Watson N, Williams DR, Waddell C. A retrospective review of adenocarcinoma-*in-situ* and glandular atypia of the uterine cervix. *Br J Obstet Gynaecol* 1987; **94**: 699–703.

66 Ostor AG, Pagano R, Davoren RA, Fortune DW, Chanen W, Rome R. Adenocarcinoma *in situ* of the cervix. *Int J Gynecol Pathol* 1984; **3**: 179–90.

67 Bertrand M, Lickrish GM, Colgan TJ. The anatomic distribution of cervical adenocarcinoma *in situ*: implications for treatment. *Am J Obstet Gynecol* 1987; **157**: 21–5.

68 Luesley DM, McCrum A, Terry PB, et al. Complications of cone biopsy related to the dimensions of the cone and the influence of prior colposcopic assessment. *Br J Obstet Gynaecol* 1985; **92**: 158–64.

69 Ronnett BM, Manos MM, Ransley JE, et al. Atypical glandular cells of undetermined significance (AGUS): cytopathologic features, histopathologic results, and human papillomavirus DNA detection. *Hum Pathol* 1999; **30**: 816–25.

70 Petrilli ES, Townsend DE, Morrow CP, Nakao CY. Vaginal intraepithelial neoplasia: biologic aspects and treatment with topical 5-fluorouracil and the carbon dioxide laser. *Am J Obstet Gynecol* 1980; **138**: 321–8.

71 Schmidt C, Pretorius RG, Bonin M, Hanson L, Semrad N, Watring W. Invasive cervical cancer following cryotherapy for cervical intraepithelial neoplasia or human papillomavirus infection. *Obstet Gynecol* 1992; **80**: 797–800.

72 Falcone T, Ferenczy A. Cervical intraepithelial neoplasia and condyloma: an analysis of diagnostic accuracy of posttreatment follow-up methods. *Am J Obstet Gynecol* 1986; **154**: 260–4.

73 Ho GY, Bierman R, Beardsley L, Chang CJ, Burk RD. Natural history of cervicovaginal papillomavirus infection in young women. *N Engl J Med* 1998; **338**: 423–8.

74 Nobbenhuis MA, Walboomers JM, Helmerhorst TJ, et al. Relation of human papillomavirus status to cervical lesions and consequences for cervical-cancer screening: a prospective study. *Lancet* 1999; **354**: 20–5.

75 Ismail SM, Colclough AB, Dinnen JS, et al. Reporting cervical intra-epithelial neoplasia (CIN): intra- and interpathologist variation and factors associated with disagreement. *Histopathology* 1990; **16**: 371–6.

76 Robertson AJ, Anderson JM, Beck JS, et al. Observer variability in histopathological reporting of cervical biopsy specimens. *J Clin Pathol* 1989; **42**: 231–8.

77 Binder MA, Cates GW, Emson HE, et al. The changing concepts of condyloma. A retrospective study of colposcopically directed cervical biopsies. *Am J Obstet Gynecol* 1985; **151**: 213–19.

78 Campion MJ, McCance DJ, Cuzick J, Singer A. Progressive potential of mild cervical atypia: prospective cytological, colposcopic, and virological study. *Lancet* 1986; **ii**: 237–40.

79 Kataja V, Syrjanen K, Mantyjarvi R, et al. Prospective follow-up of cervical HPV infections: life table analysis of histopathological, cytological and colposcopic data. *Eur J Epidemiol* 1989; **5**: 1–7.

80 Nasiell K, Roger V, Nasiell M. Behavior of mild cervical dysplasia during long-term follow-up. *Obstet Gynecol* 1986; **67**: 665–9.

81 Franco EL, Villa LL, Sobrinho JP, et al. Epidemiology of acquisition and clearance of cervical human papillomavirus infection in women from a high-risk area for cervical cancer. *J Infect Dis* 1999; **180**: 1415–23.

82 Wallin KL, Wiklund F, Angstrom T, et al. Type-specific persistence of human papillomavirus DNA before the development of invasive cervical cancer. *N Engl J Med* 1999; **341**: 1633–8.

83 Bekassy Z, Ahlgren M, Eriksson M, Lindh E. Carbon dioxide laser miniconization for treatment of human papillomavirus infection associated with cervical intraepithelial neoplasia. *Acta Obstet Gynecol Scand* 1995; **74**: 822–6.

84 Sesti F, De Santis L, Farne C, Mantenuto L, Piccione E. Efficacy of CO_2 laser surgery in treating squamous intraepithelial lesions. An analysis of clinical and virologic results. *J Reprod Med* 1994; **39**: 441–4.

85 Kiviat N. Natural history of cervical neoplasia: overview and update. *Am J Obstet Gynecol* 1996; **175**: 1099–104.

86 Ward KA, Houston JR, Lowry BE, Maw RD, Dinsmore WW. The role of early colposcopy in the management of females with first episode anogenital warts. *Int J STD AIDS* 1994; **5**: 343–5.

87 Raisi O, Ghirardini C, Aloisi P, Cermelli C, Portolani M. HPV typing of cervical squamous lesions by *in situ* HPV DNA hybridization: influence of HPV type and therapy on the follow-up of low-grade squamous cervical disease. *Diagn Cytopathol* 1994; **11**: 28–32.

88 Hopkins MP, Roberts JA, Schmidt RW. Cervical adenocarcinoma *in situ*. *Obstet Gynecol* 1988; **71**: 842–4.

89 Muntz HG, Bell DA, Lage JM, Goff BA, Feldman S, Rice LW. Adenocarcinoma *in situ* of the uterine cervix. *Obstet Gynecol* 1992; **80**: 935–9.

90 Poynor EA, Barakat RR, Hoskins WJ. Management and follow-up of patients with adenocarcinoma *in situ* of the uterine cervix. *Gynecol Oncol* 1995; **57**: 158–64.

91 Im DD, Duska LR, Rosenshein NB. Adequacy of conization margins in adenocarcinoma *in situ* of the cervix as a predictor of residual disease. *Gynecol Oncol* 1995; **59**: 179–82.

3

Automation

JORGE L GONZALEZ, R SHAWN UNDERWOOD

INTRODUCTION

The methods for preparing and screening Pap smears have essentially remained unchanged since its inception. As the decreasing trend of incidence and mortality rate of cervical cancer has reached a plateau, the attention on Pap smears has been shifted from its use to its accuracy. As a response to the once short supply of cytotechnologists and the concerns over false-negative rates accompanied by the advancement of computer sciences, automation of the Pap smear has proceeded rapidly in the last decade. The research and development of Pap smear automation has been primarily along two lines: to improve the preparation and to replace, at least to some extent, manual screening. The efforts along the first line were initially to facilitate automated screening.

Sampling and preparation problems, and to a lesser extent screening and interpretation errors, have been identified as the major sources of false-negative diagnoses.[1–5] Suboptimal specimens resulting from poor fixation, inflammation, excessive cellular overlapping, and/or obscuring blood are closely associated with false-negative rates.[6] Recent studies have also indicated that only a small proportion of the cells collected from the cervix are manually transferred to the glass slide of conventionally prepared Pap smears,[7–9] and that these are not always a representative subset of the original sample.[8,9] Two comparable but distinct methods of preparing thin-layer slides (Cytyc Corporation, Boxborough, MA, USA, and TriPath Imaging, Inc., Burlington, NC, USA) emerged to address the concerns raised about inadequate sampling and suboptimal preparation of conventional Pap smears. In an effort to supplement and reduce manual screening to improve accuracy, automated screening systems were developed. Currently, the AutoPap System (TriPath Imaging, Inc.) is the only screening system that has been approved by the Food and Drug Administration (FDA) as an automated primary screening system. Process control devices have also been invented to monitor the process of manual screening to ensure thoroughness and to improve the efficiency of the process.

THIN-LAYER PREPARATIONS VERSUS CONVENTIONAL PAP SMEARS

It was previously assumed that sampling error is entirely attributable to the health-care worker obtaining a poor sample. However, another source of sampling error derives from the fact that a significant proportion of the sampled material is not transferred to the glass slide during the manual preparation of a direct smear, but is instead discarded along with the collection device.[8] Flow cytometry studies have shown that, depending on the sampler used, up to 90 per cent of the cervical material sampled is discarded with the sampling device.[8] In a 1994 study by Hutchinson et al., the amount of cells transferred by a manual direct smear to the glass slide ranged from 6.5 to 62.5 per cent.[10] Therefore, a manual direct smear preparation may not contain the most diagnostic cells from the lesion sampled.[8] By rinsing all of the cellular material from the biosampler or ejecting the head of the biosampler into a fluid transport/storage medium, virtually none of the material is discarded and all of the cells should be well preserved.

The thin-layer preparation process disaggregates large cell clumps, and significantly reduces cervical mucus, blood, neutrophils, and cellular debris. Several studies have suggested that this would result in an increased cell harvest, with a more representative sample transferred to the glass slide, a reduction in inadequate specimens, and an increase in the detection of abnormal cells.[8,10,11]

Thin-layer technologies evolved from an effort to standardize cytology preparations and to help minimize conditions that may compromise interpretation. Early efforts in developing these technologies took place predominantly in Europe, in Germany and The Netherlands. At first they were intended for use with automatic screening devices with the goal of a single cell suspension. Subsequently, it became evident that disruption of all cell aggregates into single cells was not necessary. Thin-layer preparations produced by the current technologies retain small cell aggregates as well as single cells.

Thin-layer preparations employ a fluid-based cytology collection method. The cells are sampled by conventional methods and are then rinsed into a preservative solution either along with or without the sampling device. Health-care providers, who perform the sampling, do not prepare smears. This significantly reduces the artifacts that often occur during the preparation of such smears. The cells that are suspended in the preservative solution are then collected in a cell processor and a representative portion transferred to the center of a glass slide as a circular thin layer of cells and cell groups. The screening area is reduced by at least 75 per cent compared with conventional smears and the cells are mainly in one focal plane when screening with a ×10 objective. Since the cells arrive at the laboratory in a preservative solution, the sample can be stored for a period of time. In addition, more than one thin-layer slide can be prepared and additional tests or studies can be performed from a single sample, either at the time of the original processing or at a later date. HPV-typing, and the detection of *Chlamydia* and gonococcus by DNA probes are possible using the cells that remain in the vial after routine preparation of a thin-layer slide. In a recent study by Sherman et al.,[12] Hybrid Capture testing for human papillomavirus (HPV) DNA was successfully performed from the cervico-vaginal cellular material collected in the ThinPrep preservative. (Please refer to Chapters 2 and 6 for details on incorporating HPV-typing in the triage and management of patients with abnormal Pap smears.) HPV-typing by DNA probes is FDA-approved for the PreservCyt Solution (Cytyc) and is being sought for the CytoRich Preservative Fluid (TriPath). Although technically possible, the detection of both *Chlamydia* and gonococcus using DNA probes is not yet FDA-approved for either fixative.

Processing large numbers of cervicovaginal samples in a timely and cost-effective manner requires the development of systems that employ computerization and robotics. The two companies that have commercially available thin-layer preparation systems, the Cytyc Corporation and TriPath Corporation (formerly AutoCyte, Inc.) have addressed this need.

The ThinPrep 2000 processor manufactured by the Cytyc Corporation was the first FDA-approved system for thin-layer preparations of cervicovaginal (GYN) specimens. Approval was granted in May 1996. The TriPath Corporation has also developed a comparable but distinct system (AutoCyte) and obtained FDA approval in 1999. Since the Cytyc Corporation helped pioneer the computer technology for the thin-layer preparation of GYN cell samples and was the first to submit clinical trial results to the FDA, there are greater numbers of studies in the literature that compare the ThinPrep method with the conventional Pap smear. Both companies also have FDA approval for processing non-gynecological (NON-GYN) specimens.

Initially, there were concerns that small organisms such as *Trichomonas vaginalis* would be lost in thin-layer processing. Studies have since shown that infectious organisms are not only retained but may be more easily recognized because of the better cellular preservation.[2,13]

Another source of concern was that the loss or significant decrease of familiar patterns in thin-layer preparations, such as a background diathesis, might negatively impact diagnostic accuracy. However, studies comparing thin-layer preparations with conventional Pap smears do not support this notion. It should also be noted that both companies emphasize that cytotechnologists/cytopathologists require additional training and experience before they are fully proficient in assessing GYN thin-layer preparations. Thin-layer slides with scant cellularity can be particularly difficult to accurately screen and interpret. Differences in nuclear morphology have been reported with the ThinPrep, which uses a methanol-based fixative rather than the ethanol fixation of conventional smears. The AutoCyte system uses an ethanol-based fixative. As the familiarity and experience with thin-layer preparations of the screener increases, the detection of abnormal cells should be at least as good as conventional smears and most likely will be enhanced by the better cellular preservation and cleaner background.

ThinPrep processor

The Cytyc ThinPrep Processor uses a methanol-based antibacterial preservative called PreservCyt Solution that will preserve cells for up to 3 weeks at temperatures between 4 and 37°C. The Cervex-Brush, cytobrushes, and plastic spatulas are approved sampling devices. Wooden spatulas and cotton swabs should not be used because their porous nature tends to entrap the cells within the collection device. The slide preparation technique consists of three phases: dispersion, cell collection and cell transfer.

The processor employs a rotary drive mechanism to gently disperse the cell samples. In the dispersion phase, a cylinder with a smooth, flat, porous and biologically neutral polycarbonate filter (TransCyt Filter) at one end is rotated in the preservative solution to create shear forces of sufficient magnitude to separate randomly adherent clumps and to disperse cervical mucus without harming the cell sample.

In the cell collection phase, a slight vacuum pressure is applied to the cylinder with the attached TransCyt Filter. The cells adhere to the filter on one plane and are then ready for cell transfer. The cell collection phase is computer-controlled by software that analyzes the pressure in the cylinder. The rate of flow through the TransCyt Filter is constantly monitored to prevent too scant or too dense a cell population from ultimately being transferred to the glass slide.

The cells that adhere to the filter are then transferred to the slide by applying a pulse of air through the filter, aided by the electrostatic charge of the slide since the cells have a higher natural affinity for the glass slide than for the polycarbonate membrane.

The end result is a circular thin-layer of cells measuring 20 mm in diameter in the center of the glass slide, with a decreased amount of cervical mucus and cellular debris compared with conventional Pap smears. The filter can be used only once and must subsequently be discarded. The prepared slide is automatically deposited into a fixative solution and is ready for staining with the Papanicolaou stain by standard methods.

The first Cytyc processor that was approved for GYN specimens was the ThinPrep 2000 Processor (T-2000); it can also process NON-GYN samples. It is a single-load system – only one cervicovaginal sample can be processed at a time – which requires constant monitoring. It takes approximately 3–4 min to set up and prepare a single sample prior to staining. The Cytyc Corporation has also developed a multiload system (T-3000) which can process up to 80 specimens at one time and loads the unstained thin-layer preparations into a standard staining-rack that is compatible with most automated staining systems. It is fully automated with 'walk-away' capability and can process approximately 140 000 specimens per year. The specimens are bar-coded to ensure an automatic chain of custody verification throughout processing. The T-3000 model was approved by the FDA in the spring of 2000. Unlike the T-2000, which can process both GYN and NON-GYN specimens, the T-3000 is strictly for GYN samples and does not require constant monitoring during processing.

A prospective multicenter study involving six centers (three screening centers and three hospitals with high-risk populations) evaluated the performance of the T-2000 and compared it with that of the conventional Pap smear in detecting both epithelial cell abnormalities and benign cellular changes, as outlined in the Bethesda System.[14] A conventional Pap smear was prepared first by directly smearing the cells onto a slide. The residual material that was retained on the biosampler, which normally would have been discarded, was submitted in Cytyc preservative solution for processing by the T-2000. One pathologist served as an independent reviewer for all sites submitting samples. Two additional studies were conducted to evaluate specimen adequacy, in which all of the material collected with the biosampler was submitted for processing by the T-2000 (direct-to-vial studies). The original results, as well as those of other studies, showed that the ThinPrep smears were at least as good as conventional Pap smears in identifying both benign cellular changes and epithelial cell abnormalities (Tables 3.1–3.3).[14–18] Subsequent review of the split-sample data and additional direct-to-vial studies have demonstrated an increased detection rate of squamous intraepithelial lesions with the ThinPrep method.[19–21]

In the original split-sample study,[14] transformation-zone elements (endocervical and/ or metaplastic cells) were seen less frequently in the ThinPrep preparations than in conventional Pap smears, particularly in specimens with scant cellularity. A specimen with a lack of transformation-zone elements has traditionally been considered 'satisfactory but limited'.

Table 3.1 *Results by site, low-grade squamous intraepithelial lesions (LSIL) and more severe lesions*

Site	Cases	ThinPrep LSIL+	Conventional LSIL+
S1	1336	46	25
S2	1563	78	45
S3	1058	67	40
H1	971	125	96
H2	1010	111	130
H3	809	210	196
All sites	6474	637	538

Reproduced from the introduction to the *ThinPrep Operator's Manual* with permission from the Cytyc Corporation.[15]

Table 3.2 *Results by site, atypical squamous cells of undetermined significance (ASCUS)/atypical glandular cells of undetermined significance (AGUS) and more severe lesions*[a]

Site	Cases	ThinPrep ASCUS+	Conventional ASCUS+
S1	1336	117	93
S2	1563	124	80
S3	1058	123	81
H1	971	204	173
H2	1010	259	282
H3	809	327	359
All sites	6474	1154	1068

[a]Reproduced from the introduction to the *ThinPrep Operator's Manual* with permission from the Cytyc Corporation.[15]

Table 3.3 *Summary of descriptive diagnosis (number of patients = 6747)*[a]

Descriptive diagnosis[b]	ThinPrep		Conventional	
	n	%	*n*	%
Benign cellular changes	1592	23.6	1591	23.6
Infection:				
Trichomonas vaginalis	136	2.0	185	2.7
Candida spp.	406	6.0	259	3.8
Coccobacilli	690	10.2	608	9.0
Actinomyces spp.	2	0.0	3	0.0
Herpes	3	0.0	8	0.1
Other	155	2.3	285	4.2
Reactive cellular changes associated with:				
Inflammation	353	5.2	385	5.7
Atrophic vaginitis	32	0.5	48	0.7
Radiation	2	0.0	1	0.0
Other	25	0.4	37	0.5
Epithelial cell abnormalities	1159	17.2	1077	16.0
Squamous cell:				
ASCUS	501	7.4	521	7.7
Favor reactive	128	1.9	131	1.9
Favor neoplastic	161	2.4	140	2.1
Undetermined	213	3.2	250	3.7
LSIL	469	7.0	367	5.4
HSIL	167	2.5	167	2.5
Carcinoma	1	0.0	3	0.0
Glandular cell:				
Benign endometrial cells in postmenopausal women	7	0.1	10	0.1
Atypical glandular cells (AGUS)	21	0.3	9	0.1
Favor reactive	9	0.1	4	0.1
Favor neoplastic	0	0.0	3	0.0
Undetermined	12	0.2	2	0.0
Endocervical adenocarcinoma	0	0.0	1	0.0

[a]Reproduced from the introduction to the *ThinPrep Operator's Manual* with permission from the Cytyc Corporation.[15]
[b]Abbreviations: ASCUS, atypical squamous cells of undetermined significance; LSIL, low-grade squamous intraepithelial lesions; HSIL, high-grade squamous intraepithelial lesions; AGUS, atypical glandular cells of undetermined significance.

Table 3.4 *Summary of direct-to-vial studies*[a]

Study[c]	Number of evaluable patients	SBLB[b] due to no endocervical component	Comparable conventional Pap smear percentage
Direct-to-vial feasibility	299	9.36%	9.43%
Direct-to-vial clinical study	484	4.96%	4.38%

[a]Reproduced from the introduction to the *ThinPrep Operator's Manual* with permission from the Cytyc Corporation.[15,23]
[b]SBLB, 'satisfactory but limited by'.
[c]Direct-to-vial feasibility study compared overall clinical investigation Pap smear SBLB – no endocervical component rate. Direct-to-vial clinical study compared with site S2 clinical investigation Pap smear SBLB – no endocervical component rate.

This phenomenon was also noted in similar but independent studies that used a split-sample collection technique.[22] However, in the direct-to-vial studies, in which all of the material collected was submitted for ThinPrep processing, there were no significant differences in the percentage of cases lacking transformation-zone elements compared with rates seen in historical or parallel conventional Pap smears (Table 3.4).[15,23]

The cleaner background and the confinement of cells to a particular region of the slide has reportedly facilitated screening, including reducing screening times, and has decreased the numbers of limited specimens secondary to obscuring mucus or extensive cellular overlapping. In a split-sample study comprised of specimens from 365 patients, the ThinPrep interpretation time was 1 min and 23 s shorter, on average, per slide compared with the conventional Pap smear. In addition, over 20 per cent of the conventional Pap smears took 5–10 min to be screened while only 1.4 per cent of the ThinPrep preparations took longer than 5 min to be screened, and none of the ThinPreps took longer than 7 min.[22] Other studies have shown even greater reductions in screening times.[17,24]

AutoCyte PREP

The AutoCyte system is a semi-automated density-gradient centrifugation-based method of preparing thin-layer slides. A cervicovaginal sample is collected with an approved biosampler and is placed directly into an ethanol-based transport medium (CytoRich Preservative Fluid) for processing in the laboratory. Samples can be stored for future use in refrigerated preservative fluid at 2–8°C. This contrasts with storage at room temperature for specimens preserved in PreservCyt Solution (Cytyc). The Cervex-Brush samplers are supplied as part of the system and are currently the only FDA-approved sampling devices to be used with the system. However, approval for use of cytobrushes and plastic spatulas is being sought. The use of wooden spatulas or cotton swabs for specimen collection is discouraged. When using a Cervex-Brush, the head of the sampler is ejected into the collection vial, which is then capped and sent to the laboratory for processing. The properties of the CytoRich Preservative Fluid are such that the cells do not bond to the collection device and are easily dislodged. In addition, the preservative lyses red blood cells and liquefies cervical mucus.

In the laboratory, the sample is first manually vortexed to create shear forces that disaggregate cell clumps. A multiload, fully automated, self-contained vortexer that can process 25 specimens at a time is commercially available. The cell suspension is then aspirated through a syringe-like device developed by the former AutoCyte Corporation, called the CyRinge, into a separate tube containing the CytoRich Density Reagent. The CyRinge has a small orifice that further helps disaggregate cell clumps. The sample then undergoes centrifugal density sedimentation through the density reagent to help reduce debris, cell fragments, and neutrophils. At least 50 per cent or more of the inflammatory cells and debris are removed and the epithelial cells are concentrated. Therefore, the relative percentage of the epithelial cells comprising the sample is increased (known as the 'cell enrichment phase'). After centrifugation, the CytoRich Density Reagent tubes are placed into the AutoCyte processor (AutoCyte PREP). The processor has a programmable pipette and delivery system that transfers samples of the suspended cell concentrate to small plastic chambers mounted on cationic-coated microscope slides. The cells settle onto the slide by normal gravity. The slides are then automatically Pap stained within individual and separate chambers to prevent cross-contamination. After staining, the chambers are removed and the slides contained are ready for cover-slipping.

The CyRinge phase of the preparation is manual and therefore labor-intensive. TriPath Imaging, Inc., has since developed an adjuvant system known as the Prep Mate which is intended to automate this portion of the specimen processing has been approved recently by the FDA. Up to 12 vials can be placed into the Prep Mate at one time. The Prep Mate then aspirates the samples after piercing a circular portion of foil that is embedded in the cap of the collection vial. Each of the samples is then automatically transferred to a tube containing the density reagent. The remainder of the processing remains the same.

The processor is robotic, semi-automated, and computer-controlled. It is a multiload instrument that can prepare up to 48 specimens per run and can process six batches per 8-hour workday. Because the specimens are batched, free periods of operation ranging from 30 to 45 min occur during a run, depending on the size of the batch.

The end result is a representative and evenly distributed Pap-stained circular thin-layer of cells measuring 13 mm in diameter in the center of the glass slide. Approximately 40 000–70 000 cells are present within the thin-layer, which is well above the minimum number required to make a definitive diagnosis.[25]

Like the ThinPrep slides, the AutoCyte preparation also appears to be at least as good as conventional Pap smears for detecting both benign cellular changes and epithelial abnormalities[8,11,13] and is associated with a decrease in screening times.[8] The number of suboptimal specimens is reportedly reduced with the AutoCyte system compared with conventional smears.[2,13,26] In two studies using split-sample protocols, one involving six different clinical sites and 286 patients and the other containing 2032 paired samples, the AutoCyte method diagnosed more cases of squamous intraepithelial lesions (SIL) than did the conventional smears.[13,27] A recent direct-to-vial study by Vassilakos et al.[28] demonstrated an increased detection rate for both low-grade and high-grade SIL with AutoCyte thin-layer preparations.

In another study comparing 560 pairs of conventional smears and AutoCyte preparations, the AutoCyte method significantly reduced the number of poor quality, and therefore, suboptimal specimens (28.3 per cent for conventional smears versus 8.4 per cent for AutoCyte).[11] In addition, a greater number of cases were identified as either an intraepithelial lesion or an invasive carcinoma compared with conventional Pap smears. There was a decrease in the number of cases identified as atypical squamous cells of undetermined significance (ASCUS) or atypical glandular cells of undetermined significance (AGUS). This latter result was considered to be due to better cellular preservation and elimination of obscuring factors by the AutoCyte method, allowing more accurate categorization of the cellular changes as either neoplastic or reactive and thus removing cases from the more ambiguous categories of ASCUS/AGUS.[11]

COMPUTER-BASED AUTOMATED SCREENING SYSTEMS

Computers and software with the power and capability to scan and classify complex images with sufficient accuracy and speed are a relatively recent development. The advantages of computerized screening systems include their ability to analyze all of the cells on a slide without omission or fatigue affecting the process, and the ability of some systems to provide objective measurements to supplement the visual presentations.

The first FDA-approved systems that were formerly available consisted of two separate and distinct technologies developed by Neuromedical Systems, Inc. (PAPNET), and Neopath (now TriPath Imaging), Inc., respectively. These systems were originally intended for rescreening negative Pap smears only (i.e. secondary screeners). The PAPNET rescreener did not prove cost-effective or gain enough support among cytology laboratories to remain viable. The system (AutoPap) developed by Neopath (TriPath Imaging) Inc., was transformed into a primary screener and is the only FDA-approved computerized screening system that is currently available on the market. An AutoCyte SCREEN screening system that was originally developed by Roche and later acquired by TriPath never received approval from the FDA and is not being further developed at this time.

PAPNET

The PAPNET system is no longer in routine use but the neural net technology developed by Neuromedical Systems, Inc., was subsequently purchased by TriPath Imaging, Inc. A review of the original system is included in this section.

Early attempts to develop automated computerized screening systems for conventional Pap smears were essentially unsuccessful because of the marked degree of variability in preparation, staining, cell distribution, obscuring debris, etc., present on the smears. With the development of artificial intelligence systems (neural network technology), computer screening of conventional smears became a possibility. Neural network computers are uniquely suited for complex pattern recognition,[29,30] since they are modeled on the network of neurons in the human brain and emulate the parallel-processing capabilities of the brain. Neural network systems are 'taught' rather than programmed. They can learn by example and then generalize this information. The neural networks of the PAPNET system were 'taught' by viewing thousands of examples of cells and cell clusters and a variety of staining variables, making the system tolerant of variations in staining and preparation.[29,31]

PAPNET was a computerized system that used neural network technology to recognize potentially abnormal cells and/or cell clusters in conventionally prepared Pap smears and did not require thin-layer preparations.[29,30,32] The abnormal cells were displayed and subsequently reviewed by cytotechnologists and/or cytopathologists to render a diagnosis. Therefore, the system was intended to facilitate and assist in screening but did not directly interpret a smear as either negative or abnormal. It was marketed as a rescreening device designed to supplement conventional microscopy.

PAPNET consisted of two substations, one for scanning the smear and the other for reviewing the captured images. The scanning station had an automated microscope that was programmed to scan the smear and to capture cell images for computer processing on digital tape. The system used internal algorithms to recognize a set of potentially abnormal areas in the smear, and neural network processing to recognize the potentially abnormal cells. A total of 128 most abnormal areas of the slide ('cell scenes') were chosen by the PAPNET system from a smear to be stored on a digital tape. The scanning process took less than 10 min per smear, depending on the cellularity and the quality of the smear preparation.[32] This tape was then sent to the laboratory from which the smears originated. A cytotechnologist in the laboratory then reviewed these neural network-selected areas on the tape on a high-resolution color video monitor connected to a personal computer (PC) with a tape drive for reading the digitally recorded images. The most abnormal cell scenes could be tagged and collated for display as a summary of the most significant cytological abnormalities in the Pap smear. Using this method, abnormal cells in various parts of the smear were brought together for review. The images were displayed as two separate pages of 64 single-cell scenes and 64 cell-cluster scenes.[29] It took approximately 1 min to review and collate an average Pap smear.[30] If abnormal cells were noted on the video monitor, then the case was selected for an additional manual rescreen. The review station provided slide coordinates to facilitate the location of the abnormal cells on the glass slide. The final diagnosis was made by direct review of the glass slide by a cytotechnologist and a pathologist based on information obtained from the PAPNET display. If no abnormal cells were identified in the digitized images by the cytotechnologist, then the smear was classified as negative.

In November 1995, the FDA granted pre-market approval for PAPNET to be used in the USA as a rescreening device. Approval was obtained after a review of the data submitted during the previous year from a multicenter study containing true negative controls and women who had initially negative conventional smears with subsequent biopsy-confirmed squamous intraepithelial lesions or invasive carcinomas. By January 1996, more than 400 000 cervical smears had been rescreened by the PAPNET system worldwide and it was in routine clinical use in 15 countries as a supplemental test to conventional cervical Pap smears.[29]

A mean sensitivity of approximately 97 per cent was reported for PAPNET in recognizing significant cytological atypia, including SIL and malignancy.[29,32,33] In a 1995 study, over 35 000 smears were screened with PAPNET and over 42 000 were conventionally screened. Scores were calculated for high-grade lesions including severe dysplasia, carcinoma *in situ* (CIS) and invasive carcinoma, as percentages of the screened women.[29,34] The scores for PAPNET screening for CIS and invasive carcinoma were higher than those for conventional screening.

In a study at a laboratory in The Netherlands the PAPNET system was used to evaluate smears that included abnormalities that were repeatedly overlooked on manual rescreens.[35,36] According to the reports PAPNET detected abnormal cells on all of these cases. PAPNET may have been particularly useful when there was a paucity of abnormal cells or when the abnormality consisted of very small cells representing high-grade squamous intraepithelial lesions (HSIL) or carcinoma.[35–39]

The PAPNET system was intended as a rescreening device for negative conventional Pap smears, and therefore its primary focus was the identification of potentially abnormal epithelial cells. Nonetheless, a study was performed by Ashfaq et al.[40] to evaluate how effectively infectious organisms could be identified on the PAPNET-generated computer images. A total of 249 previously screened Pap smears that contained infectious organisms were rescreened using PAPNET. High-resolution images were examined for the presence of coccobacilli, trichomonads, *Candida* and Herpes simplex viral inclusions. The detection of infectious organisms compared with manual screening was 70 per cent, with a 30 per cent false-negative rate. With the PAPNET system, 60 per cent of the cases with *Candida* organisms, 77 per cent of the cases with trichomonads, and 59 per cent of the cases with herpetic viral inclusions were identified. Manual screening therefore has a greater sensitivity for the detection of infectious organisms than PAPNET.

AutoPap

NeoPath, Inc. was founded in 1989 by Dr Alan Nelson with the University of Washington's Center for Imaging Systems Optimization and the Boeing High Technology Center. It has since merged with AutoCyte, Inc., to form TriPath Imaging, Inc. NeoPath, Inc. developed the AutoPap 300 QC automatic Pap screener designed to automatically screen conventional Pap smears. The device is self-contained and can operate both continuously and unattended.

The system was initially approved as a quality control rescreening device of all smears categorized as negative and satisfactory by a cytotechnologist. Each smear was assigned an AutoPap quality control (QC) ranking. A cytotechnologist then rescreened those cases that had the highest AutoPap QC rankings. Preliminary studies obtained from nine participating commercial laboratories[41] indicated that 80 per cent of the false negative smears were contained within the 20 per cent of the smears that had the highest AutoPap QC ranking (20 per cent QC selection mode). Since all negative Pap smears would be rescreened by the AutoPap system, compared with only 10 per cent of randomly selected negatives as required by Clinical Laboratory Improvement Amendments 1988 (CLIA'88) regulations, a greater number of false-negative smears would be identified to allow a more accurate assessment of the performance of the cytotechnologists and to effectively lower the numbers of false-negative smears reported by a laboratory. Other studies have supported similar findings.[42,43]

The AutoPap system has subsequently been approved by the FDA as a primary screening system and is no longer being used as a quality control rescreening device for negative Pap smears. The current system processes only conventional Pap smears and is intended to detect slides with evidence of squamous cell carcinoma, adenocarcinoma, and/or the usual precursor lesions. To date, primary screening of liquid-based AutoCyte thin-layer preparations with the AutoPap system is still awaiting FDA approval.

The slides to be screened are affixed with a barcode and up to 36 trays containing eight slides per tray are processed at a rate of 6–8 min per slide with an automatic calibration check of approximately 8 min between trays. For each successfully processed slide, the device reports 'No Further Review' or 'Review'. 'Review' slides include those that have a potential abnormality, are unsatisfactory, or those that could not be analyzed because of insufficient cellularity. The FDA has approved the AutoPap to classify up to, but no more than, 25 per cent of all successfully processed slides in a given run as 'No Further Review' and these slides can be directly archived as within normal limits. The remaining 75 per cent or more of the smears that are designated as 'Review' require manual screening by a cytotechnologist. For quality control purposes, the AutoPap system classifies at least 15 per cent of all successfully processed 'Review' slides as eligible for rescreening. Slides within this group that are classified as negative after manual screening by a cytotechnologist are the most likely to have missed abnormal cells. This 15 per cent of AutoPap-selected slides may be used as a substitute for the random 10 per cent review of negative Pap smears, which is the current QC standard, for manual rescreening.

A high-speed automated video microscope that is capable of acquiring 25 images per second scans the smears submitted to the system. The captured images are transferred to an array of 15 field of view (FOV) computers connected to shared memory modules. Each FOV computer is a multifunction processor capable of more than one billion calculations per second. The FOV computers analyze the images using a series of internal algorithms based on a variety of parameters and then pass these results to the host computer, which collates the data and determines the composite results for a smear. Each Pap smear that is successfully processed and classified as 'Review' is individually ranked from 1 to n, where 1 indicates the slide most likely to contain an abnormality and n the least likely (n = total number of slides). Each slide is also assigned a group ranking from 1 to 5, where 1 is the group most likely to contain abnormal cells. In addition, information about the adequacy of a smear is provided.

A prospective, intended use study was conducted at five cytology laboratories comparing AutoPap-assisted screening (at least 75 per cent AutoPap-assisted manual screening and 15 per cent AutoPap-assisted manual rescreening) with 100 per cent manual screening and 10 per cent random rescreening.[44] A total of 25 124 Pap smears were included in this study

Table 3.5 *AutoPAP assisted screening vs. manual rescreening (total cases = 25 124)*[a]

	AutoPap	**100% Manual screening**
WNL	23 788	23 885
ASCUS	835	766
AGUS	43	42
LSIL	253	233
HSIL	66	64
AIS	0	1
Carcinoma	2	0
UNSAT	137	133
ASCUS+	1 199	1 106

[a]ASCUS+ includes atypical squamous cells of undetermined significance (ASCUS), low-grade squamous intraepithelial lesions (LSIL), high-grade squamous intraepithelial lesions (HSIL), and invasive carcinoma. WNL, within normal limits; AGUS, atypical glandular cells of undetermined significance; AIS, adenocarcinoma *in situ*. Based on data in Wilbur et al.[44]

that showed a greater number of abnormal smears identified by the AutoPap system than by the traditional methods (Table 3.5).

The AutoCyte SCREEN

AutoCyte, Inc. was originally a division of the Roche Corporation. The AutoCyte thin-layer preparation system (AutoCyte PREP) was developed for optional use with the Roche AUTOCyte computerized screening system (AutoCyte SCREEN). The standardized preparation and staining achieved with AutoCyte thin-layers was expected to eliminate inconsistencies between samples and allow more rapid and accurate computer screening compared with conventional smears. Subsequently, AutoCyte became a separate company and then merged with Neopath, Inc. to form TriPath Imaging, Inc., which had developed its own primary screening system (AutoPap).

The Roche AUTOCyte SCREEN is a fully automated screening system that can be used as an adjunct test to conventional Pap smears.[45] It has an automated microscope and slide handler driven by a powerful multiprocessor-based computer that reads barcodes for positive specimen identification. The slide handler holds 10 cassettes with 40 slides each, for a total of 400 slides, and the cassettes can be added or removed without disturbing the system during operation. No attendant is required, the AUTOCyte system can screen up to 300 slides in a 24-hour period.

High-resolution images representing 120 of the most significant cellular changes are captured and displayed on a computer screen, coupled with six additional large overview fields containing multiple cells. Cell selection is based on a series of internal algorithms. Most debris, blood cells, and normal cells are ignored by the system. Malignant, dysplastic, atypical and HPV-associated cellular changes, together with endocervical cells and diagnostically relevant cell clusters, are selectively displayed.

Although the system requires all the images to be reviewed by a cytotechnologist, it does present its own computer evaluation based on a cell population histogram analysis.[22] The review can be performed either at the AUTOCyte computer or at a separate workstation linked through a network. Stored cellular coordinates make it possible to automatically relocate a particular area of the glass slide for direct examination through the microscope. All abnormal cases are reevaluated by conventional microscopy (Fig. 3.1). In theory, the dual strategy of an expert human opinion coupled with an unbiased computer analysis may result in a greater

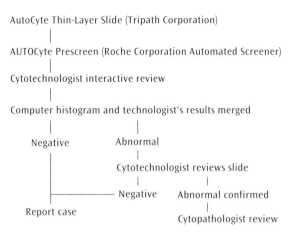

AutoCyte Thin-Layer Slide (Tripath Corporation)

AUTOCyte Prescreen (Roche Corporation Automated Screener)

Cytotechnologist interactive review

Computer histogram and technologist's results merged

Negative   Abnormal

Cytotechnologist reviews slide

Negative   Abnormal confirmed

Report case   Cytopathologist review

Figure 3.1 *Roche AUTOCyte automatic screening system flow chart.*

sensitivity for the detection of cervicovaginal cytologic abnormalities. A recent evaluation of the AutoCyte SCREEN system did show superior sensitivity by the system (85 per cent) over manually screening cervical smears (80 per cent), with comparable specificity (97 per cent).[46] However, this system has never received approval from FDA and is not being further developed by TriPath at this time.

ThinPrep imaging system

The ThinPrep imaging system is an interactive computer-assisted screening system that is still under development by the Cytyc Corporation. It consists of a PC-based, expandable image processor and a review station comprising a standard microscope with a motorized stage and electronic dotting capabilities. The system is capable of screening 100 000 slides per year at a rate of one shift per workday. In a ThinPrep slide the cells are deposited within a 20 mm-diameter circular area. It takes approximately 120 fields of view with a ×10 objective to fully screen a ThinPrep slide. The image processor automatically screens a batch of slides at a rate of 3 min per slide and selects a predetermined number of fields of view, which contain the most abnormal cells, and stores the x–y coordinates of these areas within the computer. The feasibility of using a total of 30 fields of view per slide is being examined. At the review station, the system reads the slide identification number and proceeds to the stored coordinates for that particular case. A cytotechnologist reviews the selected fields, electronically marks any fields of interest and physically dots the slide. If there are any atypical cells within the selected 30 fields of view, then the entire slide is manually screened by a cytotechnologist and, if appropriate, sent to a pathologist for review. If no atypical cells are identified within the 30 fields of view selected, then no further review is required.

Using the rate of 80 slides per day and 120 fields of view per slide, a cytotechnologist would review 9600 fields of view per day if 100 per cent of the slides were manually screened. With the ThinPrep Imaging System only 30 fields of view per slide would initially be reviewed (80 slides at 30 fields of view per slide = 2400 fields of view). Assuming a 10 per cent atypia rate, eight of the 80 slides would require 100 per cent manual screening (eight slides at 120 fields of view per slide = 960 fields of view). Therefore, a cytotechnologist screening 80 slides per day would review a total of 3360 fields of view with the ThinPrep Imaging System as opposed to 9600 fields of view with 100 per cent manual screening of all slides. This results, theoretically, in a 66 per cent reduction in screening time.

PROCESS CONTROL DEVICES

Process control devices are designed to monitor the process of manual screening to ensure thoroughness and to improve the efficiency of the process. Two such systems are Pathfinder and the AcCell workstation.

Pathfinder

The Pathfinder system was originally developed by the CompuCyte Corporation and was subsequently purchased by what is now the TriPath Corporation. A comparable but newer version of the system called Slide Wizard, which interacts with the AutoPap Primary Screener, is intended eventually to replace the existing one. Since the AutoPap Primary Screener stores the locations of the most abnormal areas of a slide, this information can be made available to the screening cytotechnologist and potentially decreases the number of fields of view per slide that have to be reviewed for those cases that the AutoPap designates as 'Review'.

Pathfinder is a microscope–computer combination that shows the screening pattern of every slide. It consists of a compact, adjustable, high-resolution video monitor attached to a base that contains a PC equipped with a floppy disk drive and is barcode and network ready. Special position sensors can be mounted on any microscope stage to determine the x and y coordinates of the stage and the field of view. The microscope is placed on top of the Pathfinder base with the position sensors attached. The electronic data can be stored on a floppy disk or the Pathfinder workstations can be networked to a server and the information can be stored centrally.

As a slide is manually screened, Pathfinder automatically displays a visual track of the areas covered on the slide and any areas that were missed. Any cells of interest can be electronically marked and coded with the attached keyboard which provides symbols to code up to 10 different cell types. Cytotechnologists can easily check their work on the video monitor and return to those areas that were missed during screening.

The system displays the time spent on each slide and the extent to which the fields overlap during screening to assist in teaching screening to cytotechnologists in training and to refine the technique of more experienced ones. Digital coding and marking of abnormal cells can help to enhance the pathologist's case review.

For each cytotechnologist, Pathfinder can generate quality control reports containing a list of all the slides screened, time spent screening, coverage, amount of field overlap and whether diagnostic cells were marked. This type of information is useful in managing productivity, assuring quality and comparing the work output between different cytotechnologists.

AcCell and TracCell

The AcCell cytology workstation was developed by the AccuMed Corporation. It consists of a motorized microscope attached to a computer. The entire workstation is accessed by a mouse that controls focus, slide movement, electronic marking of cells of interest and diagnostic reporting.

The slides are loaded into the system and are automatically transferred under the microscope objectives for screening. Once the slide is on the stage, the barcode reader identifies the slide and can access all patient data from an integrated data management system. The motorized stage automatically moves the slide under the objectives in overlapping fields of view. The cytotechnologist observes the cells through the microscope, and focus and speed are controlled with the mouse. Automatic movement can be interrupted at any time and the slide can be moved manually using the mouse (i.e. all mouse movements are transferred to the slide's movement).

Any cells of interest are marked electronically and the coordinates as well as the focus position of the marked area are stored in the computer. The system will then automatically return the user to the last area screened and commence automated movement. Before the slide is ejected from the stage, it is physically dotted by the system using AcCell's dotter mechanism, thus eliminating the need for conventional dotting by the cytotechnologists. Once a slide is screened, the mouse automatically serves as a conventional computer mouse controlling the data management system and allowing for paperless entry of diagnoses into the system.

The TracCell 2000 slide-mapping system is integrated into the AcCell workstation and automatically prescreens 100 per cent of each slide and maps it into presented and excluded areas of view. Excluded areas contain nothing of diagnostic significance – empty space, debris, etc. The cytotechnologist will be certain to see all of the cellular material present in the fewest possible fields of view. It received FDA clearance for conventional Pap smears in 1997 and for ThinPrep slides in 1998.

INHERENT COSTS

The new technologies will no doubt increase the cost of a Pap test, particularly if automated systems are used to rescreen negative Pap smears. The use of primary computerized screening systems should, in theory, decrease the ratio of the cytotechnologist's screening time to the total volume of GYN cases processed by a laboratory, and may prove more cost-effective.[47]

Thin-layer preparations

In addition to the initial investment in hardware, software, and the retraining of pathologists and cytotechnologists in the interpretation of thin-layer preparations, there are the costs of consumables per test and costs related to productivity and manpower necessitated by the more labor-intensive preparation of thin-layer slides compared with conventional smears. This is partly offset by the significant decrease in screening time per slide once the cytotechnologists become familiar and experienced with assessing thin-layer preparations. A decrease in the number of suboptimal specimens should also decrease the rate of repeat Pap smears after short intervals, which result from the designation of 'satisfactory, but limited by'.

Another consideration is specimen storage and disposal. For conventional Pap smears only a glass slide or slides are submitted to the laboratory for processing, interpreting and storage. For thin-layer preparations the specimen is received in a preservative solution and is not entirely consumed during processing. How long should the unprocessed portion of a specimen be stored? In high-volume laboratories or in laboratories where storage space is limited, specimen storage could become problematic, particularly if refrigeration is required, as in the case of CytoRich Preservative Fluid for the AutoCyte PREP system. Cost is also a consideration in the management and disposal of the stored specimens.

In 2001, the Cytyc ThinPrep 2000 processor cost in the region of $54 900 and list price of consumables was $5 625.00 per ThinPrep Pap-Test Package, which includes enough materials for 500 tests. Therefore, the estimated cost of consumables per ThinPrep Pap test is $11.25, which does not include the cost of staining. As stated previously, the T-2000 is a single-load system (only one specimen can be processed at a time) and would require proportionally greater numbers of staff as the volume of specimens increase. Processing requires constant monitoring, so there is no 'free time' during specimen preparation. A TransCyt Filter can be used only once. Thus, if the cellular density of a specimen is too great and the specimen has to be diluted and repeated, or if a filter fails during processing, a new filter must be employed, adding to the cost of processing. Once the thin-layer slide is prepared, it must still be stained.

The Cytyc ThinPrep 3000 Processor currently costs in the region of $195 000 and is a multiload system designed to batch process only GYN specimens. It is fully automated with 'walk-away' capability and can process up to 80 vials per cycle and approximately 140 000 Pap tests per year. The unstained thin-layer preparations are automatically deposited into a standard staining rack that is compatible with most automated stainers. This system eliminates the need for constant monitoring during processing.

The AutoCyte processor is a multiload system that can process up to 48 specimens per batch and can run 6 batches per 8-hour workday. The current processor costs around $55 000. Each test kit for GYN specimens is $6.95 and that for NON-GYN is $3.95. There is also a reagent rental program in which the TriPath Corporation installs and maintains the processor free of charge and the user purchases at least 480 tests per month at $7.95 per test. The thin-layer slides are stained automatically by the processor. Labor cost involved in preparing each specimen would decrease with increasing volumes. Periods, ranging from 30 to 45 min, of 'free time' occur during a run. The initial manual preparation steps are tedious in the AutoCyte System. To address this issue, the TriPath Corporation has developed the Prep Mate as described previously as well as a multiload, automated, self-contained vortexer. The list prices of the Prep Mate and multiload vortexer are $11 200 and $2000, respectively.

Both the Cytyc and TriPath Corporations emphasize that cytotechnologists require additional training and experience before they are fully proficient in assessing thin-layer preparations. Thin-layer slides with scant cellularity can be particularly difficult to screen and interpret accurately. Differences in nuclear morphology have been reported with the ThinPrep preparations, which use a methanol-based fixative as compared with the ethanol fixation of conventional smears. Both companies offer training courses.

Computer-based automated screening systems

Before the commercial use of PAPNET was discontinued, laboratories using the system were required to purchase a review station to view and collate the digitized images. The cost of the hardware and software was approximately $12 000. The laboratory shipped the negative Pap smears to a central station of PAPNET for rescreening with an approximate 4-day turnaround time. Therefore, the costs of organizing and managing the shipping and return of slides to and from the PAPNET central station had to be included in estimating the overall cost of the system. The price of rescreening was $18.00 per slide. The laboratory received a digital tape of the screened slides and PAPNET returned the original Pap smears. The laboratory personnel were trained by PAPNET in the correct use of the system, however, this also came at a price.

Since the AUTOCyte screening system (AutoCyte SCREEN) is not approved by the FDA, its list price is not available. If direct purchasing of the system is an option, then the estimated cost is in excess of $200 000. Another possible scenario is that the system will be installed in the laboratory and the user will pay a certain amount to the company per slide screened. However, this system is not being developed further at this time.

The prior AutoPap 300 QC Automatic Pap Screener by NeoPath was in the region of $365 000 plus $1500–2000 for shipping. The current model (TriPath Corporation) is a primary screening system that lists for $450 000. If the laboratory purchases the hardware and software, then after 1 year there is an additional $45 000 per year cost for the software license and support of the system. However, most users of the system are paying a dollar amount per slide (generally $4.00 to $5.00 depending on the total volume of the laboratory) screened to the TriPath Corporation. Based on a volume of 40 000 slides per year, the current list price is $4.00 per slide screened. With this latter option, the TriPath Corporation installs and maintains the system for no additional charge. Training in the use of the system is included in the price of all of the listed options.

In a 1996 editorial in *Acta Cytologica*, a mathematical model was developed to measure the cost per additional abnormal case discovered comparing AutoPap and PAPNET to no rescreening, 10 per cent random rescreening, directed rescreening of high-risk patients, 100 per cent manual rescreening, and rapid manual rescreening.[46] The model was based on a $5.00 per slide rate for conventional manual screening, which was the upper end of the average cost to manually screen a Pap smear in the USA. All methods of rescreening, whether manual or automated, add cost to a laboratory.

The use of AutoPap at a 10 per cent QC mode was $5.00 per slide for all the negative Pap smears in addition to the $5.00 cost of manual rescreening of the 10 per cent selected by the AutoPap, resulting in an increase in sensitivity of 9.8 per cent compared with a 10 per cent random manual rescreen. The projected cost of processing all negative slides with the AutoPap 300 QC System was greater than manually rescreening 100 per cent of all negative smears.[46]

The cost of rescreening negative slides at a central facility of PAPNET was approximately $10.00 per slide at the time the editorial was published. In 1997, the cost for rescreening was $18.00 per slide. Excluding the costs of the image review by a cytotechnologist in the laboratory and the costs of organizing and managing the shipping and return of slides to and from the PAPNET central station, the estimated cost was four times that of manually rescreening 100 per cent of negative smears (based on a $10.00 per slide screen rate), with an estimated increase in sensitivity of 9.9 per cent compared with a 10 per cent random manual rescreen.[46]

The greatest sensitivity was achieved with 100 per cent manual rescreening (22.4 per cent increase in sensitivity compared with a 10 per cent random manual rescreen).[46] The cost of each additional abnormal case discovered by 100 per cent manual rescreen was estimated at $1049 compared with $267 for detecting an abnormal case on the first screen. For PAPNET, the estimated figure was $4486 per additional detected abnormal case (based on a $10.00/slide screening rate) and for AutoPap it was $2197. The cost-to-benefit ratio for 100 per cent manual rescreening is significantly less than those of computerized systems. Therefore, computerized systems are no longer being used in the USA to rescreen negative Pap smears because they did not prove to be cost-effective.

Conversely, when used for primary screening, computer-based automated screening systems should, in theory, decrease the amount of time cytotechnologists spend screening slides relative to the total GYN volume in a laboratory. With the AutoPap system up to 25 per cent of the cases can be directly filed without having to be screened by a cytotechnologist, thus allowing for greater volumes to be processed by a laboratory with the same personnel, and without sacrificing quality. Systems that identify and store the locations of abnormal cells also have the potential of decreasing the review time per slide by a cytotechnologist and thus increasing productivity.

REIMBURSEMENT

Thin-layer preparations and automated screening will increase the cost of Pap smears, at least at the current cost levels. These new technologies are being marketed in an era of managed care and increasing cost consciousness. The current part A (technical) Medicare reimbursement for a Pap smear is $15.30.

The consumers and the manufacturers of thin-layer processors have been successful in increasing the insurance reimbursement for thin-layer preparations. Consequently, those cytology laboratories that have shifted predominantly or exclusively to thin-layer processing of GYN specimens have become profitable after finding this a 'loss leader' in the laboratories for decades. Increased reimbursement for computer-based automated screening is being sought. These scientific and financial developments represent advancements in cervical cytology. However, dysplasias and carcinomas of the cervix are known to be associated with a low socioeconomic status. Poor, uninsured women may not be able to afford a more costly Pap test. Ironically, it is these groups of women who would benefit the most from having annual Pap tests. In some parts of the USA, it has become a challenge to find a cytology laboratory that accepts and processes the less expensive conventional Pap smears. It would truly be unfortunate if the Pap test prices itself out of the reach of those women who need them the most. It is therefore crucial to maintain the accessibility and affordability of annual Pap tests for all women.

SUMMARY

New technologies have provided an alternative to virtually all elements of the conventional Pap test. Thin-layer preparation has been approved and found to be a superior substitute for conventional preparation by smearing, although retraining of personnel is necessary for this method to be adopted into routine use. Since not all of the material in a specimen is consumed in liquid-based systems, additional tests can be performed from a single sample. HPV-typing using DNA probes holds particular promise for triaging ASCUS cases. Automated screening systems, such as the current version of the AutoPap, have been approved to partly replace manual screening, allowing increased productivity. Devices to assure the quality of the screening process itself have also been made available. A logical, and probably inevitable, outcome of these technologies is the combination of automated screeners capable of primary screening with the cleaner and more uniform thin-layer preparations. FDA approval for use of the AutoPap for screening AutoCyte thin-layer preparations is pending. It is reasonable that if the current automated screening systems are capable of identifying abnormal cells in conventional smears, with all of their inconsistencies in preparation, standardized thin-layer preparations, which are more likely to contain diagnostic cells and have a much smaller screening area, should enhance and accelerate the screening capabilities and improve the performance of these computerized screening systems. However, all new technologies currently threaten to increase the cost of Pap smears. In order to maintain the accessibility and affordability of Pap tests for all women, an effort must be made to decrease the costs of these new technologies. The ultimate goal should be to use these new technologies efficiently and effectively to decrease the cost as well as increase the accuracy of Pap tests.

REFERENCES

1 Gay JD, Donaldson LD, Goellner JR. False-negative results in cervical cytologic studies. *Acta Cytol* 1985; **29**: 1043–6.
2 Hutchinson ML, Cassin CM, Ball HGD. The efficacy of an automated preparation device for cervical cytology. *Am J Clin Pathol* 1991; **96**: 300–5.
3 Joseph MG, Cragg F, Wright VC, Kontozoglou TE, Downing P, Marks FR. Cyto-histological correlates in a colposcopic clinic: a 1-year prospective study. *Diagn Cytopathol* 1991; **7**: 477–81.

4 Koss LG. The Papanicolaou test for cervical cancer detection. A triumph and a tragedy [see comments]. *JAMA* 1989; **261**: 737–43.

5 Kristensen GB, Skyggebjerg KD, Holund B, Holm K, Hansen MK. Analysis of cervical smears obtained within three years of the diagnosis of invasive cervical cancer. *Acta Cytol* 1991; **35**: 47–50.

6 McLachlan N, Patwardhan JR, Ayer B, Pacey NF. Management of suboptimal cytologic smears. Persistent inflammatory smears [see comments]. *Acta Cytol* 1994; **38**: 531–6.

7 Hutchinson ML, Patten FW, Stelzer GT, Hurley AA, Zahniser DJ, Douglass KL. Study of cell loss in the conventional Papanicolaou smear. *Acta Cytol* 1992; **36**: 577.

8 McGoogan E, Reith A. Would monolayers provide more representative samples and improved preparations for cervical screening? Overview and evaluation of systems available. *Acta Cytol* 1996; **40**: 107–19.

9 Tezuka F, Shuki H, Oikawa H, Higashiiwai H. Numerical counts of epithelial cells collected, smeared and lost in the conventional Papanicolaou smear preparation [letter]. *Acta Cytol* 1995; **39**: 837–8.

10 Hutchinson ML, Isenstein LM, Goodman A, et al. Homogeneous sampling accounts for the increased diagnostic accuracy using the ThinPrep Processor [see comments]. *Am J Clin Pathol* 1994; **101**: 215–19.

11 Vassilakos P, Cossali D, Albe X, Alonso L, Hohener R, Puget E. Efficacy of monolayer preparations for cervical cytology: emphasis on suboptimal specimens. *Acta Cytol* 1996; **40**: 496–500.

12 Sherman ME, Schiffman MH, Lorincz AT, et al. Cervical specimens collected in liquid buffer are suitable for both cytologic screening and ancillary human papillomavirus testing. *Cancer* 1997; **81**: 89–97.

13 Wilbur DC, Facik MS, Rutkowski MA, Mulford DK, Atkison KM. Clinical trials of the CytoRich specimen-preparation device for cervical cytology. Preliminary results. *Acta Cytol* 1997; **41**: 24–9.

14 Lee KR, Ashfaq R, Birdsong GG, Corkill ME, McIntosh KM, Inhorn SL. Comparison of conventional Papanicolaou smears and a fluid-based, thin-layer system for cervical cancer screening. *Obstet Gynecol* 1997; **90**: 278–84.

15 Cytyc Corporation. *Introduction to the ThinPrep 2000 operator's manual.* Boxborough, MA: Cytyc Corporation, 1996.

16 Awen C, Hathway S, Eddy W, Voskuil R, Janes C. Efficacy of ThinPrep preparation of cervical smears: a 1,000-case, investigator-sponsored study. *Diagn Cytopathol* 1994; **11**: 33–6.

17 Tezuka F, Oikawa H, Shuki H, Higashiiwai H. Diagnostic efficacy and validity of the ThinPrep method in cervical cytology. *Acta Cytol* 1996; **40**: 513–18.

18 Wilbur DC, Dubeshter B, Angel C, Atkison KM. Use of thin-layer preparations for gynecologic smears with emphasis on the cytomorphology of high-grade intraepithelial lesions and carcinomas. *Diagn Cytopathol* 1996; **14**: 201–11.

19 Austin RM, Ramzy I. Increased detection of epithelial cell abnormalities by liquid-based gynecologic cytology preparations. A review of accumulated data. *Acta Cytol* 1998; **42**: 178–84.

20 Carpenter AB, Davey DD. ThinPrep Pap Test: performance and biopsy follow-up in a university hospital. *Cancer* 1999; **87**: 105–12.

21 Diaz-Rosario LA, Kabawat SE. Performance of a fluid-based, thin-layer Papanicolaou smear method in the clinical setting of an independent laboratory and an outpatient screening population in New England. *Arch Pathol Lab Med* 1999; **123**: 817–21.

22 Ferenczy A, Robitaille J, Franco E, Arseneau J, Richart RM, Wright TC. Conventional cervical cytologic smears vs. ThinPrep smears. A paired comparison study on cervical cytology. *Acta Cytol* 1996; **40**: 1136–42.

23 Corkill M, Knapp D, Martin J, Hutchinson ML. Specimen adequacy of ThinPrep sample preparations in a direct-to-vial study. *Acta Cytol* 1997; **41**: 39–44.

24 Bur M, Knowles K, Pekow P, Corral O, Donovan J. Comparison of ThinPrep preparations with conventional cervicovaginal smears. Practical considerations. *Acta Cytol* 1995; **39**: 631–42.

25 Schwarz G, Schwarz M, Schenck U. Effect of the special properties of monolayer cell preparations for automated cervical cytology on visual evaluation and classification. With an estimation of the number of cells required to be screened. *Anal Quant Cytol* 1983; **5**: 189–93.

26 Vassilakos P, Saurel J, Rondez R. Direct-to-vial use of the AutoCyte PREP liquid-based preparation for cervical-vaginal specimens in three European laboratories. *Acta Cytol* 1999; **43**: 65–8.

27 Bishop JW. Comparison of the CytoRich system with conventional cervical cytology. Preliminary data on 2,032 cases from a clinical trial site. *Acta Cytol* 1997; **41**: 15–23.

28 Vassilakos P, Schwartz D, de Marval F, et al. Biopsy-based comparison of liquid-based, thin-layer preparations to conventional Pap smears. *J Reprod Med* 2000; **45**: 11–16.

29 Mango LJ. Neuromedical Systems, Inc. *Acta Cytol* 1996; **40**: 53–9.

30 Rosenthal DL, Acosta D, Peters RK. Computer-assisted rescreening of clinically important false negative cervical smears using the PAPNET Testing System. *Acta Cytol* 1996; **40**: 120–6.

31 Koss LG, Lin E, Schreiber K, Elgert P, Mango L. Evaluation of the PAPNET cytologic screening system for quality control of cervical smears. *Am J Clin Pathol* 1994; **101**: 220–9.

32 Mango LJ. Computer-assisted cervical cancer screening using neural networks. *Cancer Lett* 1994; **77**: 155–62.

33 Mango LJ, Herriman JM. The PAPNET cytologic screening system. In: Wied GL, Bartels PH, Rosenthal DL, Schenck U, eds. *Compendium on the computerized cytology and histology laboratory*. Chicago, IL: Tutorials of Cytology, 1994: 320–34.

34 Boon ME, Kok LP, Beck S. Histologic validation of neural network-assisted cervical screening: Comparison with the conventional procedure. *Cell Vision* 1995; **2**: 23–7.

35 Boon ME, Kok LP, Nygaard-Nielsen M, Holm K, Holund B. Neural network processing of cervical smears can lead to a decrease in diagnostic variability and an increase in screening efficacy: a study of 63 false-negative smears. *Mod Pathol* 1994; **7**: 957–61.

36 Boon ME, Kok LP. Neural network processing can provide means to catch errors that slip through human screening of Pap smears. *Diagn Cytopathol* 1993; **9**: 411–16.

37 Sherman ME, Mango LJ, Kelly D, et al. PAPNET analysis of reportedly negative smears preceding the diagnosis of a high-grade squamous intraepithelial lesion or carcinoma. *Mod Pathol* 1994; **7**: 578–81.

38 Hatem F, Wilbur DC. High grade squamous cervical lesions following negative Papanicolaou smears: false-negative cervical cytology or rapid progression. *Diagn Cytopathol* 1995; **12**: 135–41.

39 Robertson JH, Woodend B. Negative cytology preceding cervical cancer: causes and prevention [see comments]. *J Clin Pathol* 1993; **46**: 700–2.

40 Ashfaq R, Thomas S, Saboorian MH. Efficiency of PAPNET in detecting infectious organisms in cervicovaginal smears. *Acta Cytol* 1996; **40**: 885–8.

41 Anderson TL, Nelson AC. Quality control and proficiency testing of cytologic smear screening. An integrated approach using automation. In: Wied GL, Keebler CM, Rosenthal DL, Schenck U, Somrak TM, Vooijs GP, eds. *Compendium on quality assurance, proficiency testing and workload limitations in clinical cytology*. Chicago, IL: Tutorials of Cytology, 1995: 283–6.

42 Patten Jr SF, Lee JS. Detection of true false-negative slides by the NeoPath AutoPap 300 QC system. Comparison with random rescreen. In: Wied GL, Keebler CM, Rosenthal DL, Schenck U, Somrak TM, Vooijs GP, eds. *Compendium on quality assurance, proficiency testing and workload limitations in clinical cytology*. Chicago, IL: Tutorials of Cytology, 1995: 167–9.

43 Wilbur DC, Bonfiglio TA, Rutkowski MA, et al. Sensitivity of the AutoPap 300 QC System for cervical cytologic abnormalities. Biopsy data confirmation. *Acta Cytol* 1996; **40**: 127–32.

44 Wilbur DC, Prey MU, Miller WM, Pawlick GF, Colgan TJ. The AutoPap system for primary screening in cervical cytology. Comparing the results of a prospective, intended-use study with routine manual practice. *Acta Cytol* 1998; **42**: 214–20.

45 Knesel EA, Jr. Roche Image Analysis Systems, Inc. *Acta Cytol* 1996; **40**: 60–6.

46 Bishop JW, Cheuvront DA, Sims KL. Evaluation of the AutoCyte SCREEN system in a clinical cytopathology laboratory. *Acta Cytol* 2000; **44**: 128–36.

47 Hutchinson ML. Assessing the costs and benefits of alternative rescreening strategies [editorial] [see comments]. *Acta Cytol* 1996; **40**: 4–8.

4

Quality assurance

CATHERINE S ABENDROTH

INTRODUCTION

Quality assurance (QA) in gynecological cytology implies the detection and avoidance of 'false negatives' to most people. QA is much more than this, however.[1] A comprehensive program of 'quality assurance' in any setting (industrial, medical, or educational) includes control of mechanical, environmental, technical and human factors, ongoing efforts to improve operations, and some method of assessing the program to ensure adherence to the desired quality standards. Terms that emphasize the comprehensive and open-ended nature of these efforts include total quality management (TQM), quality systems, and continuous quality improvement (CQI). W. Edwards Deming pioneered continuous quality improvement in American industry in the 1930s; the principles of CQI have been applied to health care only relatively recently.[2] The revised Standards of the Joint Commission on Accreditation of Healthcare Organizations (JCAHO) emphasize actual performance, rather than simply the capacity to perform (1995 Manual). The Standards now emphasize achieving the desired patient outcomes (patient care functions) while making the most efficient use of resources (management functions). These performance-based, functionally organized standards (as opposed to provider-specific standards) provide a useful strategy for designing a high-quality gynecological cytology service.

A fear of admitting to less than perfect performance impedes efforts to improve quality. Professionals, and physicians in particular, find it difficult to admit to errors or learn from them, as indicated by the response to the Institute of Medicine report on medical errors.[3,4] However, only by acknowledging that medicine is an imperfect science, and by identifying causes of error, can errors be reduced. The tools of several non-medical disciplines: human factors research, cognitive psychology, the sciences of systems, the sciences of learning, prediction and experiment, and statistics are extremely powerful in error analysis and prevention.[5,6] Unfortunately, many physicians are unfamiliar with, and even suspicious of, these non-biological disciplines.

Statistics is the cornerstone of process improvement. The first step in determining if a process is functioning adequately is setting a performance standard. Next, indicators of the process in question are identified and measured. The data are collected and analyzed. If performance is below standard, an action plan to improve performance is initiated. After a specified interval of time the indicators are measured again and the new data analyzed. If the desired change has occurred, data are then periodically collected to ensure this improved level of performance is maintained. Data analysis tools such as flow diagrams, cause and effect (fish-bone) diagrams, Pareto charts, histograms and run charts are useful to visualize trends and to distinguish process errors (common cause variation), to which CQI efforts should be addressed, from isolated incidents (special cause variation), which are not an appropriate focus of CQI activity.

The ultimate desired outcome of a gynecological cytology service is prevention of cervical cancer. A successful gynecological cytology CQI program must take into account all of the functions contributing to this goal, including pretest variables (access to screening, screening interval and sample collection), test-phase variables (specimen preparation, screening, interpretation and reporting), and post-test variables (related to follow-up care). In a TQM approach, this effort is multidisciplinary and includes patient participation. However, some of these variables are beyond the immediate control of the laboratory, the clinician or the patient. For example, access to screening for many women is dependent on social and economic policy. A truly comprehensive quality plan would include strategy to address these issues.

CONTINUOUS QUALITY IMPROVEMENT PROGRAM

The development of a laboratory's CQI plan requires input from all individuals playing a role in the process: the medical director, other cytopathologists, cytotechnologists, processing technicians and clerical personnel.[7,8] Involvement of clinicians can provide valuable insight at the initial stages and at subsequent reviews.[9] The director of CQI must be knowledgeable in cytology and the principles and tools of QA, must have adequate resources (time and an adequate system of information storage and retrieval), and must be skilled in human relations (to encourage participation in data collection and effectively implement changes based on data analysis).

Most cytology laboratories have similar components in their QA plans. The least controversial components are safety, instrumentation calibration and maintenance, stain quality, personnel qualifications, on-site screening, hierarchical review, and policy and procedure manuals. Other components are subject to greater controversy.

Pre-test variables

SCREENING INTERVAL

Recommendations for the appropriate interval for Pap smear testing should take into account the rate of progression of disease, the occurrence of false negative tests and failure to appear for screening. Many physicians perform more frequent screening than published guidelines require.[10] There is, in fact, no consensus among the various published guidelines as to the appropriate interval. Morell et al.[11] used data from a large health plan to evaluate the American Cancer Society's recommendation of cervical cytological screening every 3 years. They estimated the percentage of missed cases to be 1.2 per cent if screening were offered yearly, 3.5 per cent at 2-year intervals, 10.6 per cent at 3-year intervals, and 20 per cent at 4-year intervals.

The most common practice in the USA, and that recommended by the Laboratory Testing Strategy Task Force of the College of American Pathologists (CAP), is annual cervicovaginal screening.[12] Chapter 2 includes a clinician's perspective and discussion on this subject.

SAMPLING

Despite widespread awareness of the impact of sampling on Pap smear quality and accuracy, laboratories generally do not address this pretest component in their CQI plan, perhaps because they feel that this is in the domain of the clinician. However, CQI is a multidisciplinary effort and the smear quality has a direct effect on the performance of the cytology laboratory. Instructions for smear collection, such as *Guidelines on Papanicolaou Technique* published by the National Committee for Clinical Laboratory Standards (NCCLS#GP15-A), may be provided directly to clients submitting Pap smears.[13] Feedback on smear quality may also positively affect performance, e.g. a report on the percentage of smears with 'lack of endo-cervical cells' according to individual provider.

SPECIMEN REJECTION CRITERIA

A laboratory should have written criteria for specimen acceptance or rejection based on the condition of the specimen (e.g. slide breakage) and the adequacy of demographic and clinical information. Federal regulations specify that, at a minimum, the patient name or other unique identifier, age or date of birth, last menstrual period (LMP), history of previous abnormal report(s), biopsy or treatment, provider identification, specimen source, and collection date be provided on the specimen requisition [Federal register (FR) 493.1105].[14] A survey of 84 pathologists revealed that 40 per cent of the responding laboratories had no minimal data requirement, and approximately two-thirds required only patient name, provider name and source.[15] Is this apparent disregard for the regulations a reflection of the difficulty in obtaining this information, or skepticism about the need for these data? The authors of this study achieved a rate of <1 per cent of specimens with incomplete information after implementation of a Specimen Acceptance Policy. Therefore, it is likely that laboratories are not requiring information that they do not feel is crucial. No one would argue that unique patient identifiers are necessary. Noting an abnormal history may direct the specimen for hierarchical review or targeted rescreening. The requirement for the LMP may be questioned, since it is no longer recommended that the presence of endometrial cells be reported in premenopausal women.[16] Like many regulations and inspection criteria, these specimen acceptance criteria were adopted without any testing of their efficacy, i.e. whether adherence to these criteria would positively affect intended outcomes.

DEFINITION OF HIGH RISK

Increased scrutiny may be justified for a patient at increased risk for dysplasia. This may include shortened interval for screening, more time devoted to screening her smear, hier-archical review even with negative primary screening, targeted rescreening, repeat smear for a 'satisfactory but limited by' (SBLB) diagnosis and more aggressive management, such as colposcopy for diagnosis of atypical squamous cells of undetermined significance (ASCUS). How are high-risk women identified? Important indicators that place a woman at increased risk of cervical dysplasia (early onset of sexual activity, multiple sexual partners, history of sexually transmitted disease and immunosuppression) may not be available to the clinician and let alone to the laboratory. What may be available to the laboratory, from either the provider or the laboratory information system (LIS), is a history of abnormal cytology or biopsy results. If more than one provider has cared for the patient and her specimens sent to more than one laboratory, then even such information may be incomplete or unavailable. Thus false-negative Pap smears with disastrous consequences may occur in patients who are not suspected to be at high risk. Perhaps it would be a good idea to apply 'universal precautions' to Pap smear testing with all smears examined with the same intensity regardless of the history.

Test-phase variables

PERSONNEL QUALIFICATIONS

The internal quality improvement program should ensure minimum qualifications for laboratory personnel and provide means by which these personnel can improve both the quality of their work and their job satisfaction (which are related). Minimum entry qualifications are ensured by requiring adequate training and certification and through a comprehensive new employee orientation program. The performance of processing personnel can be improved with feedback on slide quality, benchmarking data on slide quality, educational sessions on processing techniques and upgrading processing equipment. Cytotechnologists' screening performance may be positively impacted by improvements in the screening environment. Cytotechnologists' and pathologists' diagnostic skills can be sharpened through immediate feedback at daily sign-out, microscopic review sessions,[17] correlation conferences,[7] sharing of aggregate and trended data on diagnostic categories, including undercalls (under diagnoses) and overcalls (over diagnoses),[17] and continuing medical education (CME) activities such as independent study, journal clubs, teleconferences, scientific meetings, workshops, the American Society of Clinical Pathologists (ASCP) CheckSample program and self-assessment exercises,[18] and the College of American Pathologists Interlaboratory Comparison Program in Cervicovaginal Cytology (CAP-PAP).[19]

PROCESSING

There is little controversy about the recommended checks of stain quality, equipment maintenance, and other processing variables. The new Thin-layer technology is discussed in Chapter 3.

SCREENING AND WORKLOAD LIMITATIONS

Screening should be performed by qualified individuals in a quiet, comfortable environment free of distractions. According to cognitive psychology, errors in a skill-based activity, such as screening, occur when there is a break in the routine while attention is diverted.[6] Environmental distractions (noise, temperature and physical stimuli) are frequent causes of slips in skill-based behaviors. Physiological factors (fatigue and illness) and psychological factors (stress and anxiety) can also interfere with concentration. Design of the physical environment of the cytology laboratory and determination of slide limits should take these factors into account.

Slide limits must be reviewed and adjusted, if necessary, semi-annually (FR 493.1451(c)(3)).[14] Although cytotechnologists ideally would have 'line authority' (the authority for an individual with direct responsibility for a function to make decisions about that function)[20] to adjust their slide limits downward on days they are not capable of maximum performance due to stress or other factors, this is probably not practical in today's cost- and productivity-driven laboratory. Slide limits have been the subject of many debates in the cytology community and among regulators. Is the current limit of 100 slides per 24-hour day (FR 493.1257(b)) reasonable? Some experienced cytotechnologists screening predominantly normal smears may well be capable of screening more than this number. However, less experienced cytotechnologists, those with multiple responsibilities, and those dealing with a higher prevalence of abnormal smears probably should screen fewer. A survey of cytotechnologists in academic medical center cytology laboratories revealed an average of 45–55 slides per day.[21] There is a real danger that this maximum limit will be construed as a minimum number of slides that each cytotechnologist is expected to complete.[21] While it seems reasonable to assume that the error rate for screening is inversely related to screening time, there is no good data to support this assumption. In a rare report on this topic, faster screening had no negative impact on diagnostic accuracy.[22]

Thin-layer preparations have introduced another controversy: these count as one-half slide in determining total slides reviewed according to federal regulations (FR 493.1257(b)(2)).[14] Do we know that thin-layer cervicovaginal smears can be screened accurately in half the time of conventional smears? The manufacturers of these preparation devices wisely have not published performance data on this.

SPECIMEN ADEQUACY

The 1988 National Cancer Institute Bethesda workshop on terminology in cervicovaginal cytology reporting recommended that all Pap smear reports include a statement of specimen adequacy.[23] Criteria for the assessment of adequacy were formulated during a second workshop in April 1991.[16] A CAP-PAP questionnaire survey of specimen adequacy practices in 1990 found that 35 per cent of laboratories routinely reported specimen adequacy; surveys in 1991 and 1992 showed that this number had increased to 66 per cent and 85 per cent, respectively.[24] In the 1991 survey, despite a fairly high level of compliance, respondents identified specimen adequacy categorization as the most difficult element of The Bethesda System (TBS) to implement. Spires et al.[25] examined inter-observer and intra-observer reproducibility of the adequacy statement using the TBS criteria and found very good inter-observer agreement for the 'satisfactory' category ($k = 0.73$, concordance of 82 per cent), good agreement for 'unsatisfactory' ($k = 0.63$, concordance of 73 per cent), and only fair agreement for SBLB ($k = 0.48$, concordance of 65 per cent). The degree of concordance found by these authors was far better than the 20 per cent found by Yobs et al.[26] in an inter-laboratory study; Spires et al.[25] noted that the earlier study preceded the publication of TBS and emphasized that having specific criteria was important to interpretive reproducibility. A study[27] using adequacy terminology from the 1988 Bethesda conference but not the specific criteria from the 1991 conference reinforces this. This study showed poor agreement for all adequacy categories: $k = 0.27$ for 'satisfactory', $k = 0.11$ for 'less than optimal', and $k = 0.42$ for 'unsatisfactory'. Problems noted by Spires et al.[25] included quantification of per cent of cells obscured by blood or inflammation, assessment of adequacy in smears with more than one limiting factor, and quantification of the per cent of the smear covered by squamous epithelial cells. Estimates of the proportion of the slide covered by squamous epithelial cells are neither accurate nor reproducible.[28] Interestingly, although many laboratories use a diagnosis of SBLB scant squamous epithelial cells, there are no criteria for a scant squamous component.

The importance of sampling the transformation zone (TZ) is intuitively obvious, as it is generally accepted that dysplasias and carcinomas arise at this junction. Thus TBS defines cervical smears lacking an endocervical component as 'SBLB a lack of endocervical cells'.[16] However, the data on the relationship between the presence of TZ and the accuracy of the result is conflicting. On one hand, cross-sectional studies show a higher rate of abnormalities in smears with an endocervical component compared with those lacking endocervical cells.[29,30] Positive smears from women with high-grade squamous intraepithelial lesions (HSIL) and carcinoma are more likely to have an endocervical component than negative smears from these same patients.[31] On the other hand, longitudinal studies of women with an index smear lacking endocervical cells do not show a higher rate of abnormalities in subsequent smears, which might be expected if the 'limited' smears had a higher rate of false-negative results.[32,33] The published minimum criteria for what represents an adequate sampling of the TZ ('two clusters of well-preserved endocervical and/or squamous metaplastic cells, with each cluster composed of at least five appropriate cells') appear arbitrary.[16] Some cytopathologists have suggested that the cervical mucus plug represents an adequate sampling of the TZ and may not require endocervical glandular cells or metaplastic cells.[34] Further discussion of this subject is included in Chapter 2.

TBS also specifies that a fully satisfactory specimen be submitted with relevant clinical information. Yet in the aforementioned CAP surveys, insufficient clinical information rarely was cited as a reason for characterizing a specimen as unsatisfactory or SBLB.[24]

HIERARCHICAL REVIEW

Clinical Laboratory Improvement Amendments, 1988 (CLIA'88) states that gynecological smears showing reactive or reparative change, atypia, pre-malignant or malignant features should be reviewed by a technical supervisor in cytology (FR 493.1257(c)(1)).[14] Undoubtedly, smears showing ASCUS or atypical glandular cells of undetermined significance (AGUS), or a higher level of abnormality, should be confirmed by pathologist review. Pathologist review of smears showing reactive/reparative change is more controversial. A survey of 170 cytology laboratories[35] revealed that 21 per cent created more stringent criteria for the reactive/reparative diagnosis after implementation of CLIA'88, thus limiting the number of cases that must be reviewed by a pathologist. Four per cent of the laboratories surveyed did not use the reactive/reparative terminology at all to avoid forwarding such cases for hierarchical review. Although a recent study reported that 3.9 per cent of patients with reactive cellular change on their Pap smear and 1.6 per cent of patients with normal smears showed squamous intra-epithelial lesions (SIL) on follow-up smears,[36] one could reasonably argue that most Pap smears showing reactive cellular changes fall within the spectrum of normal. This is the approach followed by the CAP-PAP. Similarly, TBS and the companion atlas define and illustrate reactive changes as benign cellular changes.[37] Reactive cellular change covers a wide spectrum. At one extreme, i.e. atypical repair, it perhaps is best considered ASCUS. This distinction, however, is not made in the CLIA'88 regulations.

Post-test variables

RECOMMENDATIONS

The efficacy of the Pap test ultimately is dependent on appropriate follow-up. An interdisciplinary approach could conceivably involve the pathologist in post-test management, such as including a recommendation in the report and follow-up tracking. However, one of the most controversial aspects of the original Bethesda proposals was the statement that the 'diagnostic report should include a recommendation for further patient evaluation when appropriate'.[23] In response to criticism of this perceived intrusion into the clinician's domain, the participants of the second Bethesda conference[16] agreed that recommendations should be limited to suggestions for obtaining additional tissue to clarify uncertain pathological changes, or to address an adequacy problem (e.g. estrogen therapy in cases of ASCUS associated with atrophy). In addition, a qualifying phrase such as 'if clinically indicated' should be appended to allow the clinician to exercise their clinical judgment as to the appropriateness of the recommendation.

Recommendation for a short-interval repeat Pap smear prompted by the absence of endocervical cells is controversial. Some authors insist that these less than fully adequate smears warrant repeat.[38] Others feel that this is unnecessary owing to the lack of evidence of increased risk in these women,[32,33] unless it is clinically indicated because of a suspicious lesion or high-risk factors.

TBS does not require recommendations. They may be used at the discretion of the pathologist. Some institutions allow individual clinicians to indicate whether they prefer to receive recommendations or not.[24,39]

ERROR DETECTION

The laboratory must seek out errors, not for punitive purposes but rather to learn from these errors (a crucial distinction that too often is lost in the current litigious climate). The subject of false negatives and error detection is covered in depth in a later section (see the topic False Negatives in the section entitled Accuracy of Pap Smear Results).

BENCHMARKING

In addition to these internal aspects of CQI, the laboratory needs external standards against which to measure its own performance. Benchmarking data for cytology laboratories are available in the form of CAP Q-Probes (voluntary quality assurance program),[40] CAP-PAP summary reports,[41,42] and practice surveys,[19] other inter-laboratory surveys and comparisons,[15,35] and intramural programs in large laboratories.[7,17,22,43] The use of this benchmarking data may require careful analysis and selective extrapolation, as the criteria reported might not be defined and measured the same way in different laboratories. In particular, comparing 'false-negative' rates among different institutions is fraught with problems because of variation in definition (see the topic False Negatives in the section entitled Accuracy of Pap Smear Results).

Cost

A comprehensive CQI program undoubtedly increases the cost of Pap smears. However, improved accuracy in Pap smear testing leads to earlier treatment and lives saved, which may result in cost-saving in the long term. Neither the cost-effectiveness nor the medical effectiveness of cervical screening has been validated by prospective, randomized trials.[44–46] Any such studies would have to weigh the positive economic benefits of early detection and treatment against the added costs of overtreatment of lesions with limited potential for progression and of false positives. Because of the long preclinical detectable phase of cervical neoplasia, a somewhat lower sensitivity is acceptable in Pap smear screening compared with other screening programs. Any CQI efforts aimed at increasing sensitivity at the expense of decreased specificity for the absence of significant cervical disease are sure to be costly[31,39] but not necessarily cost effective.

Some estimates of the costs of pathology CQI activities have been made. A CAP Q-Probe of quality improvement programs in anatomical and clinical pathology revealed a median time investment of 40 hours/month on manual data collection and analysis mostly by a pathologist.[47] The labor costs for three quality-assurance monitors used by a large community hospital (10 per cent random rescreen, cytology–histology correlation, and 18-month directed retrospective review in patients with new diagnoses of dysplasia) were compared.[48] The directed retrospective review was 10 times as sensitive as the random 10 per cent review, while consuming only 15 per cent of the labor hours required for the 10 per cent rescreen. The 10 per cent random rescreen may cost a laboratory from 250 to 350 hours/year,[48,49] and is performed by a cytotechnologist in 65 per cent of the laboratories that responded to a survey conducted by the International Academy of Cytology.[38] Allen et al.[35] estimated the additional costs incurred by pathologists' reviewing all 'reactive/reparative' smears as required by CLIA to range from $4.5 million to $40 million depending on the percentage of such cases.

It is important to remember that spending more on quality improvement may have a negative impact on the outcome. Helfand et al.[50] used a mathematical model to predict the effects of the CLIA'88 regulations on the incidence of invasive cervical carcinoma. Predicting decreased access to screening because of an increase in the cost of a Pap smear, the model showed that a small increase in sensitivity (5 per cent or less) at the cost of a 50 per cent increase in the price of a Pap smear would result in an increase of 23 cases of invasive carcinomas per 100 000 women. Unlike quality improvement activities in industry, which usually result in cost-savings or increased earnings,[16] the benefit of improved quality in the health-care industry cannot be measured in terms of expenses or revenues and will be realized only with long-term commitment. In the face of fierce competition for health-care dollars, a successful screening program requires a sound foundation in finance, business management, and strategic planning as well as in quality health care.[20]

CLINICAL LABORATORIES IMPROVEMENT ACT

History

Cytology and pathology professional organizations have been aware of the need for QA in the laboratory since the use of the Pap smear became widespread in the 1950s, and there was legislative interest in quality standards two decades prior to the well-known *Wall Street Journal* articles of 1987.

Proficiency testing (PT) for independent cytology laboratories in the state of Wisconsin[51] was initiated in August, 1967 following the passage of the Social Security Act–Health Insurance for the Aged (Medicare) in 1966 and the Clinical Laboratories Improvement Act of 1967 (CLIA'67) (CLIA '67 is Section 353 of the Public Health Service Act and applies to laboratories engaged in interstate commerce). The Medicare legislation did not require PT of cytology laboratories, but those laboratories licensed by CLIA'67 were required to participate in PT. The Wisconsin program consisted originally of surveys of three cases bimonthly; in the third year of the program this was changed to surveys of four cases quarterly. The test cases included gynecological and non-gynecological materials. Acceptable performance was set at 90 per cent. The program evaluated diagnostic accuracy, trends and reproducibility. Ten out of 15 laboratories had achieved an acceptable level of performance after 16 surveys. These results were presented at the 18th Symposium Meeting of the American Society of Cytology in November 1970.[51,52] The report concluded that this type of survey instrument could not adequately assess the overall performance of a laboratory, that the use of different terminology hindered evaluation and that a comprehensive internal QA program must accompany external evaluation. Nonetheless, the PT instrument was felt to be useful in providing benchmark data for individual laboratories to measure their own performance against.

In 1968, New York initiated a program 'to test and record the performance of cytotechnologists and tabulate their qualifications and experience'.[53] This program differs from the Wisconsin one and the current philosophy of PT in that the focus was on individual rather than laboratory performance, on the premise that 'variability in personal interpretation as well as accuracy and reproducibility of results are an integral part of cytodiagnosis'. The test consisted of three Pap smears and two sputum specimens. Differences in terminology were dealt with by allowing only three responses: positive, negative and suspicious.

Acceptable performance was 80 per cent responses correct. The test cases were accompanied by a personal questionnaire. Results after the first year of the program showed a pass rate of 85 per cent. Recent graduates had a higher pass rate, and cytotechnologists performed better than supervisors. There was no relationship between performance and training, professional status, membership in professional societies or attendance of scientific meetings. Both the New York and Wisconsin programs recommended additional education rather than punitive measures for laboratories or individuals failing to meet satisfactory performance levels.[51,52]

The Centers for Disease Control (CDC) field-tested two pilot programs of performance evaluation in cytology in the 1970s.[54] Field tests of on-site PT in 1972–73 and 1978 showed that overall the target diagnosis was made in 64 per cent of test cases, with approximately equal significant undercalls (7.5 per cent) and overcalls (8.9 per cent). In contrast to the results of the New York program, professional certification did correlate with better performance, and performance improved after 1 year of experience but leveled off thereafter. Cytotechnologists performed better than pathologists. A retrospective rescreening model was field tested in 1979. The necessity to rescreen large numbers of cases prospectively in order to detect errors in a population with a low prevalence of disease was recognized as a problem even then.

In 1977, Senator Jacob Javits (Republican, NY) attempted without success to introduce the Clinical Laboratory Improvement Act of 1977 to amend Section 353 of the Public Health Service Act (CLIA'67)[55] and to impose a uniform set of standards on all clinical laboratories. Senator Javits subsequently attempted to introduce CLIA'79, with accompanying House bills introduced by Congressmen Waxman (Democrat, CA) and Leland (Democrat, TX). At the same time, Congressman Rangel (Democrat, NY) proposed the Medicare and Medicaid Amendments of 1979 (known as the mini-CLIA) with the same goal of unifying clinical laboratory quality standards under both the Social Security Act and the Public Health Service Act. All of these bills failed at various points in the legislative process.

Investigations of and closures of cytology laboratories in the 1970s prompted the CDC to draft more comprehensive standards, which were presented in 1980 to the American Society of Cytology (ASC) as 'Quality Control Standards for Cytology'.[55] Many of these provisions were ultimately incorporated into CLIA'88, including requirements for requisition and report forms, record management, statistical analyses, histological correlation, workload limitations, evaluation of cytotechnologist diagnostic accuracy and retrospective rescreening. PT was required also, as in CLIA'67. In 1981, Health Care Financing Administration (HCFA) awarded a non-competitive contract to the Laboratory Accreditation Committee of the ASC[55] to develop guidelines for quality standards in cytology practice and cytology laboratory inspection. This committee proposed further refinements of CLIA'67 regulations and the CDC draft standards to include 10 per cent rescreening of cytotechnologists and pathologists, 5-year instead of 2-year slide retention, and mandatory continuing medical education (CME) for all personnel.[55]

In 1985, the Department of Health and Human Services (DHHS, formerly the Department of Health, Education, and Welfare) contracted Macro Systems, Inc., a consulting firm, to evaluate the current laboratory standards of DHHS.[55] They recommended uniformity in standards for all laboratories, recognized the importance of process standards, discouraged the focus on restrictive personnel standards, recommended that regulations be based on the degree of test complexity, suggested more focus on outcome measures (PT was considered to be one), and emphasized regulations based on empirical studies, which was not the case for the current regulations. Thus, DHHS began revisions of the quality standards for laboratories regulated under Medicare and Medicaid and CLIA'67. Ironically (so it now seems), their goals included reduction of the regulatory burden, removal of inconsistencies and elimination of unnecessary credentialing requirements.[55]

In November of 1987, the now famous articles by Walt Bogdanich appeared in the *Wall Street Journal*[57] raising concern about 'Pap mills' and the danger they presented to women's health. 'Deadly Mistakes', a television series produced by Lea Thompson, a Washington, DC, newscaster, was also aired in November 1987. These sensational media reports prompted several congressional hearings. Seven separate bills resulted and ultimately were merged into one – H.R. 5471. The final bill included workload limits, standards for rescreening, unannounced PT, rules for handling inadequate smears and requirements for on-site screening, slide retention and periodic inspection by persons experienced in cytology. President Reagan signed this bill, which amended Section 353 of the Public Health Service Act (CLIA'67), into law on October 31, 1988. Thus, Public Law 100–578 became CLIA'88.[14]

During this period, revisions of CLIA'67 were ongoing. These preceded passage of CLIA'88, and were initiated by the cytology community, in contrast to the legislative-driven CLIA'88. HCFA, the CDC, and the National Institutes of Health (NIH) cosponsored a conference on the 'State of the Art in Quality Control Measures for Diagnostic Cytology Laboratories' in Atlanta, Georgia, USA, in March 1988. The conference participants, representing several pathology and cytology professional organizations, were asked to prepare recommendations for quality control and assurance in cytology laboratories, specifically in the areas of PT, workload limitations and personnel qualification standards. HCFA, under a deadline imposed by the Secretary of the DHHS, asked for these recommendations by May 1988. Representatives from the American Society of Cytotechnologists (ASCT), ASC, and CAP met with CDC representatives in May 1988 to try to arrive at a consensus on these issues. A Notice of Proposed Rulemaking (NPRM) was published in August 1988 with a 90-day comment period. A second 'State of the Art in Quality Control Measures for Diagnostic Cytology Laboratories' conference was held in September 1988 so that the proceedings could be submitted in response to the NPRM within the 90-day comment period. This comment period ended 3 days after CLIA'88 became law on October 31.[55] The Final Rule for the revisions of CLIA'67 was published on March 14, 1990, and became effective on September 10, 1990. The NPRM for CLIA'88 was published on May 21, 1990, and the Final Rule for CLIA'88 was published on February 28, 1992, effective September 1, 1992 (except for PT, see below), supplanting the revised CLIA'67. The most controversial requirement of CLIA'88 – proficiency testing – is discussed in detail below.

Proficiency testing

HISTORY

PT in clinical laboratory medicine began over 50 years ago, as an educational, self-assessment, inter-laboratory comparison program.[59] The Final Rule for CLIA'67 required that laboratories be enrolled in an approved PT program by January 1, 1991,[58] and under CLIA'88 the deadline was January 1, 1994 (FR 493.855(a)).[14] The regulations specified that all individuals examining gynecology preparations (cytotechnologists and pathologists) must be tested at least once a year. Testing could be announced or unannounced, would be on-site and would consist of a set of 10 glass slides. The passing score would be 90 per cent, with retesting required for any individual failing the primary testing event. No approved PT program existed at the time of the Final Rule, however, and further, a Request for Proposal (RFP) for PT programs issued in the fall of 1992 and again in the spring of 1993 drew no responses.[60] Finally, in 1994, the state of Wisconsin implemented a 1-year voluntary glass slide PT program.[61] The program met all federal requirements including penalties for failure on PT. Testing began in July 1994 but immediately came under attack by individuals concerned about being bound by federal regulations while the rest of the country was not. The program lasted less than a year.

A symposium on PT, sponsored by the CDC, CAP and Cytopathology Education Consortium (with representation from the ASCP, ASC and ASCT) was held in Atlanta in November, 1993. The Clinical Laboratory Improvement Advisory Committee (CLIAC), established concurrently with CLIA'88 (FR, Vol. 57, No. 40, 2/28/92, pg 6832), subsequently made several recommendations, including: (1) a national glass slide PT program is unfeasible logistically and financially; (2) PT should be applied to the laboratory, not to the individual; and (3) research, including outcomes studies, is needed to assess the effectiveness and costs of PT for quality assurance in gynecological cytology. Phased implementation and investigation of alternative testing methodologies was suggested.[62] In a December 6, 1994, Federal Register notice, HCFA extended the effective date for enrollment in a PT program to January 1, 1995, and accepted CLIAC's recommendation to accept testing media other than glass slides.[63]

CONTROVERSIES OVER FORMAT AND CONTENT

Alternatives to a glass slide proficiency test are worth considering, given the logistical and economic difficulty in obtaining sufficient quantities of validated, comparable glass slides. The state of Pennsylvania piloted a videotape proficiency test in 1992, which was loudly rejected by the local cytopathology community. Although most individuals in our Pennsylvania laboratory found the test format uncomfortable, test scores were high. A more common alternative to glass slide PT is digitized (computerized) images. A CDC-sponsored study[64] that compared performance by 82 screeners on computerized PT, glass slide PT and the screener's work performance found a weak correlation (0.24) between computerized PT and work performance and also glass slide PT and work performance. Mean scores on the glass slide test were 93 per cent; mean scores on computerized PT were only 83 per cent (CLIA'88 defines failure as <90 per cent). An ASCP pilot program of computerized PT showed a 27 per cent discrepancy between glass slide and computerized PT.[65] One potential advantage to computerized PT is that the number of challenges per examination can be increased, which increases test reliability. However, these tests de-emphasize the importance of locator skills in screening. Computer technology could be useful in testing screening by comparing the marks made by a screener with the coordinates indicated by a computerized screening device, or by measuring completeness of slide coverage by the screener using a stage-drive device. Thin-layer methodology offers the potential of a glass slide test without the limitations of conventional glass slide testing since multiple slides can be prepared from the same specimen, thus providing comparable diagnostic material.

While vendors and professional societies struggle to devise a reliable, affordable method of PT to satisfy CLIA regulations, others have asserted that the rules for implementation of these regulations are too lax. Two public watchdog groups, the Consumer Federation of America and Public Citizen, charged DHHS with failing to comply with the statutory mandate of CLIA'88 that PT take place to the extent practicable, under normal working conditions.[66] According to this, the time allowed for a PT event should equal the time it would normally take to screen the same number of slides under normal working conditions. Assuming the maximum allowed screening rate of 4.5 min per slide (100 slides per 8 hours screening), no more than 45 min should be allowed for a 10-slide PT. The US District Court for the District of Columbia decided this suit in favor of the plaintiffs in August, 1995. In compliance with this decision, HCFA published a new rule in the November 30, 1995, Federal Register to shorten the time for PT from 2 hours to 45 min while appealing the district court decision. The US Circuit Court of Appeals for the District of Columbia upheld the ruling of the District Court on May 21, 1996, on the basis that the Final Rule for CLIA'88 does not offer a sufficient explanation of why the rate for PT should be less than the maximum allowable screening rate. HCFA was offered the choice of articulating a convincing rationale for this difference or to continue the rule-making process. In effect, only the latter option was viable. HCFA had offered, during the appeal process, the explanation that PT should be afforded a longer time because PT events include a higher proportion of abnormal slides than does routine screening. The appeals court refused to consider what it defined as an entirely new theory, however, since this was presented only at the district court stage rather than during the rule-making process.[66]

This rather bizarre scenario highlights the public's lack of understanding of Pap smear testing at many levels. PT should not be a video game-like competition (increasing level of play with a harder mix of cases and lose points if not fast enough!). Furthermore, CLIA mandates that the PT samples 'must be examined or tested with the laboratory's regular patient workload by personnel who routinely perform the testing in the laboratory, using the laboratory's routine methods'(FR 493.801(b)).[14] Can PT ever satisfy these mandates? It is difficult to integrate test slides into the screening stream without the cytotechnologists' awareness. Once a cytotechnologist is aware that the slide is a test slide, there is no hope that it truly will be screened as would a routine smear; test slides are inevitably scrutinized more than routine Pap smears.[67] Along these lines, should the test include the same percentage of abnormal slides as the laboratory's normal workload? The same arguments against the 10 per cent rescreen for detection of substandard screening (see next section on Accuracy of Pap Smear Results) apply here[68] and therefore necessitate a higher percentage of abnormal smears on a proficiency test.

The diagnostic categories for cytology PT as defined by CLIA'88 are unsatisfactory, normal/benign, low-grade squamous intraepithelial lesion (LSIL), and HSIL. The scoring system penalizes wrong responses in proportion to their distance from the target response. However, there is documented significant inter-observer,[69,70] intra-observer,[71] and inter-laboratory[26] variability in the diagnosis of LSIL versus HSIL. It does not seem fair to penalize an individual who 'misdiagnoses' LSIL as HSIL or vice versa on PT.

The next question involves whether PT should be directed at individuals or laboratories. If simulating normal working conditions, PT should test the performance of the laboratory. Under normal working conditions, informal sharing of cases, hierarchical review and review of previous Pap smears and corresponding histopathology contribute to increased accuracy in Pap smear reporting. An individual member of the laboratory is unlikely to render an opinion on a smear with questionable findings without input from someone else. Thus, judging an individual's performance on a proficiency test, while denying them this routine practice, is a poor indicator of the overall quality of the laboratory. Since satisfactory performance on PT is necessary for licensure renewal and accreditation, to assess the quality of the laboratory instead of the individual should be the aim of external review. Locator skills and diagnostic accuracy of individuals also should be assessed as they contribute to overall laboratory performance, although these are among the goals of the internal quality assurance program.

CURRENT 'EQUIVALENTS' OF PROFICIENCY TESTS

Although a CLIA-approved PT is currently available only in Maryland, a number of inter-laboratory comparison programs are available for a laboratory to implement external review and quality assurance. The largest, with 2089 laboratory subscribers in 1997, is the CAP-PAP program.[69] This program, piloted in 1989 with 207 laboratories, was recognized in 1996 as a CAP Survey. Laboratories accredited by the CAP Laboratory Accreditation Program (LAP, granted deemed status by HCFA in 1994) must participate in PAP or an equivalent glass slide PT program for successful accreditation in cytopathology. The program is based on firm educational principles. Five referenced slides are mailed to and reviewed by the participating laboratories quarterly. A fax option for laboratory responses and feedback on reference diagnoses allows review of the cases again, if necessary, while the slides are still in the laboratory. Each laboratory also receives a summary of peer interpretations on these same slides, as well as an annual summary report. The program includes validated graded slide sets and educational non-graded sets. Response categories are broader than those defined by CLIA (series 100 includes normal/reactive, series 200 includes all malignant/premalignant changes) and circumvent the problem of inter-observer variability discussed above. Workshops, slide seminars, and practice proficiency tests offered at many professional meetings are additional opportunities for PT. Large cytology laboratories may have their own in-house glass slide PT program.[22]

COST AND BENEFIT

Despite all the controversy and discussion on the content and implementation of PT, data on its efficacy (meaning the degree to which the test produces the desired effect or result) are still lacking. Is the intent of cytology PT to remove incompetent practitioners from the field, or to improve the quality of an individual's or a laboratory's work? Test performance may improve with more experience in taking proficiency tests,[72] but this does not necessarily mean that the diagnostic work of the laboratory has improved. Is poor performance on PT a valid indication of incompetency? Cytology PT, as currently proposed, fails to meet most measures of test validity.[65,72] Estimates of the financial resources necessary for a national PT program have been made based on data from the Maryland State Proficiency Testing Program.[73] Under a 2-hour PT model, the first test event would currently cost $5–7 million. A 45-min test would save $3–4 million. However, assuming a higher fail rate with the shorter test, more repeat tests would be necessary, as would retraining after three failures, for an overall increased cost of $0.5–1.6 million above the original projections.

ACCURACY OF PAP SMEAR RESULTS

'False negatives'

'False negative' in cytopathology has become a 'buzz word' that raises both angst and ire. It is a term that is misunderstood and misused by the cytology community nearly as often as by the lay public, or, more ominously, those in the legal system. Yet these are – as so well put by Naryshkin and Davey[74] with apologies to Steve Martin and the movie 'Roxanne' – just 'worms', unless we have a common understanding of this term and its meaning in assessing the value of a test to society, or the quality of the laboratory performing the test. False-negative results in Pap smears can be attributed to sampling error, screening error and interpretive error. Before discussing these, however, certain attributes of measurement must be understood.

SENSITIVITY, SPECIFICITY, POSITIVE AND NEGATIVE PREDICTIVE VALUES

A false-negative result is simply a negative test result in a person with the disease that the test is intended to test for. The false-negative rate (FNR) of a test is obtained by subtracting the sensitivity of the test from 100 per cent. Other measures of the performance of a test include specificity, positive and negative predictive values. Sensitivity is the relative ability of a test to detect disease (true positive results) among all those with disease, whether they tested positive (TP) or falsely negative (FN). Specificity is the ability of a test to exclude disease in persons who do not have disease. In other words it is the proportion of truly negative test results among all those without disease, whether they tested negative (TN) or falsely positive (FP). Positive (or negative) predictive values (PV+ and PV−, respectively), which are probably of more interest to a user of the test (clinician), indicate the proportion of patients with positive (or negative) test results who actually have the disease (or no disease). Their relationships are illustrated in Table 4.1.

Unfortunately, it is virtually impossible to measure directly the sensitivity and specificity of cervical cytology (and thus impossible to calculate the FNR), since patients with negative test results do not usually have confirmatory colposcopy and biopsy. The PV+ is more readily measured, since most positive tests will be followed by biopsy or repeat cytology. Soost et al.[75] calculated the PV for 71 566 cervicovaginal smears using a strict validation procedure of histological follow-up for all positive results. They also attempted to determine the sensitivity by ruling out false-negative results with a minimum of two follow-up smears within 2 years of negative smears. Based on these methods, they estimated sensitivity and specificity of cervical screening for the entire population of 274 297 women screened by the Cytological Institute of the Bavarian Cancer Society from 1971 to 1980 to be 80 per cent and 99.95 per cent, respectively. The PV− in their population was 99.8 per cent and PV+ ranged from 90 per cent to 95.5 per cent for severe dysplasia through invasive carcinoma. The PV+ was lower for mild-moderate dysplasia (73 per cent).

Sensitivity can be measured directly only if there is some means to identify accurately all cases of disease in a certain population. Mitchell et al.[76] used the Victorian Cancer Registry database of all women with cervical cancer during 1983 to calculate a sensitivity of 96 per cent for the detection of cervical carcinoma. A different methodology of comparing observed to expected cases of carcinoma yielded an estimated sensitivity of 93 per cent. Histological follow-up on 483 women with cytological diagnoses of cervical intraepithelial neoplasia (CIN) III in 1985 showed a PV+ of 93 per cent. PV− was estimated by random rescreening of 1791 slides to be 98 per cent. Sensitivity, specificity, and PV+ from a Q-Probe study of cytological–histological correlation yielded values of 89 per cent, 65 per cent and 89 per cent, respectively.[42]

It should be pointed out that the predictive values of a test depend on its sensitivity and specificity as well as on the prevalence rate of the disease being tested for in the population. Table 4.2 illustrates this point.[75] The sensitivity and specificity of the test remain 95 per cent and 95 per cent, respectively, in both circumstances.

Table 4.1 *Definition and relationship of commonly used terms in quality assurance*

Test	Disease present	Disease absent	Total
Positive	TP	FP	TP + FP
Negative	FN	TN	FN + TN
Total	TP + FN	FP + TN	TP + TN + FN + FP

TP, tested positive; FN, tested falsely negative; TN, tested negative; FP, tested falsely positive.
Sensitivity = TP/(TP + FN).
Specificity = TN/(TN + FP).
Positive predictive value (PV+) = TP/(TP + FP).
Negative predictive value (PV−) = TN/(TN + FN).

Table 4.2 *Predictive values of a test*[a]

Prevalence rate (%)	Positive predictive value (%)	Negative predictive value (%)
50	95	95
1	16	99.9

[a]Data from Soost et al.[75]

For a disease with a low prevalence rate (e.g. cervical carcinoma), the positive predictive value is low even when the test has an excellent sensitivity and specificity. The prevalence of cervical dysplasia/carcinoma is increased in a high-risk population, and so is the PV+ of the Pap smear. Therefore, it is important for the clinician to be aware of the woman's risk status when interpreting a Pap smear result. This may be difficult in a managed care environment, where patients may receive care from different providers and information transfer may be suboptimal.[77]

OTHER MEASUREMENTS OF ACCURACY OF PAP TESTS

The measurements described above work well for data that can be dichotomized. However, this is not the case for cervicovaginal cytology. Pap smear results include negative and several degrees of positivity. Likelihood ratio (LR) and receiver operator characteristic (ROC) curves, which can be applied to an ordinal spectrum of diagnostic categories (normal → dysplastic → invasive carcinoma), can be used to assess accuracy of cytological diagnosis.[78] LR is the probability of a given test result (e.g. ASCUS) if that disease is present divided by the probability of the same test result if disease is absent. LR can be calculated for each diagnostic category and then multiplied by the pretest clinical odds of disease (prevalence and risk factors) to estimate the post-test odds of disease. Therefore, for each Pap diagnosis, the clinician could estimate the odds that the patient actually had that diagnosis. The ROC curves are created by plotting the true positive rate (sensitivity) on the y-axis against the false positive rate $(1 -$ specificity) on the x-axis for varying diagnostic criteria. Each point along the curve corresponds to an LR, and represents the trade-off between specificity and sensitivity.

COMPARING FALSE-NEGATIVE RATES

Much of the confusion in the literature about the accuracy of Pap smears stems from the improper use of the statistics for dichotomized data and the diversity of ways that different authors define a positive test result. As long as the definitions are variable, reports by different authors will be incomparable. Pap smear results can be dichotomized based on any given threshold for a 'positive' result: a narrow definition being LSIL or worse and a broad definition ASCUS/AGUS or worse.[47] Another source of confusion is in how inclusive a definition of Pap smear testing is applied, i.e. including pre- and post-test variables versus test-phase (laboratory) variables only.

Comparison of laboratory accuracy is also hindered by the different ways test results are verified. Some reports are based on directed retrospective review of smears with histological follow-up[7,11,40,48,79–88] while others have calculated FN rates from random rescreening of negative slides,[48,50,54,84] from directed rescreening of smears from high-risk patients,[17] or from a randomized recall of patients for repeat smears.[82] The denominator might be total cases reviewed, all negatives, all dysplasias, all cancers or total volume. These factors explain the wide range of false-negative rates (from 6 per cent to 94 per cent) reported in the literature.[11,81] Bosch et al.[67] illustrated the magnitude of this problem by calculating an FNR on their own laboratory data using three different formulas: the rates were 0.003 per cent, 9.5 per cent, and 70 per cent. A standard formula is needed for calculating and reporting error rates in gynecological cytology.

Screening errors

METHODS OF DETECTING SCREENING ERRORS

Directed retrospective rescreening and random rescreening of negative smears can be used to detect errors in primary screening. Both activities are required by CLIA'88. Random rescreening is the method most laboratories use to estimate their screening error rates, but it is fraught with problems in methodology, terminology, administration and interpretation.

FALSE NEGATIVE FRACTION

Krieger and Naryshkin[89] proposed the 'false negative fraction' (FNF) as an estimate of false negatives due to screening, or the percentage of positive cases missed during screening:

FNF = estimated number of false-negative cases/(total number of positive cases
+ estimated number of false-negative cases).

Nagy[90] prefers 'false negative proportion' (FNP = number of actual or estimated FN results/actual or estimated positive results) to FNF. To determine the FNF, the number of FN found during routine random rescreening is divided by the percentage of total cases rescreened to estimate total FN. The total number of positive cases is derived from laboratory statistics.

Since this rate is independent of the prevalence of the disease, it can be used to compare error rates among cytotechnologists and among cytology laboratories (benchmarking). The definition of positive result can be set at any level of abnormality but must be the same in the numerator and denominator. From several studies in which a FNF was given or could be computed, it ranged from 1.5 per cent to 20 per cent, with most around 3–5 per cent.[48,49,54,81,84] The single largest data set, comprised of over one million cases rescreened, indicates an absolute floor, or irreducible FNF, of 5 per cent.[89]

It is important to realize that the FNF depends on the threshold chosen for the calculation. The accuracy of Pap smear interpretation is poorer for lower-level abnormalities and thus the FNF will be higher. Further, if a laboratory's rescreening is not random but enriched by selecting high-risk cases, FNF, as calculated with the above formula is invalid, since it assumes that a representative sample of the entire patient population of the laboratory is rescreened. In addition, all of these studies make the assumption that the rescreening is error-free. Renshaw and colleagues[91,92] made the cogent arguments that calculation of the true FNR of primary screening must incorporate the FNR of rescreening and that to determine the FNR accurately, abnormal smears must be included in rescreening.

The percentage to be rescreened randomly can vary from 10 per cent, as required by CLIA'88, to 100 per cent. Random 10 per cent rescreening is neither cost-effective nor efficacious in identifying cytotechnologists with higher screening error rates, as discussed before. Flehinger (in Melamed)[68] determined that in a population with a prevalence of 20 out of 1000 of cervical neoplasia, it would take more than 3 years of rescreening at the 10 per cent rate to distinguish reliably a cytotechnologist missing one case out of four from a cytotechnologist missing no more than one case out of 10. A method proposed by Krieger et al.[93] takes into account the prevalence of epithelial abnormalities in a population in determining the absolute number of slides that should be rescreened, in order for random rescreening to produce statistically significant results. For example, with a prevalence of epithelial abnormality at 5 per cent, it takes a rescreening of 680 slides to detect a significant difference between an 'acceptable' FNP of 5 per cent and 'unacceptable' FNP of 15 per cent.[93]

Immediate rescreening does, however, have the advantage of identifying errors before any serious consequence occurs. This is why a new cytotechnologist is always subject to a higher percentage of immediate rescreening before it is reduced to the routine 10 per cent level. The random immediate rescreen may also help a laboratory achieve consensus on diagnostic criteria and specimen adequacy assessment, decrease transcription errors, and contribute to a downward trend in the FNF.[22]

As an alternative to 10 per cent rescreening, Farakar[94] proposed a rapid, partial rescreening of all negative smears before the report is issued. The slide is step-screened from one corner to its opposite, plus one length along the inside edge of the coverslip. Compared with primary screening, this method, which covers 15 per cent of the surface area of the slide, detected 80 per cent of the abnormalities. At 15 s/slide, the rescreening workload was estimated to approximately equal that required for the conventional 10 per cent rescreen. Using this method, the FNF for reports leaving the laboratory was calculated to be only 0.4 per cent.[95] The larger number of FN discovered by this method also provided more realistic data for judging the screening performance of individual cytotechnologists. A working party sponsored by the National Health Service, the British Society for Clinical Cytology, and the Royal College of Pathologists recommended that partial rescreening replace 10 per cent random review in the UK.[95] Renshaw et al.[96] agree that rapid rescreening is more effective than routine 10 per cent rescreening for detecting false-negative cases, and is comparable to routine rescreening for measuring the FNR of primary screening. They suggest that rapid *pre*screening may be the best method of all.[97]

Another issue concerning rescreening is who should perform the review. Federal regulatory language allows this review to be performed by a technical supervisor (pathologist), a cytology general supervisor, or a qualified cytotechnologist with three years of full-time experience (FR 493.1257 (d)(1)).[14] Automated technology has been approved for either rescreening negative smears[98] or selecting cases to be reviewed.[99] The quality and cost of each option should be considered. The new technologies are discussed in depth in Chapter 3.

Interpretive and sampling errors

The other component of laboratory error in false-negative cytology is interpretive error, which is usually identified from retrospective review of previous negative smears of patients with a newly detected high-grade abnormality and from cytological–histological correlation, as mandated by CLIA (FR 493.1257 (d)(2–3)).[14] Both provide data for the laboratory to evaluate its performance, and are more likely than the 10 per cent rescreen to provide information to improve the accuracy of cytological interpretation.[17,100] These studies also provide data for sampling error.

Before we examine the results of cytological–histological correlation studies, we need to take with a grain of salt the concept of histology as the 'gold standard' for cervical disease. All correlation studies attribute some share of the discrepancies to histology. This may include sampling error (diseased area of cervix not biopsied), misdiagnosis of the cervical biopsy, insufficient sectioning of the tissue and poor histological technique prohibiting accurate diagnosis.[7,42,43,48,82,87] Diagnostic errors in histological sections are no less common than in cytological diagnosis.[7,42,43,87] Furthermore, inter-observer variability exists in histology as in cytology.[27,48,101–103]

Three large cytological–histological correlation studies ($n = 175–2971$)[7,42,43] show remarkably similar overwhelming percentages of discrepant cases attributed to sampling error (90–93 per cent), but a smaller correlation study ($n = 69$) showed a lower percentage due to sampling error (less than 60 per cent).[87] In a large CAP Q-Probes study, insufficient sampling on the Pap smear played a role in 41.4 per cent (1230) of 2971 discordant Pap smear–biopsy pairs, and biopsy sampling error in 40.6 per cent (1205).[48] Cytology interpretive errors (both false-positive and false-negative) contributed to 122 (4.1 per cent) of the discrepancies and biopsy interpretative errors to 240 (8.1 per cent). Screening errors accounted for 160 (5.4 per cent, including 120 changes to ASCUS or AGUS and four to inadequate) of the discrepancies. Both screening and interpretive errors on cytology were noted in 14 (0.5 per cent).

Directed retrospective review (look-back) studies also confirmed that there were no atypical cells on the previous negative smears in the majority (57–83 per cent) of cases,[11,79,80,82,88,100,104] which presumably represent sampling errors, with the possible exception of cases of rapid progression.[85] Laboratory errors ranged from 15 to 38 per cent; interpretive error was more frequent than screening error.[79,80,100]

From a laboratory quality improvement aspect, the greatest value in correlation and look-back studies lies in assessing the causes of the interpretive errors and, hopefully, learning from these. This means that this 'dirty laundry' must be shared with others in the laboratory, not simply reviewed in private by the pathologist or cytotechnologist of record. Cytological misdiagnoses detected by retrospective review are equally divided between low-grade and high-grade lesions, in contrast to the histological misdiagnoses, which typically involve low-grade lesions.[7,43,81,87,101,105] At the low-grade end, it may be difficult to distinguish inflammatory cytological changes from ASCUS or LSIL. High-grade lesions can be overlooked if the cells are few, small, or bland. High-grade intraepithelial lesions may be confused with reactive glandular cells, immature squamous metaplasia, tubal metaplasia, endometriosis, stromal cells, atrophy and fragments of lower uterine segment (many of these included among the problematic 'hyperchromatic crowded groups').[81,85,106,107]

Some causes of false-negative results

The most frequent cause of screening or interpretive errors is probably scarcity of the atypical cells – an extension of sampling error.[81,85,100,107,108] There may be a limit on the number of atypical cells – 100 cells has been suggested[106] – below which we cannot expect to reliably recognize their presence. In one study,[81] 15 out of 16 false-negative smears had a very small number of abnormal cells that were detected only after prolonged screening on review. Data such as this should raise our awareness of the danger of small numbers of abnormal cells. 'Errors' detected by extraordinary measures should not imply substandard performance of a laboratory under normal working conditions.

Another common theme with FN smears is suboptimal or inadequate specimen quality due to obscuring blood or inflammation.[81,85,88,100,107] Particular care should be given to these smears, as the more severe cervical abnormalities, carcinoma in particular, may, by their destructive nature, cause these limiting factors.[88] As many as 12–14 per cent of the false-negative smears are deemed inadequate on review;[85,88] this is a sampling error compounded by an interpretive error.

The educational value and potential positive impact on patient care of the retrospective review is undeniable. The 5-year length of the required look-back period may be excessive, however. Allen et al.[79] identified 75 per cent of the FN smears within 2 years preceding the index high-grade smear, and Tabbara and Sidawy[100] identified 94 per cent within 3 years. By Pareto analysis, which helps focus QI activity by looking at the distribution of error, the most efficient approach would be to limit the look-back period to 3 years.

Other sources of errors

A small number of 'false negatives', using the broadest definition of the term, are due to disease factors, provider factors other than sampling and patient factors. There may be a form of aggressive cervical neoplasia that arises and progresses in the interval between the last negative Pap smear and the discovery of high-grade dysplasia or carcinoma, even if the interval is not excessively long.[85] Lapses in clinical management that contribute to false-negative tests include failure to follow up abnormal cytology, failure to confirm positive cytology histologically, failure to perform biopsy in women with clinical symptoms despite a negative Pap smear result and failure to recognize clinical symptoms, as related to cervical pathology.[12,83,86,104]

The patient may fail to return for follow-up or to undergo necessary diagnostic procedures[12,109] either due to limited access or other personal reasons. A significant problem involves women that do not receive screening at all: studies on invasive cervical carcinoma show that 50 per cent of these patients have never had Pap smears, or had not had one in the 5 years preceding the cancer diagnosis.[83,104,109] Older women with invasive cancer had even higher rates of non-participation in screening.[13,83,111,112]

Amended reports

Interpretation of the CLIA'88 requirement that amended reports be issued if this information would affect current patient management is very controversial. Many cytopathologists feel that the only way this would affect patient management is to prompt the patient to initiate litigation, since the index HSIL smear has already determined treatment. If it is reported, must this be a written amendment or is a verbal communication with the clinician acceptable? If the point of this CQI activity is to monitor and improve laboratory performance, there is little point in announcing individual errors to clinicians and patients. Conversely, the laboratory must not be perceived as trying to hide mistakes. Documentation of ongoing quality monitors and disclosure of errors may be of benefit to the laboratory if the patient has since developed invasive carcinoma and the case does go to litigation.

SUMMARY AND FUTURE TRENDS

In summary, every laboratory engaged in the practice of gynecological cytology should adopt some method of evaluating and monitoring false negatives, preferably a method that allows benchmarking with other laboratories. Reasons for false negatives should be identified in order to correct errors and improve the quality of service. Most importantly, laboratories and Pap smear providers must understand and acknowledge that errors do occur in order not to perpetuate the misconception that the Pap smear should have a zero error rate.

Pap smears have come a long way to assume the dubious honor of being the most regulated procedure in pathology, and perhaps in medicine. However, all the current regulations address only the quality of results. Contrary to CQI in industry, cost-effectiveness is not a consideration in the CQI regulations for Pap smears. Given the trend of cost containment for the healthcare system, efficient use of resources and efficacy of procedures in the cytology laboratories (management functions), in addition to patient care functions, will be under scrutiny sooner or later either by payers or by our non-pathologist colleagues in medicine. It will probably be inevitable for the cytopathology community to include the financial considerations in CQI instead of the current pursuit of perfecting the inherently imperfect Pap smears at any cost. Adjunct testings, such as hybrid capture human papillomavirus (HPV) testing (see Chapter 6), telomerase assays,[113] and immunoperoxidase staining for proteins regulating DNA replication,[114] will improve the detection of significant lesions but will no doubt add to the cost. It would be desirable for more cytopathology professionals to become better educated in CQI philosophy and methodology. The tools to collect, analyze and present data will certainly advance. The commercially available laboratory information systems for cytology have standard programming to generate all the necessary statistics and reports required by CLIA'88. Outcome studies and cost analyses are desperately needed to validate meaningful activities and enable us to dispose of useless monitors. Last but not least, we cannot allow increased costs of Pap smears to deny any woman access to this simple, potentially life-saving test. It is imperative that policy makers and leaders in the health-care system provide sensible directions and necessary resources for CQI to guarantee both availability and quality of Pap smear testing to all women.

REFERENCES

1 Mody DR, Davey DD, Branca M, et al. Quality assurance and risk reduction guidelines. *Acta Cytol* 2000; **44**: 496–507.

2 Berwick DM. Continuous improvement as an ideal in health care [see comments]. *N Engl J Med* 1989; **320**: 53–6.

3 Kohn LT, Corrigan JM, Donaldson M. *To err is human: building a safer health system.* Washington, DC: Institute of Medicine, 1999.

4 Leape LL. Institute of Medicine medical error figures are not exaggerated. *JAMA* 2000; **284**: 95–7.

5 Blumenthal D. Making medical errors into 'medical treasures" [editorial; comment] [see comments]. *JAMA* 1994; **272**: 1867–8.

6 Leape LL. Error in medicine [see comments]. *JAMA* 1994; **272**: 1851–7.

7 Joste NE, Crum CP, Cibas ES. Cytologic/histologic correlation for quality control in cervicovaginal cytology. Experience with 1,582 paired cases. *Am J Clin Pathol* 1995; **103**: 32–4.

8 Lachowicz C, Kline TS. Communication and cytopathology – Part III: Shared responsibility for quality improvement [editorial]. *Diagn Cytopathol* 1993; **9**: 371–2.

9 Iverson D. Quality improvement in action. *ASC Bull* 1996; **33**(6): 67.

10 Woo B, Cook EF, Weisberg M, Goldman L. Screening procedures in the asymptomatic adult. Comparison of physicians' recommendations, patients' desires, published guidelines, and actual practice. *JAMA* 1985; **254**: 1480–4.

11 Morell ND, Taylor JR, Snyder RN, Ziel HK, Saltz A, Willie S. False-negative cytology rates in patients in whom invasive cervical cancer subsequently developed. *Obstet Gynecol* 1982; **60**: 41–5.

12 Glenn GC. Practice parameter on laboratory panel testing for screening and case finding in asymptomatic adults. *Arch Pathol Laboratory Med* 1996; **120**: 929–43.

13 Gardner NM. In-house quality assurance program in a state cytology laboratory. *Acta Cytol* 1989; **33**: 487–8.

14 Federal Register Vol 57, No 40, 2-28-92. Washington, DC: US Government Printing Office, Superintendant of Documents.

15 Layfield LJ, Zaleski S, Bottles K, Cohen MB. Laboratory compliance with federal government and professional society recommendations. *Diagn Cytopathol* 1994; **11**: 85–92.

16 The Bethesda System for reporting cervical/vaginal cytologic diagnoses: revised after the second National Cancer Institute Workshop, April 29–30, 1991. *Acta Cytol* 1993; **37**: 115–24.

17 Anderson GH, Flynn KJ, Hickey LA, Le Riche JC, Matisic JP, Suen KC. A comprehensive internal quality control system for a large cytology laboratory. *Acta Cytol* 1987; **31**: 895–9.

18 Bonfiglio TA. Quality assurance in cytopathology. Recommendations and ongoing quality assurance activities of the American Society of Clinical Pathologists. *Acta Cytol* 1989; **33**: 431–3.

19 Nielsen ML. Cytopathology laboratory improvement programs of the College of American Pathologists: Laboratory Accreditation Program (CAP LAP) and Performance Improvement Program in Cervicovaginal Cytology (CAP PAP). *Arch Pathol Laboratory Med* 1997; **121**: 256–9.

20 Anthony R, Young D. *Management control in nonprofit organizations*, 5th edn. Boston, MA: Irwin, Inc., 1994: 329.

21 Mody DR, Davey DD, Kline TS. 'Workload limits' and CLIA 88 in the 1990's: how much is too much? Or too little? [editorial] [see comments]. *Diagn Cytopathol* 1997; **16**: svii–sviii.

22 Krieger PA. Strategies for reducing Papanicolaou smear screening errors: principles derived from data and experience with quality control. *Arch Pathol Laboratory Med* 1997; **121**: 277–81.

23 National Cancer Institute Workshop. The 1988 Bethesda System for reporting cervical/vaginal cytological diagnoses. *JAMA* 1989; **262**: 931–4.

24 Nielsen ML, Davey DD, Kline TS. Specimen adequacy evaluation in gynecologic cytopathology: current laboratory practice in the College of American Pathologists Interlaboratory Comparison Program and tentative guidelines for future practice. *Diagn Cytopathol* 1993; **9**: 394–403.

25 Spires SE, Banks ER, Weeks JA, Banks HW, Davey DD. Assessment of cervicovaginal smear adequacy. The Bethesda System guidelines and reproducibility. *Am J Clin Pathol* 1994; **102**: 354–9.

26 Yobs AR, Plott AE, Hicklin MD, et al. Retrospective evaluation of gynecologic cytodiagnosis. II. Interlaboratory reproducibility as shown in rescreening large consecutive samples of reported cases. *Acta Cytol* 1987; **31**: 900–10.

27 Cocchi V, Carretti D, Fanti S, et al. Intralaboratory quality assurance in cervical/vaginal cytology: evaluation of intercytologist diagnostic reproducibility. *Diagn Cytopathol* 1997; **16**: 87–92.

28 Renshaw AA, Friedman MM, Rahemtulla A, et al. Accuracy and reproducibility of estimating the adequacy of the squamous component of cervicovaginal smears. *Am J Clin Pathol* 1999; **111**: 38–42.

29 Kristensen GB, Skyggebjerg KD, Holund B, Holm K, Hansen MK. Analysis of cervical smears obtained within three years of the diagnosis of invasive cervical cancer. *Acta Cytol* 1991; **35**: 47–50.

30 Vooijs PG, Elias A, van der Graaf Y, Veling S. Relationship between the diagnosis of epithelial abnormalities and the composition of cervical smears. *Acta Cytol* 1985; **29**: 323–8.

31 Kurman RJ, Henson DE, Herbst AL, Noller KL, Schiffman MH. Interim guidelines for management of abnormal cervical cytology. The 1992 National Cancer Institute Workshop. *JAMA* 1994; **271**: 1866–9.

32 Kivlahan C, Ingram E. Papanicolaou smears without endocervical cells. Are they inadequate? *Acta Cytol* 1986; **30**: 258–60.

33 Mitchell H, Medley G. Longitudinal study of women with negative cervical smears according to endocervical status [see comments]. *Lancet* 1991; **337**: 265–7.

34 Koss LG. *Diagnostic cytology and its histopathologic bases*, 4th edn. Philadelphia: JB Lippincott Company, 1992.

35 Allen KA, Zaleski MS, Cohen MB. Laboratory use of the diagnosis 'reactive/reparative' in gynecologic smears: impact of CLIA '88. *Mod Pathol* 1995; **8**: 266–9.

36 Barr Soofer S, Sidawy MK. Reactive cellular change: is there an increased risk for squamous intraepithelial lesions? [see comments]. *Cancer* 1997; **81**: 144–7.

37 Kurman RJ, Soloman D. *The Bethesda system for reporting cervical/vaginal cytologic diagnosis: Definitions, criteria and explanatory notes for terminology and specimen adequacy*. New York: Springer-Verlag, 1994.

38 Vooijs GP. Opinion poll on quality assurance and quality control. Conducted by the Committee on Continuing Education and Quality Assurance of the International Academy of Cytology. *Acta Cytol* 1996; **40**: 14–24.

39 Herbst AL. The Bethesda system for cervical/vaginal cytologic diagnoses. *Clin Obstet Gynecol* 1992; **35**: 22–7.

40 Jones BA. Rescreening in gynecologic cytology. Rescreening of 3762 previous cases for current high-grade squamous intraepithelial lesions and carcinoma – a College of American Pathologists Q-Probes study of 312 institutions. *Arch Pathol Laboratory Med* 1995; **119**: 1097–103.

41 Davey DD, Nielsen ML, Frable WJ, Rosenstock W, Lowell DM, Kraemer BB. Improving accuracy in gynecologic cytology. Results of the College of American Pathologists Interlaboratory Comparison Program in Cervicovaginal Cytology [see comments]. *Arch Pathol Laboratory Med* 1993; **117**: 1193–8.

42 Jones BA, Novis DA. Cervical biopsy-cytology correlation. A College of American Pathologists Q-Probes study of 22 439 correlations in 348 laboratories. *Arch Pathol Laboratory Med* 1996; **120**: 523–31.

43 Ibrahim SN, Krigman HR, Coogan AC, et al. Prospective correlation of cervicovaginal cytologic and histologic specimens. *Am J Clin Pathol* 1996; **106**: 319–24.

44 Bonfiglio TA. Cervical cytology: perspectives from both sides of the Atlantic [editorial; comment] [see comments]. *Hum Pathol* 1997; **28**: 117–19.

45 Herbert A. Is cervical screening working? A cytopathologist's view from the United Kingdom [see comments]. *Hum Pathol* 1997; **28**: 120–6.

46 van der Graaf Y, Vooijs GP, Zielhuis GA. Cervical screening revisited. *Acta Cytol* 1990; **34**: 366–72.

47 Bachner P, Howanitz PJ, Lent RW. Quality improvement practices in clinical and anatomic pathology services. A College of American Pathologists Q-probes study of the program characteristics and performance in 580 institutions. *Am J Clin Pathol* 1994; **102**: 567–71.

48 Rohr LR. Quality assurance in gynecologic cytology. What is practical? *Am J Clin Pathol* 1990; **94**: 754–8.

49 Tabbara SO, Sidawy MK. Evaluation of the 10 per cent rescreen of negative gynecologic smears as a quality assurance measure [see comments]. *Diagn Cytopathol* 1996; **14**: 84–6.

50 Helfand M, O'Connor GT, Zimmer-Gembeck M, Beck JR. Effect of the Clinical Laboratory Improvement Amendments of 1988 (CLIA '88) on the incidence of invasive cervical cancer. *Med Care* 1992; **30**: 1067–82.

51 Inhorn SL, Clarke E. A state-wide proficiency testing program in cytology. *Acta Cytol* 1971; **15**: 351–6.

52 Penner DW. Quality control and quality evaluation in histopathology and cytology. *Pathol Annu* 1973; **8**: 1–19.

53 Collins DN, Kaufmann W, Albrecht R. New York State computerized proficiency testing program in exfoliative cytology: evaluation. *Acta Cytol* 1971; **15**: 468–72.

54 Yobs AR, Swanson RA, Lamotte Jr LC. Laboratory reliability of the Papanicolaou smear. *Obstet Gynecol* 1985; **65**: 235–44.

55 Ashton PR. Federal regulation of cytopathology laboratories. The American Society for Cytotechnology's perspective: 1977–1991. In: Schmidt WA, Miller TR, Katz RL, Silverman JF, Ashton PR, eds. *Cytopathology Annual.* Baltimore, MD: Williams & Wilkins, 1992: 217–27.

56 Gupta PK. American Society of Cytopathology (ASC) statement on technical devices for innovation in cervical cytology screening [special announcement]. *Diagn Cytopathol* 1996; **14**: 286.

57 Bogdanich W. Physicians carelessness with Pap tests is cited in procedure's high failure rate. *Wall Street J* 1987; Dec 29: 17.

58 Buckner S-B. Legislation and regulations governing the field of cytology: review and update. In: Schmidt WA, ed. *Cytopathology Annual.* Baltimore: Williams & Wilkins, 1992: 199–215.

59 Belk W, Sunderman FW. A survey of the accuracy of chemical analyses in clinical laboratories. By William P. Belk and F. William Sunderman, 1947 [classical article]. *Arch Pathol Laboratory Med* 1988; **112**: 320–6.

60 Henry MR. Cytology legislation and regulation: What's new? *American Society of Cytology Cytoteleconference*, Oct 26, 1993.

61 Naryshkin S. The rise and fall of HCFA PT in Wisconsin. *Focus* 1995; **2**(2): 11–13.

62 *PAP Program Newsletter.* April, 1994; 1.

63 Time extended for some CLIA elements. *Statline*. December 4, 1994; **10**(25): 3.

64 Keenlyside RA, Collins CL, Hancock JS, et al. Do proficiency test results correlate with the work performance of screeners who screen Papanicolaou smears? *Am J Clin Pathol* 1999; **112**: 769–76.

65 Vooijs GP, Davey DD, Somrak TM, et al. Computerized training and proficiency testing. International Academy of Cytology Task Force summary. Diagnostic Cytology Towards the 21st Century: An International Expert Conference and Tutorial. *Acta Cytol* 1998; **42**: 141–7.

66 Appeals court says HCFA must explain cytology PT rate or publish new rule. *Focus* 1996; **3**(2): 1–4.

67 Bosch MM, Rietveld-Scheffers PE, Boon ME. Characteristics of false-negative smears tested in the normal screening situation. *Acta Cytol* 1992; **36**: 711–16.

68 Melamed MR. Presidential address. Twentieth annual scientific meeting, American Society of Cytology. *Acta Cytol* 1973; **17**: 285–8.

69 Woodhouse SL, Stastny JF, Styer PE, Kennedy M, Praestgaard AH, Davey DD. Interobserver variability in subclassification of squamous intraepithelial lesions: results of the College of American Pathologists interlaboratory comparison program in cervicovaginal cytology [see comments]. *Arch Pathol Laboratory Med* 1999; **123**: 1079–84.

70 Young NA, Naryshkin S, Atkinson BF, et al. Interobserver variability of cervical smears with squamous-cell abnormalities: a Philadelphia study. *Diagn Cytopathol* 1994; **11**: 352–7.

71 Klinkhamer PJ, Vooijs GP, de Haan AF. Intraobserver and interobserver variability in the diagnosis of epithelial abnormalities in cervical smears. *Acta Cytol* 1988; **32**: 794–800.

72 Shahangian S. Proficiency testing in laboratory medicine: uses and limitations [see comments]. *Arch Pathol Laboratory Med* 1998; **122**: 15–30.

73 Federal and state news: United States. *Focus*, March, 1996; **3**(1): 9.

74 Naryshkin S, Davey DD. Terminology of false negative and false positive Pap smears: 'They're just worms' [editorial]. *Diagn Cytopathol* 1996; **14**: 1–3.

75 Soost HJ, Lange HJ, Lehmacher W, Ruffing-Kullmann B. The validation of cervical cytology. Sensitivity, specificity and predictive values. *Acta Cytol* 1991; **35**: 8–14.

76 Mitchell H, Medley G, Drake M. Quality control measures for cervical cytology laboratories. *Acta Cytol* 1988; **32**: 288–92.

77 Woodhouse SL, Wagner E. Managed discontinuity of care: the value and fate of cytohistologic correlation [editorial]. *Diagn Cytopathol* 1997; **16**: 105–6.

78 Raab SS. Diagnostic accuracy in cytopathology. *Diagn Cytopathol* 1994; **10**: 68–75.

79 Allen KA, Zaleski S, Cohen MB. Review of negative Papanicolaou tests. Is the retrospective 5-year review necessary? [see comments]. *Am J Clin Pathol* 1994; **101**: 19–21.

80 Gay JD, Donaldson LD, Goellner JR. False-negative results in cervical cytologic studies. *Acta Cytol* 1985; **29**: 1043–6.

81 Hatem F, Wilbur DC. High grade squamous cervical lesions following negative Papanicolaou smears: false-negative cervical cytology or rapid progression. *Diagn Cytopathol* 1995; **12**: 135–41.

82 Husain OA, Butler EB, Evans DM, Macgregor JE, Yule R. Quality control in cervical cytology. *J Clin Pathol* 1974; **27**: 935–44.

83 Janerich DT, Hadjimichael O, Schwartz PE, et al. The screening histories of women with invasive cervical cancer, Connecticut. *Am J Public Health* 1995; **85**: 791–4.

84 Koss LG. Cervical (Pap) smear. New directions. *Cancer* 1993; **71**: 1406–12.

85 Sherman ME, Kelly D. High-grade squamous intraepithelial lesions and invasive carcinoma following the report of three negative Papanicolaou smears: screening failures or rapid progression? *Mod Pathol* 1992; **5**: 337–42.

86 Slater DN, Milner PC, Radley H. Audit of deaths from cervical cancer: proposal for an essential component of the National Screening Programme [see comments]. *J Clin Pathol* 1994; **47**: 27–8.

87 Tritz DM, Weeks JA, Spires SE, et al. Etiologies for non-correlating cervical cytologies and biopsies. *Am J Clin Pathol* 1995; **103**: 594–7.

88 van der Graaf Y, Vooijs GP, Gaillard HL, Go DM. Screening errors in cervical cytologic screening. *Acta Cytol* 1987; **31**: 434–8.

89 Krieger P, Naryshkin S. Random rescreening of cytologic smears: a practical and effective component of quality assurance programs in both large and small cytology laboratories [editorial] [see comments]. *Acta Cytol* 1994; **38**: 291–8.

90 Nagy GK. False negative rate. A misnomer, misunderstood and misused [see comments]. *Acta Cytol* 1997; **41**: 778–80.

91 Renshaw AA. A practical problem with calculating the false-negative rate of Papanicolaou smear interpretation by rescreening negative cases alone [see comments]. *Cancer* 1999; **87**: 351–3.

92 Renshaw AA, DiNisco SA, Minter LJ, Cibas ES. A more accurate measure of the false-negative rate of Papanicolaou smear screening is obtained by determining the false-negative rate of the rescreening process. *Cancer* 1997; **81**: 272–6.

93 Krieger PA, Cohen T, Naryshkin S. A practical guide to Papanicolaou smear rescreens: how many slides must be reevaluated to make a statistically valid assessment of screening performance? [see comments]. *Cancer* 1998; **84**: 130–7.

94 Faraker CA. Partial rescreening as a quality assurance method [letter; comment] [see comments]. *Acta Cytol* 1996; **40**: 1323–4.

95 Faraker CA. Partial rescreening for quality assurance in gynecological cytology [letter; comment]. *Diagn Cytopathol* 1997; **16**: 191–2.

96 Renshaw AA, Bellerose B, DiNisco SA, Minter LJ, Lee KR. False negative rate of cervical cytologic smear screening as determined by rapid rescreening. *Acta Cytol* 1999; **43**: 344–50.

97 Renshaw AA, Cronin JA, Minter LJ, et al. Performance characteristics of rapid (30-second) prescreening. Implications for calculating the false-negative rate and comparison with other quality assurance techniques. *Am J Clin Pathol* 1999; **111**: 517–22.

98 Mango LJ. Neuromedical Systems, Inc. *Acta Cytol* 1996; **40**: 53–9.

99 Patten SF, Lee JS, Nelson AC. NeoPath, Inc. NeoPath AutoPap 300 Automatic Pap Screener System. *Acta Cytol* 1996; **40**: 45–52.

100 Tabbara SO, Sidawy MK. Evaluation of the 5-year review of negative cervical smears in patients with high grade squamous intraepithelial lesions. *Diagn Cytopathol* 1996; **15**: 7–10; discussion 10–11.

101 Grenko RT, Abendroth CS, Frauenhoffer EE, Ruggiero FM, Zaino RJ. Variance in the interpretation of cervical biopsy specimens obtained for atypical squamous cells of undetermined significance. *Am J Clin Pathol* 2000; **114**: 735–40.

102 Ismail SM, Colclough AB, Dinnen JS, et al. Reporting cervical intra-epithelial neoplasia (CIN): intra- and interpathologist variation and factors associated with disagreement. *Histopathology* 1990; **16**: 371–6.

103 Jones S, Thomas GD, Williamson P. Observer variation in the assessment of adequacy and neoplasia in cervical cytology. *Acta Cytol* 1996; **40**: 226–34.

104 Mobius G. Cytological early detection of cervical carcinoma: possibilities and limitations. Analysis of failures [editorial]. *J Cancer Res Clin Oncol* 1993; **119**: 513–21.

105 Robertson AJ, Anderson JM, Beck JS, et al. Observer variability in histopathological reporting of cervical biopsy specimens. *J Clin Pathol* 1989; **42**: 231–8.

106 DeMay RM. To err is human – to sue, American [editorial] [see comments]. *Diagn Cytopathol* 1996; **15**: iii–vi.

107 Robertson JH, Woodend B. Negative cytology preceding cervical cancer: causes and prevention [see comments]. *J Clin Pathol* 1993; **46**: 700–2.

108 Mitchell H, Medley G. Differences between Papanicolaou smears with correct and incorrect diagnoses [see comments]. *Cytopathology* 1995; **6**: 368–75.

109 Koss LG. The Papanicolaou test for cervical cancer detection. A triumph and a tragedy [see comments]. *JAMA* 1989; **261**: 737–43.

110 Herrero R, Brinton LA, Reeves WC, et al. Screening for cervical cancer in Latin America: a case-control study. *Int J Epidemiol* 1992; **21**: 1050–6.

111 Hayward RA, Shapiro MF, Freeman HE, Corey CR. Who gets screened for cervical and breast cancer? Results from a new national survey. *Arch Intern Med* 1988; **148**: 1177–81.

112 Nasca PC, Ellish N, Caputo TA, Saboda K, Metzger B. An epidemiologic study of Pap screening histories in women with invasive carcinomas of the uterine cervix. *NY State J Med* 1991; **91**: 152–6.

113 Kyo S, Takakura M, Ishikawa H, et al. Application of telomerase assay for the screening of cervical lesions. *Cancer Res* 1997; **57**: 1863–7.

114 Williams GH, Romanowski P, Morris L, et al. Improved cervical smear assessment using antibodies against proteins that regulate DNA replication. *Proc Natl Acad Sci USA* 1998; **95**: 14932–7.

5

Medicolegal issues

SHIRLEY E GREENING

HISTORICAL ASPECTS

The evolution of medical liability

'To err is human – to sue, American'[1] is the title of an editorial by DeMay and a succinct description of the current medical-legal climate in the USA, which has been variably attributed to greedy lawyers, self-interested expert witnesses, avaricious patients, poor doctor–patient communication or, at least from the perspective of plaintiff attorneys, negligence of health practitioners.[2] Less frequently considered but arguably more fundamental reasons for this situation may be found in the evolving philosophy and culture in the USA. Shifts in the number, role and status of medical and legal practitioners, as well as shifts in cultural and community expectations for the success of medical treatments have historically converged to fuel medical malpractice litigation.[2] The advance of science has also contributed to sometimes unrealistic expectations of medical treatment. Technological advancement carries with it a greater opportunity for errors or accidents and lawsuits occur when those new expectations are not fulfilled.[2]

The evolution of medical liability in the USA emerged in the mid-nineteenth century. Innovations in orthopedic techniques at that time greatly reduced the need for limb amputations. Reconstruction of limbs replaced limb amputation as the standard of care. As mounting expectations for perfect results were not realized, the USA entered into its first medical malpractice crisis. In the first half of the twentieth century, secularization, urbanization and the belief in 'perpetual progress' became societal norms, as did the propensity of the public to sue to redress injuries as a result of perceived negligence.[2] With societal factors entrenched and medical education and technology progressing, cyclic malpractice crises continued, although their subject matter kept changing as medical knowledge and technology advanced. With improved surgical techniques, the public (and the medical profession) grew used to surgical successes. By the mid-twentieth century, unmet expectations for surgical cures had replaced orthopedic injuries as the most common types of claims. By the 1980s, obstetrics took on this dubious distinction.[2]

The emergence of diagnostic laboratory medicine as a recognized medical specialty only served to expand the scope of potential litigation, as individuals sought redress for errors of screening and diagnostic tests that they believed should guarantee 100 per cent accuracy.[20] Thus, from the mid-nineteenth century to the present, this pattern of litigation has repeated itself. The sequence begins with the introduction of a new technology or application, moves to professional endorsement and use, and leads to public acceptance that engenders expectations for success. When successes are not achieved, the sequence culminates in a litigation crisis.[2] Such has been the history of diagnostic cytology with cervical cytology in particular following the same path. Papanicolaou smears became popular in the 1950s when the American Cancer Society began to recommend the technique for early diagnosis and treatment of cervical cancer.[3] Over the last 50 years, advocates of Pap smears have done an exemplary job of public education concerning the benefits of the Pap smear but have been less thorough in explaining its limitations. Until quite recently, cautionary statements about the potential for, much less the reality of, false-negative test results were rarely made. Women have come to expect an unattainable level of detection proficiency and diagnostic precision from a test that was originally designed to triage for further management, rather than to specifically diagnose cervical cancer and its precursors.[4]

The evolution of liability in cervical cancer screening

The story began in the late 1960s when a woman alleged that her doctor was negligent because he took an inadequate cervical specimen and did not call her back for another Pap smear. She also alleged that the cytology laboratory was negligent because it did not tell her doctor that the Pap smear was unsatisfactory and instead reported it as negative. This woman was awarded $160 000, which when adjusted for inflation was comparable to the million-dollar awards we see today.[5] In a malpractice case from the early 1970s, a physician was alleged to have been negligent for failing to oversee the work of a cytotechnologist who read the plaintiff's Pap smear at home without medical supervision. Although a jury did not find the physician negligent, the jury's decision was reversed on a technicality when the case was appealed.[6]

Cytology malpractice lawsuits were rare through the 1970s, but questions regarding substandard cytology practice were not confined to civil actions between private parties. An anonymous complaint about a cytology laboratory under contract to the United States Air Force prompted the Air Force to conduct reexamination of almost 750 000 Pap smears that the laboratory had read. By the end of the investigation eight deaths had been linked to false-negative Pap smears and at least one lawsuit had been filed. The laboratory had employed poorly trained or untrained cytologists and failed to conduct even rudimentary quality assurance procedures.[7]

Between 1985 and 1990, nine claims involving failure to act on positive Pap smears were found among 338 jury verdicts on delayed cancer diagnosis. Another eight claims in that study were based on inaction because of false-negative Pap smears.[8] Pap smears with false-negative diagnoses comprised about 25 per cent of the total claims filed with one medical malpractice insurance company between 1989 and 1992.[9] A review of 335 claims between 1993 and 1995 from the same insurance company found 56 (16.7 per cent) claims involving Pap smears.[10] Malpractice claims involving Pap smears continue to be one of the fastest growing and financially draining areas in medical liability.

CURRENT STATUS

The legal concept of negligence

Alleged negligence is the basis of all medical malpractice claims. Negligence (malpractice) does not exist until it is proved, and negligence can only be determined in the context of the litigation process. It is the plaintiff's responsibility to prove the four essential elements of a negligence claim. These elements are: (1) the cytologist and/or laboratory owed a duty to the plaintiff; (2) the cytologist and/or laboratory was not practicing within an acceptable standard of care; (3) the plaintiff has been injured because of the substandard practice; and (4) the false-negative Pap smear was the cause of the patient's injury.

As worthy of sympathy as cervical cancer patients are, it is difficult for plaintiffs and their attorneys to convince a jury that all four of these elements are present. This is the reason why so few patient complaints actually result in lawsuits and why the majority of malpractice claims are won by medical defendants.[11,12]

Negligence as a legal determination and false-negative Pap smears as an unavoidable reality of cytology practice are not two sides of the same coin. Cytologists may indeed make a number of detection or diagnostic errors, but the vast majority of these errors do not harm patients. Even if a cytologist is disciplined in their employment setting because too many abnormal cases have been misread, this still is not negligence in the legal sense. It may be poor practice, but it is not legally sufficient negligence. A detailed discussion of the legal concepts and litigation process concerning Pap smears can be found in the International Academy of Cytology Task Force summary on medicolegal affairs.[13]

Standard of care

STANDARDS FOR INDIVIDUAL PRACTITIONERS

The legal standard for a cytologist's conduct is based on the concept of reasonableness. Conduct is deemed reasonable when it conforms to the degree of skill, proficiency, knowledge and care ordinarily possessed and employed by members in good standing in the profession. This legal definition of the 'reasonable, prudent practitioner' does not mean that a cytologist must exceed commonly accepted standards or be the best practitioner, but neither does it permit substandard conduct without liability.

From a legal standpoint, a cytotechnologist's role is to detect and mark non-negative cells for further review. To do this with ordinary knowledge and skill, the cytotechnologist is expected to be aware of commonly recognized laboratory procedures and practices and to comply with regulatory requirements such as workload limits. The reasonable cytotechnologist standard does not include the ability to diagnose accurately an abnormality because practice acts generally do not permit individuals other than physicians to make medical diagnoses.

A pathologist or cytopathologist is judged by standards applicable to their medical specialty. The standard for reasonable conduct for a pathologist encompasses both diagnostic accuracy and responsibility for the direction/supervision of laboratory personnel and protocols. The latter is usually the standard that applies to the pathologist in malpractice claims on false-negative Pap smears, since slides reported as negative are rarely seen by pathologists.

As a defense, cytologists often make the point that all cytologists make detection or diagnostic errors and that an honest mistake is within accepted standards.[14] The law's 'reasonable practitioner' standard also assumes that misjudgments occur. Reasonable errors of judgment are recognized under the umbrella of standard practice, and are not negligent. However, the burden is on the cytology defendants to convince a jury that their misjudgments are in fact reasonable.

Attorneys who litigate cytology malpractice cases are aware that variation of practice exists in cytology. In legal terms, these are called community standards or 'respectable minority' standards. However, in their roles as client advocates, it is the plaintiff attorneys' job to prove to a judge or jury that the way a defendant cytologist practiced did not meet accepted cytology practice standards.

PROFESSIONAL STANDARDS AS THE BASIS FOR THE LEGAL STANDARD OF CARE

Judges and juries involved in the litigation of cytology malpractice claims rely on the profession to promulgate standards that are scientifically defensible and appropriate for the discipline. In other words, this standard-setting role in the legal context is deferred to members of the cytology profession.[15] Legal proof of a cytology practice standard must relate to and be established by professional standards and scientific sources that are contemporaneous with the alleged negligence. Standards promulgated today will apply prospectively but may not be applicable to past events.

Virtually every cytology malpractice lawsuit is framed as an unreasonable mistake that injured a woman. Characteristically, this includes an assertion that a false-negative diagnosis delayed treatment of a patient's cervical cancer leading to a shortened or lost chance of survival or a diminished quality of life. However, while cytology malpractice cases may seem generally similar, the legal system treats each case as a unique set of circumstances particular to each patient/plaintiff. Each malpractice claim requires an independent fact-finding process in which evidence concerning cytology standards of practice is presented in the form of exhibits, opinion letters, affidavits, depositions and live testimony at trial.

Materials most commonly used to establish cytology practice standards are the regulations of the Clinical Laboratory Improvement Amendments (either CLIA'88 or its predecessor CLIA'67), laboratory accreditation guidelines, and cytology books and journals. Certification eligibility guidelines, professional competency statements, codes of ethics, laboratory protocols and personnel policies are also potential sources from which to establish applicable standards of practice for individual cytologists. They provide the basis for determining what a cytologist in a specific legal case should have done or known.[16]

The cytology quality control provisions in CLIA'88 are not practice standards *per se*, and regulatory compliance does not in itself prove that the actions of a laboratory were reasonable.[17] Minimum regulatory compliance may not be a sufficient defense when laboratory personnel should have taken more comprehensive actions for a specific type of slide, diagnosis or patient/plaintiff. Conversely, non-compliance with a regulatory provision does not necessarily prove that a laboratory procedure or protocol was substandard.

Laboratory accreditation programs are designed to help laboratories improve their practices by showing that they adhere to acceptable laboratory quality control and quality assurance indicators. Voluntary enrollment in such programs can create a presumption that a laboratory is operating according to the profession's standards. However, there are no current accreditation programs that also monitor the competence of individual practitioners. In a legal inquiry, if a laboratory passes an accreditation survey or inspection, this fact will not guarantee immunity from legal action for an individual cytologist.

Journals and textbooks, often referred to as learned treatises, can be used to show the body of knowledge that was available at the time a slide was misread. Commonly used texts can provide evidence of what a cytologist should have known or done as they read a slide. Published practice guidelines can also be admitted into evidence as learned treatises.[17]

LABORATORY PROCEDURES AND RECORDS AS EVIDENCE OF PRACTICE

Cytologists may be asked to produce their laboratory procedure manuals, quality control (QC) and quality assurance (QA) records, workload records and employee time records. The laboratory must be able to demonstrate that cytotechnologists and other staff members have complied with the laboratory's protocols. Those protocols will also be measured against existing professional and regulatory standards. A number of cytology malpractice claims have involved cytotechnologists that exceeded workload limits or were not familiar with, or even aware that the laboratory had, a procedure manual. These situations should serve as reminders that the laboratory must attend to and document all pre-analytical, analytical and post-analytical QC/QA procedures.

When patient slides and records are appropriately discarded after federal, State or professional retention guidelines have been met, laboratories are not liable for these materials. However, if slides and records are retained for longer periods than federal, State or professional guidelines require, the laboratory can be compelled to produce them for review during the discovery phase of litigation.

THE ROLE OF CONSULTANTS AND EXPERT WITNESSES IN CYTOLOGY MALPRACTICE LITIGATION

Both plaintiff and defense attorneys obviously need the consultation of cytologists to understand cytological terms and to interpret clinical information as they prepare their cases. In addition to reviewing slides and rendering non-binding opinions, consultants advise attorneys on questions to ask during depositions, relevant literature to read, and whom to invite as expert witnesses. A consultant may also serve as an expert witness, in which case their opinions will appear on the record in the form of testimony.

State and federal rules of evidence prescribe the qualifications that experts must possess in order to testify, how expert testimony is presented, and how expert testimony may be impeached.[18] Expert witness rules require that expert witnesses meet the legal test for substantially similar practice. Therefore, in Pap smear litigation, cytopathologists should provide expert testimony on standards for cytopathologists and cytotechnologists should provide expert testimony on the standard of practice for cytotechnologists, especially screening and detection functions. Experts can explain the facts and state their opinions regarding whether a practitioner's conduct is standard or substandard. Unless a jurisdiction has a law to the contrary, expert witnesses are not required to explain what facts or data they use to formulate their opinions. To balance this inconsistency, an expert's credentials and the credibility are subject to cross-examination by the opposing attorney and their opinions are often challenged by the testimony of experts from the opposing party.

The current legal system in the USA is based on advocacy, which is designed to allow opposing sides to present their best case and ultimately to achieve justice. Attorneys customarily introduce their expert witness testimony in a manner constructed to reflect the perspective of plaintiff or defense. What may be viewed as biased expert opinion by cytologists is viewed by the legal system as advocacy. Expert testimony, however, is not law. It can only help to persuade a jury that substandard practice probably did or did not occur as relates to a particular plaintiff's circumstances. The opinions of expert witnesses can be most slanted when a profession's standards are inadequately defined or completely absent. However, even if practice standards exist, they are not conclusive in and of themselves, neither do they take the place of the facts particular to any one legal dispute. Each lawsuit is litigated individually on a case-by-case basis. Judges or juries weigh all information before them in order to determine whether a negligent act has occurred.

The role of expert witnesses is as controversial as the cytology slides in question. The plaintiff-only expert is routinely vilified as mercenary – the 'professional hired gun'. Plaintiff expert opinions are often characterized as biased because they have the benefit of the patient's clinical outcome. However, this information is also available to defense experts. Defense-only experts have their own biases to introduce that may also unduly influence the fair resolution of legal actions.[19,20] This controversy is highlighted in the disparate settings of prospective initial screening and diagnosis by laboratory personnel (potential defendants) versus retrospective review by the consultant or expert witness. Maintaining objectivity in litigation slide review is of paramount importance.[21] Whenever possible, blinded review without knowledge of ultimate clinical outcome is a preferred method of simulating conditions present during the initial slide evaluation. However, this kind of simulation may not always be feasible. Indeed, when an attorney asks a cytologist to review slides, it is usually obvious that they are a lawyer and that the slide is potentially involved in a lawsuit. A conscionable cytologist should directly state that further information, including whether the lawyer is for the plaintiff or defense, is inappropriate. Reviewers, consultants or experts should review slides with only the patient information available to the original screener and should never agree to review slides if a lawyer attempts to force the reviewer into a diagnostic corner or into an opinion that cannot be supported by morphological evidence on the slide. The majority of lawyers respect and abide by these simple guidelines.

Guidelines for Pap smear slide review in the context of litigation as well as proposals to replace individual experts with peer panels, committees, arbitration boards, blinded evidence review or other mechanisms have been supported by cytology professionals.[22] However, it is unlikely that the legal system will opt for wholesale substitution of individual expert testimony in favor of empanelled reviewers,[23] even though such proposals are designed to reduce the negative effects of unqualified or irresponsible expert witnesses.[24] To counteract perceptions of bias, it is in the profession's best interests to establish objective guidelines for experts' conduct in the context of litigation that apply non-prejudicially to both plaintiff and defense experts,[25] and to establish mechanisms that subject the testimony and opinions of expert or consultant reviewers to professional scrutiny.

Defensive cytology: minimizing the risk of malpractice liability

Cytology litigation will continue to focus on false-negative smears on a case-by-case basis for the foreseeable future, but laboratories can minimize their risk of malpractice liability by implementing the following measures.

GENERAL CYTOLOGY LABORATORY PRACTICES

Cytology malpractice litigation tends to ferret out inadequate laboratory practices as much as the misread slides.[26] Cytotechnologists that never see the cytopathologist or that are not familiar with the contents of the laboratory's procedure manual are examples of lapses in defendant laboratories' quality assurance programs. The lack of collaborative microscopic or clinical review of cases, of in-house or outside continuing education participation and of documented slide review are also considered suspect laboratory practices. Speed-screening, unsustained attention, environmental distracters and the repetitive nature of the screening process represent usual but, nonetheless, problematic areas contributing to poor laboratory performance.[27] Many prior lawsuits present striking examples of the unfortunate correlation of misdiagnosis with less than optimal environments and practices as well as with substandard quality control and assurance programs. When producing evidence of what a laboratory does or does not do to ensure screening accuracy, laboratories must provide hard data to document ongoing monitoring of performance and corrective actions when a deficiency is found. There is a strong link between sound quality assurance procedures and legal risk minimization.

LEGAL RISK MANAGEMENT STRATEGIES

Legal risk management strategies are as important as laboratory procedures and practices to prevent malpractice claims and undesirable outcomes of litigation, and should be in place before laboratories become involved in a lawsuit.[28]

1 Immediate notification to the laboratory's risk management office, insurance carrier and attorney of a potential lawsuit – laboratory staff should never attempt to resolve a legal query or dispute on their own.
2 Release slides and/or records only to the laboratory's attorney, risk management office or insurance carrier, even under court-ordered subpoena – the laboratory's attorney can always negotiate with the plaintiff's attorney for opportunities to review these materials. Since any and all slide(s) will likely be reviewed externally, it is essential to photocopy reports, requisitions and slides in their original condition. Do not remove any dots/marks that are on the slides. It is imperative to release only materials that specifically pertain to the patient in question. Laboratories that volunteer any and all materials requested run the risk of opening the door to additional allegations not even connected with a particular case, and of providing fodder for future claims. Laboratories should not surrender materials just because an attorney is asking for them.
3 If at all possible, do not review the slides in question until instructed to do so by the laboratory's attorney. The temptation to review these slides immediately is naturally great, but such retrospective reviews, conducted in an agitated state of heightened alertness, can lead to over-diagnosis and an inappropriate response.
4 If the laboratory determines that a slide was diagnosed erroneously, await instructions from the laboratory's risk manager, insurance carrier or attorney before sending out an amended report, which may help to settle a dispute quickly and out of the public eye if the detector/diagnostic error was actually below the standard of care. However, to issue an amended report as a knee-jerk reaction to potential litigation may cause the laboratory to appear negligent, even if subsequent external reviewers consider the misdiagnosis reasonable.
5 The laboratory's risk manager or corporate counsel should have a protocol in place for preparing and responding to formal legal proceedings. Never agree to undergo a deposition without adequate preparation and legal representation. Laboratory personnel may also be asked or ordered to provide written answers to questions (interrogatories, requests for admissions) from the plaintiff attorney. The attorney(s) representing the laboratory or the cytologist should review and respond to these questions.[29]
6 If a laboratory or its staff are named defendants, they are entitled to attend any depositions of other witnesses, including the patient/plaintiff.

CYTOLOGY LABORATORY PRACTICES SPECIFIC FOR LAWSUIT PREVENTION

Laboratories can also institute certain basic operational protocols to reduce the risk of malpractice claims and lawsuits.

1 Consistently reporting limited and unsatisfactory specimens. It is with trepidation in this age of curtailed reimbursement and fierce market competition to alienate clinicians/clients

by suggesting to them that their sampling and smearing techniques are less than satisfactory. However, not reporting an inadequate specimen is legally risky. The Specimen Adequacy Statement can serve as a disclaimer, alerting the clinician to a potentially compromised specimen. Laboratories have successfully defended false-negative smears in which specimen limitations were reported.

2 Discard gynecological slides over 5 years old and most QC/QA records and requisitions after 2 years (reports after 10 years). If slides with clinical histories that are more than 5 years old are used for educational purposes, these materials should be segregated from the clinical service records of the laboratory and patient identifiers removed.

3 The current CLIA '88 regulations require a 5-year retrospective review of negative slides when a current high-grade or more serious lesion is detected. An amended report is required if the revised diagnosis would affect current patient management. However, only in rare circumstances will a prior false-negative diagnosis, even if significant, affect current patient care. Laboratories are required to maintain documentation of the review, whether or not an amended report is issued. Therefore, the retrospective review process should be used primarily for education and quality assurance, and the laboratory should include a reasonable and defensible protocol for this process in its operation manual.

4 CLIA regulations currently require a pathologist to sign out all reactive-reparative cases. Some laboratories assign these cases to the 'Within Normal Limits' reporting category to minimize the number of cases a pathologist needs to review. This practice may subject laboratories to increased liability risk and a finding of regulatory non-compliance. Therefore, laboratories should include a justification for such categorization in their operation manual so that their practice is legally defensible.

INFORMED CONSENT AND CYTOLOGY REPORT DISCLAIMERS

Informed consent requires the disclosure of any risks, alternatives and benefits of a test so that a patient can make an informed decision whether they want to have or to refuse a laboratory test. While information about conventional Pap smear performance is useful, potential liability for non-disclosure of the availability of automated screening methods and liquid-based preparations was once a 'hot button' issue for cytology laboratories.[30,31] However, with increasing use of liquid-based preparations in cytology practice, the need to provide information about this screening alternative has become a less significant issue. It would appear that it might help, and certainly would not hurt, to provide information to patients about choices for cervical cancer screening tests. However, it is the clinician's duty to inform the patient about risks, benefits and alternatives. The clinician is in the best position, physically and professionally, to inform the patient and to document their consent, refusal or choice concerning which test to use. However, it is the responsibility of the laboratory to provide information to the clinician concerning alternatives, automated or otherwise, that the laboratory can reasonably provide.[32] With the appropriate information, the clinician, not the laboratory, carries the responsibility and the liability for disclosing or not disclosing this information to the patient.

Today's marketing strategies have a greater influence than ever in creating public demand for products. It might be a helpful to remember that informed consent includes disclosure of alternatives. Although a great number of alternatives exist for cervical cancer screening, such as molecular, chemiluminescent, colpographic and other techniques, in addition to automated testing and liquid-based preparations, their efficacy has not been proven and their availability is very limited. Therefore, their inclusion in the informed consent statements is probably not required with the potential exception of human papillomavirus DNA testing in the near future.

A disclaimer statement on a Pap smear requisition and/or report is not the same as informed consent, which documents a patient's active participation in the decision to use a test after their health-care provider has disclosed the risks and benefits of the test. A disclaimer will not shield a laboratory from liability if other practices of the laboratory are substandard. Disclaimers, however, do serve the purpose of educating and reminding the clinician that Pap testing carries with it a risk of error. Communicating this uncertainty when the result of a screening Pap smear is reported is a key element in the prevention of malpractice.[33] The clinician in turn can convey this information to the patient. When using a disclaimer, laboratories do not need to list every possible condition that may affect the accuracy of Pap smear testing. In fact, overly lengthy disclaimers can undermine the clinician's confidence in the laboratory's diagnosis. A combination of informed clinician–patient discussion and a short disclaimer/information statement from the laboratory, perhaps with an offer to provide additional supporting documentation at the clinician's request, should be sufficient for educational purposes.

LITIGATION CELLS

Whether in routine laboratory reviews or in the context of litigation, finding a few small, abnormal cells in a case initially diagnosed as negative is problematic. Identified largely in the context of retrospective review and often diagnosed as atypical squamous or glandular cells of undetermined significance (ASCUS or AGUS), these cells have been coined 'litigation cells' by Frable.[34] The ASCUS reporting category casts a wide interpretive net that has created both scientific and legal confusion. At one extreme, clinicians are notified of minor alterations in an otherwise benign smear. At the opposite extreme, these cells can alert clinicians to a significant cervical squamous disease. The scientific inquiry is focused on determining which of these cases represent clinically significant misses.[35] The legal inquiry is focused on determining at what point these cases represent reasonable, acceptable errors, as opposed to practice below the standard of care for detecting abnormalities on Pap smears.

It is fair to say that at least some of these 'revised' ASCUS cases do fall within the range of reasonable error. However, an assessment of reasonableness is particularly case-dependent. Many variables, such as technical and cellular adequacy, make each slide a unique circumstance. In the current litigation climate, asserting that all such missed cases are inevitable is a weak position as a legal defense strategy. Ultimately, cytology practice standards that incorporate quantitative and qualitative cytomorphological parameters could serve to minimize these errors and strengthen the defense of such cases.

Other litigated Pap smear cases have involved clearly identifiable malignant cells but were diagnosed as negative.[36] The defensibility of such cases depends on other factors. If the cells are abundant and obscuring material or other artifacts do not compromise the visualization, it is advisable to settle the claim quickly: defending such a clearly misread specimen is not a winnable proposition. Fortunately, these obvious and true false-negative cases constitute only a small percentage of all cervical cytology malpractice cases. For cases in which low numbers of malignant cells are present and/or in a technically unsatisfactory or limited specimen, the liability may lie in the laboratory's failure to report the inadequate condition of the slide. Typically, the plaintiff or their clinician argues that failure to notify the clinician about the condition of the specimen caused a delayed diagnosis of cancer.[37] Plaintiffs use this argument even when they have stipulated that there were too few malignant cells on the slide to constitute a reasonable expectation for detection and diagnosis. Laboratories expose themselves to an increased risk of liability when technically unsatisfactory or limited cell preparations are not reported. A statement describing a specimen's inadequacy can function as a risk minimization tool even when a specimen has been misdiagnosed.

Some cytology malpractice cases have focused on whether an endocervical glandular abnormality (AGUS) should have been detected. Current knowledge about how to interpret subtle morphologic cell changes across the AGUS spectrum has not yet reached a stage where cytologists can consistently and reproducibly discriminate between benign reactive and early neoplastic endocervical glandular processes.[38] Missed or misdiagnosed cases at the two extremes of this spectrum, i.e. clearly normal and clearly abnormal ones, may warrant legal resolution. Those cases in the mid-range of the spectrum, i.e. benign reactive versus AGUS, favor reactive or favor neoplasm, should probably not constitute a basis for litigation at this time.

Finally, the cytology malpractice claims that have been litigated to date address only those cases in which abnormal cells are present on Pap smear slides. Cytologists and clinicians still have not found a fail-safe solution to eliminate inadequate clinical sampling and to guarantee total access to cervical cancer screening. This will be our greatest challenge.

FUTURE DIRECTIONS

Malpractice/tort reform

Realizing that blanket immunity for medical mistakes is unlikely, the medical community has put its support behind tort reform measures designed to change the way the legal system addresses medical injury claims. A number of state-based tort reforms are in effect. They fall generally into the categories of attorney fees, statutes of limitation, collateral source rules, joint and several liability, limits on damage awards, periodic payment of damage awards, and alternatives to litigation.[39] All states have statutes that govern medical malpractice claims. However, the extent to which the methods or costs of litigation are limited are quite variable. Malpractice litigation is usually funded through contingency fee arrangements between the plaintiff and her attorney. Most states require that attorney fees be 'reasonable'. No state forbids the use of contingency fee arrangements by plaintiff lawyers.

Statutes of limitation limit the period of time during which a plaintiff may file a lawsuit. For cancer misdiagnosis cases, most statutes begin at the time when the plaintiff learns that she has cancer and end (or toll) after 2 or 3 years.

Traditionally, a successful plaintiff could recover money from a defendant even if the plaintiff had been reimbursed by her own insurance or by government benefits (the collateral source). Most states now require that a plaintiff's damage award be offset by these reimbursements.

Joint and several liability rules allow plaintiffs to sue multiple defendants in hopes of finding the 'deepest pocket'. This is occasionally seen in cytology malpractice cases in which the cytotechnologist, the cytopathologist, the clinician, one or more laboratories, the hospital, the corporation, etc., are all sued. Most states now limit a plaintiff's ability to recover money from multiple defendants by requiring a determination of each defendant's proportional responsibility for the injury.

Many states have enacted legislation that limits the non-economic (e.g. payment for emotional distress, pain and suffering, loss of enjoyment of life or loss of consortium) and punitive damages (i.e. payments that are intended to make an example of a grossly negligent defendant in an effort to deter similar conduct by others) that juries may award to a plaintiff. For example, several states limit non-economic damage awards to $250 000. Other states limit punitive damages to a percentage of a defendant's gross income or allow punitive damages only when a defendant's conduct has been willfully negligent or reckless. No state currently limits economic damages, but some states allow for the payment of damages over a period of years rather than as a lump sum.

Finally, alternative dispute resolution methods such as arbitration and mediation have been proposed as ways to reduce or eliminate the use of Courts to resolve malpractice litigation. Arbitration is conducted in the presence of an impartial third party whose decision is usually binding. Mediation uses a third party as a facilitator rather than as a decision-maker. If the parties to the mediation cannot reach an agreement, they can go forward through the Court system.

Better defined standards: the value of consensus conferences and practice guidelines

To minimize continued legal challenges, the cytology community has focused its efforts on developing consensus statements and practice guidelines that will convey to patients, clinicians, attorneys and cytologists the current status of and reasonable expectations for Pap test performance. Such statements and guidelines must be coupled with a vigorous public and professional education effort to counteract public perceptions built on the success of 50 years of cervical cancer screening.[40]

Owing to variability of practice and philosophy within the cytology community, consensus conferences provide a valuable forum for reconciling diverse opinions and achieving uniformly acceptable standards. Guidelines for reporting terminology, laboratory quality assurance and clinical management have been developed by consensus and form the basis of cytology practice standards on which legal determinations are now based.[41,42]

A principal legal function of consensus conference recommendations is to reflect the 'standard of care' in a particular area. However, the application of codified standards to a specific set of circumstances, as in the context of malpractice litigation, may be difficult since a number of other determinants enter into the equation, not the least of which is the relative persuasiveness of opposing expert witnesses. The credibility of consensus conference results will depend on the degree to which legitimate differing views of experts are discussed openly and included in the consensus recommendations.[43]

The primary value of practice guidelines is not their use in litigation but their use in practice.[43] Cytology practice guidelines can determine the legal standard of care if the key legal players (parties, lawyers, judges and payers/insurers) perceive them to be convincing statements of proper standards that have been defined outside the context of litigation by respected and disinterested parties.[44] Jutras suggests that guidelines are unlikely to influence the legal standard of care unless they first settle debates within the cytology profession about what does and what does not constitute reasonable practice.[44] Furthermore, if practice guidelines describe only minimum acceptable practices, allow for any and all exceptions, and recognize a wide range of acceptable practices or, if they are not updated regularly, they could be viewed as not meeting the legal standard of care and would therefore not play a decisive role in litigation. Each of these situations would leave room for legal argument, because qualified scientific statements need to be transformed into unqualified legal conclusions in order to serve as standards of care in court.

As Lewis noted, clinical practice guidelines produced exclusively by a specialty society or a single profession may be acceptable legally.[45] If clinical practice guidelines extend in influence and affect resource allocation and other public policy decisions, there will be pressures to open the process of development to other stakeholders. The ultimate consumers of clinical practice guidelines are not providers but the public, which is interested in their validity and not their origin.[45]

Until indisputable cytology practice standards and performance benchmarks to which both plaintiffs and defendants can stipulate are established, courts will continue to rely on expert witnesses from both sides to sort out why variability of practice exists, what those variable practices are and how they relate to individual malpractice cases. The legal system will still provide a venue to determine the particulars of the slide, circumstance or patient that account for a missed diagnosis, and will decide whether each case represents a reasonable error that is excusable.

Automated cytology – the new 'standard of care'?

The cytology profession is currently in a period of rapid change in which old and new methods and technologies are competing not only for market share but also for the public's trust. The decision to offer automated preparation or screening of Pap smears to laboratory clients is based as much on economic choices as it is on scientific evidence.[46] If laboratories decide to offer automated tests, they will be responsible for the results of those tests. Potential liability for automated cytology may extend beyond the laboratory actually housing the systems and processing test results. It can also apply to laboratories that merely provide information about the availability of automated testing and to the manufacturer of the system (see discussion below).

The threat of liability may deter laboratories from using expert systems that can reduce false negatives and may lead to higher insurance costs and professional fees. These costs would likely be passed on to the public. If the weight of clinical studies suggests that automated cytology is useful in minimizing clinically significant screening errors, the cytology community will be obligated to reassess its position that the use of these emerging technologies does not now represent a practice standard.[47] Integration of automated preparation and screening systems into cytology practice may also create future legal obligations for laboratories. Cytology laboratories will have to consider at what point clients and patients must be notified of the availability of automated screening and at what point the scientific evidence actually requires the use of an automated system as a standard practice.[48] For cytology laboratories and cytologists, negligence and product liability risk assessments will be fundamentally similar regardless of whether an automated cytology screening system is recommended by or used in the laboratory. Miller and colleagues[49] have cautioned that automated systems should not be adopted simply because they exist. '[They] should be used only when [they] perform a given task at a higher level of reliability or quality than the current manual system and do so at an acceptable cost in time and expense. A program that merely maintains an existing standard of quality should be used only when it does so at a decreased cost in time or expense compared to the existing system'.[49] Manufacturers of automated cytology systems can also be held liable for their systems under product liability laws. These laws, in general, require the manufacturer to compensate buyers or users of their products when it is found that a defect in that product caused an injury. Manufacturers usually counter claims of alleged defects with the 'FDA defense' or the 'State-of-the-Art Defense.' The 'FDA Defense' in product liability cases is a manufacturer's assertion that compliance with existing Food and Drug Administration (FDA) regulations and standards at the time of FDA approval is a valid defense to plaintiff claims of defective devices or negligence in the design, operation or clinical use of a medical device. 'State of the Art' is the point at which scientific or technological knowledge existed with respect to a product at the time of its manufacture, design or use. Defendant manufacturers or laboratories are usually allowed to present evidence that a product's design was the safest, best, most commonly available or in use at the time of an alleged failure. However, laboratories are not required to have and use cutting-edge technology simply because it exists.[50]

If and when automated systems meet the standards suggested by Miller et al.,[49] as described above, a number of defenses are available to manufacturers and laboratories in product liability law just as they are in traditional tort law. Defenses include contributory negligence or assumption of risk by the plaintiff, comparative negligence, statutes of limitation, learned intermediary doctrines and federal preemption of state claims.

REFERENCES

1 DeMay RM. To err is human – to sue, American [editorial] [see comments]. *Diagn Cytopathol* 1996; **15**: iii–vi.

2 De Ville K. Medical malpractice in twentieth century United States. The interaction of technology, law and culture. *Int J Technol Assess Health Care* 1998; **14**: 197–211.

3 Koss LG. A quarter of a century of cytology. *Acta Cytol* 1977; **21**: 639–42.

4 Dehner LP. Cervicovaginal cytology, false-negative results, and standards of practice. *Am J Clin Pathol* 1993; **99**: 45–7.

5 Cornell V. Central Medical Clinic, et al., CA Sup. Court Case No. NC C 3 792 G. (1971).

6 Devine V. Murrietta, 49 Cal. App. 3d 855, 122 Cal. Rptr. 847 (1975).

7 New Papanicolaou tests suggested for Air Force dependants. *US Med*; Aug 1978: 1.

8 Kern KA. Medicolegal analysis of the delayed diagnosis of cancer in 338 cases in the United States. *Arch Surg* 1994; **129**: 397–403; discussion x–4.

9 Troxel DB, Sabella JD. Problem areas in pathology practice. Uncovered by a review of malpractice claims [see comments]. *Am J Surg Pathol* 1994; **18**: 821–31.

10 Scott MD. Liability issues with the Papanicolaou smear: an insurance industry perspective. *Arch Pathol Lab Med* 1997; **121**: 239–40.

11 Huycke LI, Huycke MM. Characteristics of potential plaintiffs in malpractice litigation. *Ann Intern Med* 1994; **120**: 792–8.

12 Palmmisano D. *Risk management in a capsule. The 'Big A' and the '25 C's'*. 1995; Access Year: 1999. Available at: www.intrepidresources.com/html/risk.html

13 Frable WJ, Austin RM, Greening SE, et al. Medicolegal affairs. International Academy of Cytology Task Force summary. Diagnostic Cytology Towards the 21st Century: An International Expert Conference and Tutorial [see comments]. *Acta Cytol* 1998; **42**: 76–119; discussion 20–132.

14 Austin RM. Pap smear liability [letter response]. *CAP Today* 1995; **9**: 6–10.

15 *Medical experts and establishing standards of care in malpractice cases*. Lectric Law Library, 1998; Access Year: 1999. Available at: www.lectlaw.com/files/exp23.html.

16 Department of Health and Human Services, Health Care Financing Administration, Public Health Service, 42 CFR *et seq.*, 57FR 7002–7186, February 28, 1992 [revising regulations applicable to laboratories and implementing provisions of the Clinical Laboratory Improvement Amendments of 1988, P.L. 100–578].

17 Bierig JR, Hirshfeld EB, Kelly JT, Raskin RD. Practice parameters: malpractice liability considerations for physicians. *Leg Med* **1991**: 207–25.

18 FED. R. EVID., as amended. Rules 702–705. St Paul, MN: West Publishing, 1987.

19 Fisher CW, Dombrowski MP, Jaszczak SE, Cook CD, Sokol RJ. The expert witness: real issues and suggestions [see comments]. *Am J Obstet Gynecol* 1995; **172**: 1792–7; discussion 7–1800.

20 Skoumal SM, Maygarden SJ. Malpractice in gynecologic cytology: a need for expert witness guidelines. *Mod Pathol* 1997; **10**: 267–9.

21 Austin RM. Results of blinded rescreening of Papanicolaou smears versus biased retrospective review. *Arch Pathol Lab Med* 1997; **121**: 311–14.

22 Stastny JF, Spires S, Austin RM. Pap litigation: where do we go from here? [editorial]. *Diagn Cytopathol* 1998; **19**: 235–7.

23 Hyams AL, Brandenburg JA, Lipsitz SR, Shapiro DW, Brennan TA. Practice guidelines and malpractice litigation: a two-way street [see comments]. *Ann Intern Med* 1995; **122**: 450–5.

24 Brent RL. The irresponsible expert witness: a failure of biomedical graduate education and professional accountability. *Pediatrics* 1982; **70**: 754–62.

25 Frable WJ. Guidelines for experts reviewing Papanicolaou smear litigation cases. *Arch Pathol Lab Med* 1997; **121**: 331–4.

26 Derman H. Quality and liability issues with the Papanicolaou smear: lessons from the science of error prevention [see comments]. *Arch Pathol Lab Med* 1997; **121**: 287–91.

27 Jones D, Cibas ES. Still better than a computer: Human visual perception in cytology. *ASC Bull* 1996; **33**: 51–2.

28 Pelehach L. The Pap smear on trial. *Lab Med* 1997; **28**: 509–16.

29 *Your lab in court*. American Society for Clinical Laboratory Science, Access Year: 1999. Available at: www.ascls.org.

30 Bierig JR, Weber SA. Pap smear liability: do computer-assisted rescreening devices affect the standard of care? *CAP Today* 1997; **11**: 32–4.

31 Godfrey SE. The Pap smear, automated rescreening, and negligent nondisclosure [see comments]. *Am J Clin Pathol* 1999; **111**: 14–17.

32 McCoy DR, Sidoti MS. The Pap smear liability crisis [letter; comment]. *Am J Clin Pathol* 1999; **112**: 274–80.

33 Skoumal SM, Florell SR, Bydalek MK, Hunter WJ, 3rd. Malpractice protection: communication of diagnostic uncertainty. *Diagn Cytopathol* 1996; **14**: 385–9.

34 Frable W. Litigation cells: definition and observations on a cell type in cervical vaginal smears not addressed by the Bethesda System [editorial]. *Diagn Cytopathol* 1994; **11**: 213–15.

35 Frankel K. ASCUS diagnosis [letter to the editor]. *CAP Today* 1996; **10**: 9.

36 Greening SE, Somrak T. Medicolegal issues in cytology: Legal principles and liability outlook. In: Schmidt W, ed. *Cytopathology Annual*. Chicago: ASCP Press, 1994: 65–81.

37 Berg V. Footer, LLR 1996. DC. 81.

38 Wilbur DC. An approach to the 'atypical' endocervical cell. Cytopathology Review (Syllabus) of American Society of Cytopathology. Columbus, OH, April, 1999.

39 Compendium of selected state laws governing medical injury claims: US Department of Health and Human Services, Public Health Service, Agency for Health Care Policy and Research; 1996 March. AHCPR Publ No. 96–0006.

40 Cockburn J, Redman S, Hill D, Henry E. Public understanding of medical screening. *J Med Screen* 1995; **2**: 224–7.

41 Committee on gynecologic practice: recommendations on the frequency of Pap test screening. ACOG Committee Opinion Number 152, March 1995.

42 Kurman RJ, Soloman D. *The Bethesda system for reporting cervical/vaginal cytologic diagnosis: definitions, criteria and explanatory notes for terminology and specimen adequacy*. New York: Springer-Verlag, 1994.

43 McIntyre KM. Medicolegal implications of consensus statements. *Chest* 1995; **108**: 502S–5S.

44 Jutras D. Clinical practice guidelines as legal norms. *CMAJ* 1993; **148**: 905–8.

45 Lewis S. Paradox, process and perception: the role of organizations in clinical practice guidelines development [see comments]. *CMAJ* 1995; **153**: 1073–7.

46 Kluge EH. Physicians, limited resources and liability [see comments]. *CMAJ* 1996; **155**: 778–9.

47 Statement on technical devices for innovation in cervical cytology screening [editorial]. *Am J Clin Pathol* 1996; **106**: 441.
48 Cannataci JA. Liability for medical expert systems: an introduction to the legal implications. *Med Inform (Lond)* 1989; **14**: 229–41.
49 Miller RA, Schaffner KF, Meisel A. Ethical and legal issues related to the use of computer programs in clinical medicine. *Ann Intern Med* 1985; **102**: 529–37.
50 Lauro V. Travelers Insurance Company, La. App. 262 So2d 787 (1972).

6

Human papillomaviruses

CHRISTINA ISACSON, MARK E SHERMAN

INTRODUCTION

Advances in our understanding of the biology and natural history of human papillomavirus (HPV) infections have had a major impact on cervical cytology practice and this influence will undoubtedly increase. Multidisciplinary studies combining pathology, epidemiology and molecular biology have provided unified evidence that HPV is the etiologic agent of nearly all cervical squamous intraepithelial lesions (SIL) and carcinomas. The prevalence of genital HPV infections in developed countries has increased since the 1960s, suggesting that HPV now represents the most common sexually transmitted viral disease.[1] Fortunately, most new HPV infections in young women are transient and resolve without significant clinical sequel.[2] Only a small minority of HPV infections progress to an immediate cancer precursor (high-grade SIL) if untreated. Therefore, HPV infection approaches the criteria for a necessary cause of cervical cancer, but it is not a sufficient cause. The cofactors that lead to progression from HPV infection to cancer are not known. Nonetheless, the identification of specific HPV types as etiologic agents of cervical cancer indicates that knowledge of the biology and natural history of HPV infection is important in diagnosis, clinical management and prevention of cervical disease.

The goal of this chapter is to provide a brief overview of the biology and classification of HPV, the epidemiology and natural history of HPV infection, and molecular methods for detecting HPV. The final section of the chapter is on the potential clinical applications of HPV testing and its future trends.

BIOLOGY OF HPV

Structure and gene function

Human papillomaviruses are small, epitheliotropic DNA viruses that measure 55 nm in diameter and consist of a polyhedral capsid enclosing a circular genome consisting of 7900 base pairs (bp). The double-stranded HPV genome is divisible into three regions: an early (E) region, a late (L) region and a non-coding region. The E region codes for non-structural proteins, the L region codes for proteins that form the viral capsid and the non-coding region (also known as the upstream regulatory region) contains the viral promoter, the origin of HPV replication and other controlling elements.

Briefly, the early genes *E6* and *E7* encode proteins capable of inducing cellular proliferation and are expressed in all grades of HPV-associated lesions. Other early genes include *E1*, which seems to be involved in viral DNA replication and plasmid maintenance, and *E2*, which regulates transcription of *E6* and *E7*. *L1* and *L2* are highly conserved genes involved in production of the major and minor capsid proteins, respectively. The non-coding region is upstream of the early genes and includes a steroid-responsive promoter as well as binding sites for *E2* and other molecules involved in regulation of early gene transcription.

Viral transcription and replication are linked to the degree of squamous epithelial cell differentiation.[3] E-region genes are expressed in the basal layers and L-region genes are expressed in the differentiated superficial cells.[4] Consequently, when squamous maturation is present, such as in condylomata, many *L1* and *L2* proteins are present; whereas in less differentiated lesions, such as high-grade squamous intraepithelial lesions (HSIL), there is little or no capsid protein expression, and fewer whole HPV virions are produced per infected cell.

Classification

Over 90 different HPV types have been described and characterization of new candidate types is ongoing. New HPV types are identified by DNA sequence analysis of the entire viral genome. A new type should share <90 per cent sequence homology with conserved regions of known viral types.[5]

Human papillomaviruses may be divided into two broad groups based on tissue tropism: cutaneous (skin) and anogenital. There are about 30 different anogenital HPV types and these are often further subclassified according to oncogenic potential (Table 6.1). Low-risk types confer little, if any, risk for the development of invasive cancer and are identified primarily in condylomata acuminata and some low-grade squamous intraepithelial lesions (LSIL). Low-risk types are rarely found in the absence of other HPV types in HSIL. The most

Table 6.1 *Anogenital human papillomaviruses. Bold numbers indicate predominant type*

Oncogenic risk	HPV types	Associated lesions[a]
Low	**6, 11**, 42–44, 53–55, 62, 66, 70	Condylomata acuminata, LSIL
Intermediate	**31**, 33, 35, 39, 51, 52, 54, 58, 59, 61, 66–68	LSIL, HSIL, carcinoma
High	**16, 18, 45**, 56	LSIL, HSIL, carcinoma

[a]LSIL, low-grade squamous intraepithelial lesion; HSIL, high-grade squamous intraepithelial lesion.

common low-risk types are HPV 6 and 11. HPV types in the intermediate-risk group are rarely found in condylomata, but are associated with flat LSIL, HSIL and some invasive cancers. High-risk types are often identified in LSIL and represent the overwhelmingly predominant HPV types found in HSIL and carcinomas. Some clinical researchers consider the intermediate- and high-risk types together as one group, called either 'oncogenic' or 'cancer-associated', as they account for the vast proportion of significant lesions (HSIL and carcinoma). There are approximately 15–20 oncogenic anogenital types of HPV and the numerically predominant types in cancer are HPV types 16, 18, 31 and 45.[6]

Molecular pathogenesis

Introduction of cloned *E6* and *E7* DNA of the high-risk types HPV 16 and 18 can immortalize cells in culture[7] and these genes are, therefore, considered to be oncogenes. The E6 and E7 oncoproteins contribute to dysregulated growth by promoting the degradation of two key cell cycle regulatory proteins, p53 and pRb.[8,9] Degradation of p53 is mediated through the binding of high-risk E6 to a ubiquitin ligase, called E6-associated protein (E6-AP).[10] The E7 oncoprotein forms complexes with several host proteins, including the retinoblastoma tumor suppressor gene product, pRb. When pRb is bound by E7, it disrupts an inhibitory pathway for transactivation of genes, resulting in increased transcription of growth-related proteins.[11] The low-risk HPV E6 and E7 proteins exhibit a much weaker association with p53 and pRb.[10,12] These findings provide molecular support for the division of viral types into low-risk and oncogenic groups. By analogy with the clinical observation that infection with oncogenic HPV types alone is insufficient to produce carcinoma, it has been shown that expression of oncogenic *E6* or *E7* does not by itself lead to transformation of cells in culture.

The physical state of the virus is related to the pathogenesis of various disease states. In condylomas and most SIL, HPV replicates as an extrachromosomal circular plasmid within the host cell nucleus, whereas in malignant lesions the virus is often integrated into the host genome.[13] To date, specific sites within the human genome that are 'hotspots' for HPV integration have not been identified and it is possible that integration sites occur randomly.[14] In contrast, integration consistently results in a break in the viral genome at the *E1/E2* region with the *E6* and *E7* regions remaining intact.[15] Loss of function of the *E1/E2* genes following integration is thought to lead to deregulated transcription of the *E6* and *E7* oncogenes, promoting cellular transformation. This theory is supported by *in vitro* studies demonstrating a selective growth advantage of cervical epithelial cells with integrated HPV 16 DNA.[16] However, in SIL and cancers, individual cells may contain both integrated and episomal HPV, which further complicates our understanding of viral integration. The association between clonal HPV integration and clinically significant lesions (HSIL and cancers) suggests that tests for HPV integration could be clinically useful if technically feasible.

Despite significant advances, the biological properties of HPV have been difficult to study because the virus cannot be cultured in the laboratory with standard techniques. Animal models for HPV-associated oncogenesis are also limited, as papillomaviruses (PV) are species-specific. Recent studies have utilized transgenic and severe combined immunodeficiency (SCID) mice models. Transgenic mice expressing HPV 16 *E6* and *E7* have been shown to develop squamous carcinomas of the vagina and cervix with chronic estrogen exposure.[17] Recently, human xenografts of cervical epithelium in SCID mice have been shown to maintain a dysplastic morphology with high-dose estrogen exposure and introduction of high-risk HPV types through recombinant adenovirus infection.[18] Further development of these models may provide insights into the molecular pathogenesis of SIL and cancers, including the mechanisms that lead to progression of HPV infection to HSIL and the process of invasion.

Finally, a variety of host factors may affect the outcome of HPV infections. A recent study has suggested that specific p53 polymorphisms may be more susceptible to HPV E6-mediated degradation and confer increased cancer risk.[19] However other reports have contradicted these findings.[20–23] Host immune responses are also related to the outcome of HPV infections and may be partly dictated by inheritable factors, such as human leukocyte antigen (HLA) type.

EPIDEMIOLOGY OF HPV

Establishing HPV as a cause of cervical SIL and cancer

Sexual behavior has long been recognized as the main risk factor for cervical cancer and its precursors. Specifically, onset of sexual activity before the age of 16 years and greater than five lifetime sexual partners are associated with the greatest increased risk.[24] 'High-risk' males who have a history of multiple partners and sexually transmitted disease also increase the risk of cervical cancer in their female partners in a manner analogous to a woman's own sexual behavior.[25] A sexually transmitted agent has thus been strongly suspected in the development of cervical disease. Since the 1970s, when zur Hausen et al. established a relationship between cervical cancer and HPV infection,[26] many epidemiological studies have examined the etiologic importance of HPV DNA detection. Initial studies were flawed owing to low sensitivity and low specificity of early HPV DNA assays. Once improved tests became available, epidemiological studies confirmed earlier clinical and molecular observations linking HPV to cervical SIL and cancer.[24,27,28] Other possible risk factors include use of oral contraceptives, low socioeconomic status, smoking and parity.[24] However, if one controls for the presence of HPV infection, most of these risk factors become markedly reduced in importance. Sexual activity conveys little or no risk beyond transmission of the virus. The relative and attributable risks of cervical disease conferred by HPV infection are substantial. Women with detectable HPV DNA have a relative risk of approximately 40 of having a cervical cytological abnormality and the proportion of cervical lesions attributable to HPV exceeds 90 per cent.[24]

In summary, the evidence for a causal association is overwhelming and includes the following: (1) HPV DNA is detected in nearly all women with cervical cancer and SIL compared with a consistently low percentage in control women;[6,24,29] (2) HPV infection precedes the development of SIL;[2,30,31] (3) HPV infection, particularly that of certain specific types, is specifically associated with the development of mucocutaneous carcinomas of the anogenital tract;[32] and (4) there is coherence with existing biological evidence and with other known epidemiological risk factors.[32]

Risk factors for HPV infection

The prevalence of HPV infection is increased in pregnant women and pregnancy may contribute to an increased viral load and cell growth through either direct or indirect (immunological or hormone-related) mechanisms.[33]

The host immune response to HPV also appears to be an important risk factor in predicting the outcome of HPV infection. An increase in prevalence and severity of HPV-related disease has been documented in human immunodeficiency virus (HIV)-positive patients as well as in other immune-related disorders. Women that are HIV-positive are four times more likely to have an HPV infection than non-infected women.[34] The increased detection rate is related to immunosuppression. It is not known, however, if this is mediated via reactivation of prior infections or facilitation of new infections. HLAs are important in the presentation of foreign antigens to the immune system. Specific HLA class II haplotypes are associated with cervical SIL and carcinoma, suggesting that certain HLA haplotypes confer an increased risk for the development of cervical neoplasia following HPV infection.[35–37] The key immune response involved in clearing HPV infection is thought to reflect cell-mediated mechanisms involving antigen presenting cells (Langerhans cells) and T-helper lymphocytes.[38,39] Viral persistence related to immunosuppression could contribute to the development of disease because persistence is a prerequisite for neoplasia.

Prevalence of HPV

Human papillomavirus infections are extremely common in the general population, but it is difficult to give a simple answer regarding the prevalence of HPV infection since it varies with the population tested, the method of sample collection and the HPV detection method used. In general, estimates range from 1–3 per cent of the population based on a cytological diagnosis of LSIL, 6–8 per cent using non-amplified HPV DNA tests and 15–30 per cent using polymerase chain reaction (PCR)-based tests.[32] For conceptual purposes, perhaps the easiest way to view the magnitude of HPV infection is to think of a pyramid formed by a combination of HPV detection and cytological/histological diagnoses (Fig. 6.1). At the top are the most severe manifestations of HPV infection: invasive carcinoma and HSIL. In the USA, there are approximately 15 000 new cases of cervical cancer each year.[40] Estimates for HSIL are difficult to obtain, but the diagnosis of HSIL appears to be approximately 20 times commoner than that of carcinoma.[41] The actual number of HSIL in the USA may be much higher than the figure listed, as these data do not reflect the large subset of women that have never been screened. Women with LSIL followed by cytologically normal women that test positive for HPV DNA by either non-amplified methods or with PCR-based methods (see HPV detection methods section below) form the base of the pyramid.

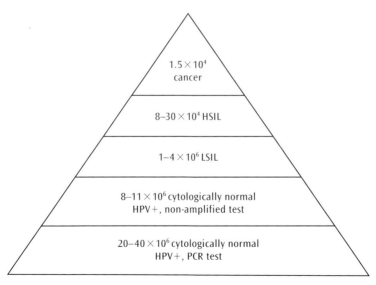

1.5×10^4 cancer

$8–30 \times 10^4$ HSIL

$1–4 \times 10^6$ LSIL

$8–11 \times 10^6$ cytologically normal HPV+, non-amplified test

$20–40 \times 10^6$ cytologically normal HPV+, PCR test

Figure 6.1 *Estimated cervical human papillomavirus (HPV) infections and HPV-related disease in the USA. HSIL, high-grade squamous intraepithelial lesion; LSIL, low-grade squamous intraepithelial lesion; PCR, polymerase chain reaction.*

Natural history of HPV infection

Most HPV infections spontaneously regress within 2–3 years, often without producing clinically detectable disease.[2,42] Multiple HPV types are detected in about 20–30 per cent of infected women.[24] The prevalence of HPV infection peaks at 16–25 years of age and then declines sharply.[24,43] Postulated reasons for this decrease with age include: (1) immunological clearance or suppression of existing infections; (2) decreased exposure to new HPV types because of fewer new sexual partners; or (3) a 'cohort effect', reflecting a population-based increase in prevalence in recent years.

Low-grade squamous intraepithelial lesions are the morphological manifestation of a productive HPV infection. As such, peak occurrence of LSIL is in young women at the same age as the HPV peak infection rate and similarly the majority regress.[44,45] The incidence of HSIL peaks in women in their late twenties to early thirties.[24] The occurrence of HSIL in an older age group may reflect the importance of persistent HPV infection in the development of HSIL. Alternatively, women infected with HPV at older ages may be at increased risk for developing high-grade lesions. The percentage of high-grade lesions that progress to invasive carcinoma, if left untreated, is very high and is perhaps over 50 per cent, if follow-up is long enough.[46] Invasive cervical cancer develops on average a decade or more later than HSIL, usually after the age of 45 years. Cervical cancer is extremely rare in women under 30 years of age.

Human papillomavirus infection precedes and predicts the development of cervical neoplasia. Results from several large prospective studies of cytologically normal women show substantially elevated relative ($>$10) and absolute ($>$30 per cent) risks of incident SIL, including HSIL, within a few years of HPV DNA detection.[2,30,31] Oncogenic HPV types are associated with a greater risk of developing lesions (both LSIL and HSIL) than are other HPV types. Interestingly, several of the studies have shown the development of HSIL without a preceding diagnosis of LSIL.[30,31] It has been questioned by some whether or not LSIL is a true precursor to HSIL.[47]

Persistent HPV infection is critical to disease development. Several prospective studies have indicated that the risk of subsequent cervical neoplasia seems to be proportional to the number of specimens testing positive over time for HPV, particularly for the 'high-risk' types.[2,30,48] In addition, persistence of HPV infection is more likely in older women (age $>$30 years) than in younger women.[42] These findings suggest that cervical cancer may arise within the subset of women with persistent HPV infection of oncogenic types.

SPECTRUM OF HPV-ASSOCIATED DISEASE

Distribution of HPV within lesions

The relative proportions of common HPV types in clinical lesions are shown in Fig. 6.2.[6,49–52] Exophytic condylomata acuminata are predominately associated with low-risk viral types: HPV 6 (two-thirds) or HPV 11 (one-third). Other low-risk viral types that are found in these lesions include HPV 26, 42–44, 53–55, 62 and 66. LSIL may contain any of the anogenital HPV types. Low-risk viral types account for only about 20 per cent of LSIL. The remainder shows a varying distribution of oncogenic viral types. 'Intermediate' risk-types account for 30 per cent (HPV types 31, 33, 35, 52, 58 and 67), classic 'high-risk' types 16 and 18 account for 15–20 per cent and other unknown risk types account for the rest.[41–51,53,54] Most recently, the baseline data from the atypical squamous cells of undetermined significance (ASCUS)/LSIL triage study (ALTS) showed that 83 per cent (95 per cent confidence interval = 80–86 per cent) of

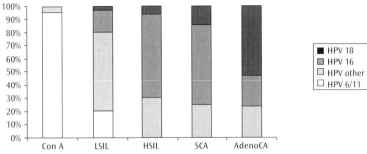
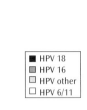

Figure 6.2 *Human papillomavirus (HPV) distribution in lesions. Con A, condyloma acuminatum; LSIL, low-grade squamous intraepithelial lesion; HSIL, high-grade squamous intraepithelial lesion; SCA, squamous carcinoma; AdenoCA, adenocarcinoma.*[6,49–52]

the 642 women referred with LSIL tested positive for the cancer-associated HPV types (types 16, 18, 31, 33, 35, 39, 45, 51, 52, 56, 58, 59, and 68) by hybrid capture II (HC II) assay (Digene Corporation, Silver Spring, MD, USA).[55] Further, it should be emphasized that it is not possible to predict the HPV type associated with an LSIL on morphology alone.[56]

High-grade squamous intraepithelial lesions and squamous carcinomas share a similar distribution of HPV types. The predominant type is HPV 16 and this is found in about 50 per cent of both lesions. Types 16, 18, 31 and 45 are found in up to 75 per cent of cervical carcinomas in most geographical regions of the world.[6] In most studies, HPV 18 predominates in adenocarcinomas, adenosquamous carcinomas and small cell carcinomas.[57–59] Less common oncogenic types include HPV types 33, 35, 39, 51, 52, 56, 58, 59 and 66–68, making a total of about 15 different HPV types responsible for the majority of cervical carcinomas. Initial studies suggesting that HPV 18 is relatively uncommon in HSIL compared with carcinoma led to the hypothesis that HPV 18 may be associated with rapid-onset carcinomas that develop rapidly from short-lived HSIL;[60,61] however, this result has not been conclusively confirmed.

Although several researchers have speculated that HPV is involved in the pathogenesis of essentially all cervical carcinomas,[29,62] there are still rare cancer cases in which HPV DNA is undetectable.[6,63] Postulated reasons for this lack of HPV detection include: (1) inadequate sampling of the tumor; (2) integration of the viral genome with disruption of the region detected by the specific assay employed; (3) failure to detect novel HPV types; and (4) false-negative HPV tests due to other causes.

The Bethesda System

The Bethesda System (TBS) follows a conceptual model for the biology of HPV-associated cervical lesions.[56,64] The terms 'koilocytotic atypia' and mild dysplasia/CIN I were combined into a single category of LSIL for the following reasons: (1) these lesions share the same distribution of HPV types; (2) patient demographics and risk factors are similar; (3) the clinical behavior of the lesions is comparable; and (4) the cytological distinction between these lesions is unreliable.[56] Moderate dysplasia/CIN II and severe dysplasia/carcinoma *in situ*/CIN III were combined into the category of HSIL because all these lesions are treated in the USA.

More importantly, HPV infection and the resulting SIL may be logically viewed as a dichotomous process with two general outcomes: LSIL are largely transient manifestations of HPV infection, whereas HSIL are more closely related to true intramucosal neoplasms with a greater likelihood of progressing to invasive carcinoma. In addition, the replacement of the words 'dysplasia' and 'neoplasia' with 'intraepithelial lesion' reflects the fact that the natural history of an individual lesion is uncertain.

It should be pointed out that the distinction between the acute infectious manifestation of HPV infection (LSIL) and the more permanent lesion resembling neoplasia (HSIL) is not simply a reflection of viral type. While low-risk types do not tend to persist and are strongly linked with transient LSIL, oncogenic types of HPV, including HPV 16, also produce transient manifestations (LSIL) most of the time. However, these viruses may persist in a minority of cases due to incompletely described factors and, in some of these cases, an HSIL may develop.

TECHNICAL ASPECTS OF HPV DETECTION METHODS

Human papillomavirus detection methods have evolved over several decades from relatively insensitive and technically demanding procedures to simpler, more rapid methods with potential clinical utility (Table 6.2). All of these assays rely upon a hybridization reaction in which there is specific recognition of HPV DNA target sequences by complementary RNA or DNA sequences called probes. There are three conceptual categories of HPV DNA assay methods: those that directly identify nucleic acids (non-amplified), those that amplify the signal produced by the hybridization reaction (signal amplification) and those that amplify the nucleic acids first and then detect the product (target amplification). The tests best suited for routine clinical use are the signal-amplified (hybrid capture system) and the target-amplified (PCR) assays.

Non-amplified methods

The Southern blot was the original reference standard for HPV detection and is briefly described here to provide a background for the current HPV tests. DNA is extracted from a cell sample and cleaved with restriction enzymes into fragments. Next, the sample is electrophoresed to separate the fragments according to size and transferred to a filter that is hybridized with DNA probes that recognize HPV DNA sequences. The filter is washed to remove any unbound probes and the remaining hybridization product is detected by autoradiography. The advantage of this technique is that it can reliably identify specific HPV types with its combination of hybridization and restriction fragment analysis. Disadvantages include the need to use multiple type-specific HPV probes, the large sample requirement because amplification techniques are not used, issues related to storing and handling radioactive probes, and achieving technical expertise.

The Dot blot is a technically simpler procedure in which extracted denatured DNA is bound to a filter and then hybridized with HPV probes. The rapidity of the test made it very popular when first introduced; however, the test, as commercially formatted, proved to be relatively insensitive, in part due to the small number of different type-specific HPV probes included in the assay.

In situ hybridization assays combine HPV detection with morphology. DNA or RNA probes recognizing one or a mixture of HPV types are applied directly to cytological or histological slides that have been pretreated to allow cell permeability and separation of DNA strands. After washing away any unbound probes, the hybridization products are visualized with either enzymatic detection methods or autoradiography. The main advantage of this assay is that it permits the localization of HPV DNA within cells and tissues. Commercially available *in situ* hybridization tests use probe cocktails for a limited number of HPV types and range in

Table 6.2 *A comparison of the different human papillomavirus (HPV) detection methods*

Test	Category	Sample type	Sensitivity	Use	Advantages	Disadvantages
Southern blot	Non-amplified	Fresh tissue	10–40 HPV/cell	Historical; detection of new HPV types; integration status	Reliable; old 'gold' standard	Requires a large amount of tissue; technically difficult
Dot blot	Non-amplified	Exfoliated cells	10–40 HPV/cell	Now combined with PCR assays	Rapid	Low sensitivity; limited probes
In situ hybridization	Non-amplified	Tissue sections or cytological preparations	10–100 HPV/cell	Detects common HPV types in large copy number	Localization of HPV within cells and tissue	Low sensitivity; limited probe groups with inability to distinguish types
Hybrid capture system (HCS)	Signal amplification	Exfoliated cells	HC I = 50 000 HPV/sample; HC II=1000 HPV/sample	Possible clinical utility; multiple applications (see text)	Rapid; easy to use; semi-quantitative	Does not provide specific typing as usually performed
Polymerase chain reaction (PCR)	Target amplification	Exfoliated cells, fresh tissue; archival material	10–100 HPV/sample	Best for research; possible clinical utility (see text)	Most sensitive; allows specific typing	Easy to contaminate; detects many clinically innocuous infections

sensitivity from 10 to 100 copies of virus per cell. In certain situations, such as in the differential diagnosis of exophytic condylomata, *in situ* techniques may be diagnostically useful.[65,66] More recent *in situ* hybridization assays are able to pick up one copy of HPV per cell;[67] however, the assays require considerable technical expertise.

Signal amplification tests

The hybrid capture system (HCS) is a non-radioactive, rapid liquid RNA–DNA hybridization technique that uses signal amplification rather than viral DNA amplification.[68] Sample DNA is denatured and mixed with cocktails of HPV RNA probes recognizing either 'low-risk' or 'high-risk' types. Duplexes consisting of HPV DNA and RNA probes are bound by monoclonal antibodies immobilized to the reaction chamber (originally a tube, now a microplate). To amplify the signal, the captured DNA–RNA hybrids are reacted with numerous secondary antibodies conjugated to multiple molecules of alkaline phosphatase and the products are detected with chemiluminescence. A luminometer reads the light output and displays the assay results as relative light units (RLU) compared with a standard positive reference provided with the kit. HCS has several features that enhance its sensitivity and specificity over the non-amplified tests: (1) the use of whole genomic probes allows recognition of the entire HPV genome; (2) RNA–DNA hybrids are more stable than DNA–DNA hybrids; (3) many conjugated secondary antibodies can coat one immobilized RNA–DNA hybrid, resulting in amplification of the signal; and (4) cleavage of the chemiluminescent substrate by alkaline phosphatase emits light proportional to the amount of target DNA in the specimen, allowing semi-quantification.

The first generation of HCS assay, HC I or tube test, identified five low-risk and 11 oncogenic HPV types (6/11, 16, 18, 31, 33, 35, 39, 42–45, 51, 52, 56 and 58). It had a detection threshold of 10 pg/mL of HPV DNA, which corresponds to approximately 50 000 copies of virus per assay. HCS has been recently modified to a microtiter plate format (HC II) with increased analytical sensitivity to a detection threshold of 1 pg/mL (or lower) of HPV DNA, which corresponds to about 1000 copies of virus per assay. In addition, the probe mix has been expanded to include oncogenic HPV types 59 and 68.[68] The HCS microtiter plate format is easy to perform and rapid. Studies have shown accuracy and inter-laboratory reliability for HPV testing with HCS and both generations are currently FDA-approved HPV DNA diagnostic kits. One limitation of HCS is that there is a lack of normalization for cellular DNA, therefore, DNA quantification can be affected by variation in cellularity and composition of the sample.

Target amplification tests

Polymerase chain reaction tests amplify the target prior to detection. DNA extracted from a sample is subjected to multiple cycles of *in vitro* DNA synthesis using target-specific DNA primer sets to achieve logarithmic amplification of a specific length of DNA. Identification of the correct-sized product is confirmed by gel electrophoresis. The PCR is an ultra-sensitive technique able to pick up as few as 10–100 targets and potentially even only one copy per reaction. Many different specimen types can be used, such as fresh tissue, smears, and cells in liquid and formalin-fixed archival material.

Variables that may influence PCR assay sensitivity and specificity include primer selection and the techniques used for product detection. The two most common HPV primer sets are MY09/MY11[69] and GP5+/GP6+.[70] Both sets of primers amplify a conserved region of the *L1* open reading frame and are called 'consensus' primers, as they are able to amplify many different HPV types, including uncharacterized types. The size of the product generated may influence the assay sensitivity. In general, PCR reactions become more efficient with decreasing target size.

Further, DNA extracted from formalin-fixed archival material can be degraded into small fragments or cross-linked to formalin, making the target inaccessible to the primers. The MY09/MY11 primers amplify a 450 bp region, whereas the GP5+/GP6+primers amplify a 150 bp region. This is leading to the development of new consensus primers that amplify smaller regions in an attempt to maximize test sensitivity.[62] In general, both the MY09/MY11 and the GP5+/GP6+ primer sets have been proven to work extremely well and identify HPV DNA in more than 90 per cent of pathologically confirmed cervical SIL and cancers. When directly compared, the sensitivity for HPV detection between the two primer sets is similar, with only some differences in the detection of specific HPV types.[71] Other primer sets, such as consensus primers for the *E1* region as well as type-specific E6 primers, have been developed,[72,73] but none are used widely.

After confirmation of the correct-sized amplicon, most PCR reaction products are detected with hybridization to either HPV cocktails or type-specific probes. Specific HPV genotyping can also be accomplished by restriction-fragment length analysis, single-strand conformation polymorphism analysis, or by direct sequencing of the PCR products. More recent techniques have been aimed at single-step typing methods such as reverse line blot hybridization[74] or assays based on enzyme-linked immunosorbent assay (ELISA).[75]

The exquisite sensitivity of PCR makes it useful in epidemiological investigations since it identifies all HPV-infected women, including those who are clinically normal and typically have low viral loads. However, this extreme level of sensitivity may reduce the potential clinical utility of the test in young women who have a high rate of transient, insignificant infections. Furthermore, PCR assays are extremely prone to contamination that can occur at any step along the way from specimen collection to detection of the products. Quality control in PCR assays, as well as all other sensitive HPV testing methods, is essential.

CLINICAL TESTING FOR HPV

Cervical cytological screening has significantly decreased the morbidity and mortality of cervical cancer. However, data suggest that cytological screening has an irreducible false-negative rate and that management of patients with equivocal results, such as ASCUS and atypical glandular cells of undetermined significance (AGUS), has become an increasing problem. Clinical testing for HPV has been suggested as a method to improve current strategies for the detection of clinically significant cervical disease. Possible uses include: (1) management triage of patients with equivocally abnormal smears (ASCUS or AGUS); (2) to provide predictive/prognostic information for the development of lesions; (3) as a quality assurance measure to validate cytological and histological diagnostic criteria; and (4) as a primary screening mechanism for cervical disease.

General aspects of clinical HPV testing

METHODS OF SAMPLE COLLECTION

The optimal method for collecting cervical cells for HPV DNA analysis has not been determined, but several techniques yield comparable results. Cells from the cervix can be removed during a gynecological examination with Dacron swabs, cotton swabs, conical brushes or broom devices. A single sample of exfoliated cells may be placed into a medium suitable for both thin-layer cytology and HPV testing or an initial sample may be prepared as a smear and then a second can be collected in a specimen transport medium useful for virological testing only. The same concerns in collecting cells for cytology apply to HPV testing. Cervical mucus should be removed from the canal prior to collection and adequate sampling of the transformation zone is essential. The broom device and conical brush may be better at cutting through cervical mucus and reach further within the cervical canal. Recently, the use of self-administered vaginal tampon specimens for HPV testing has been shown to be equivalent to the physician-directed swab.[76]

An advantage of using a liquid cytology medium for the collection of cervical specimens is that HPV DNA testing and other assays can be performed on a single sample of known cellular composition.[77,78] In addition, the single sample collection gives the cytology laboratory the opportunity to perform cytological screening first, save the unused cellular contents of the vial and then decide whether HPV testing is indicated or not based on the cytology results. Vials obtained from women with normal cytology or definite SIL would not necessarily require testing, whereas testing could be performed in equivocal cases. If a separate collection medium is used, all women would need to have two scrapes performed, or women with equivocal cytology would need to return to have a second sample collected specifically for HPV testing. The latter approach would greatly reduce the cost-effectiveness and convenience of using HPV testing. Techniques available for collecting exfoliative cells in liquid media for preparing thin-layer cytological slides of gynecological samples include the PreservCyt/ThinPrep method (Cytyc, Boxborough, MA, USA) and the CytoRich/PREP sample system (AutoCyte, Burlington, NC, USA). HPV DNA testing with HC II is FDA-approved for use with either the specimen transport medium (STM) supplied with the HCS or with PreservCyt; USA trials are planned to evaluate Cytorich.

VIRAL TYPES

The cancer risk in cervical lesions is related to the presence of oncogenic HPV types. The HCS may be used to detect low-risk and oncogenic HPV types, but further classification is not typically performed. Testing for the oncogenic types would suffice for most clinical purposes. PCR-based methods using consensus primers are potentially capable of detecting all known, as well as uncharacterized HPV types. For clinical testing purposes, it is probably sufficient to include the most common HPV types, and both HCS and PCR-based methods detect the majority of HPVs identified in cervical cancers throughout the world.[6] The utility of testing for low-risk HPV types has been questioned. In a study examining the relationship between TBS diagnoses (negative, ASCUS and SIL) and HPV typing, low-risk HPV DNA was detected in about 20 per cent of each diagnostic category for every reviewer, whereas HPV (mainly the oncogenic types) were detected in 100 per cent of the cases unanimously diagnosed as SIL.[79] If detection of HSILs is set as the benchmark for test performance, HPV testing should be for oncogenic HPV types only. Specific HPV typing may be relevant for vaccine applications but is not important for colposcopy triage because low-risk viruses are not associated with an increased risk of cancers.

POPULATION TO BE TESTED

Patient age is a significant factor to consider when applying clinical HPV testing. Because HPV DNA positivity is highly prevalent in cytologically normal women aged under 30 years, it has been argued that HPV testing would not discriminate between transient infections and true disease. However, as HPV prevalence decreases with age, the positive predictive value of finding HPV DNA should increase with age. HPV detection in older women is more likely to represent a persistent infection since these women, historically, may have had fewer new sexual partners than younger women. Further, the use and accuracy of the Pap smear declines with age owing to inadequate sampling of the receding transformation zone (false negatives) and overdiagnosis of atrophy-related changes (false positives).[80] Because of the inaccuracy of cytology in older women and the assumed low incidence of new HPV infections, it is postulated that a negative HPV test would permit significant lengthening of the screening interval with virtually no risk of cancer.

Other factors to consider in the population to be tested are patient reliability for follow-up, sexual behavior characteristics, prior history of abnormal cytological findings, the patient–physician relationship and the performance of the cytology laboratory being used for diagnosis. Monogamous, compliant patients who have a history of normal Pap smears are considered to be at low risk.[81] In addition, the diagnostic performance of cytology laboratories varies, especially in the use of equivocal categories of cellular change.[79]

Guiding the management of equivocal Pap smears

Ancillary HPV testing is being actively evaluated as a technique to detect women with equivocal cytology who harbor an underlying HSIL.

ASCUS

The category of ASCUS is the most common abnormal cervical cytological diagnosis. Briefly, ASCUS is problematic because it lacks reproducibility and is associated with highly variable outcomes (see Chapter 8). Although colposcopy would be a safe way of excluding an underlying HSIL in women with ASCUS, this approach is impractical as an estimated two to three million women receive a diagnosis of ASCUS annually in the USA.[82] Consequently, HPV testing has emerged as a potential strategy for colposcopy triage of women with ASCUS cytology. The rationale is that detection of oncogenic HPV types should identify the vast majority of the women with an underlying SIL, especially HSIL, whereas a negative result should provide reassurance that the 'atypical' cells represent an unusual reactive change. In order for HPV-mediated clinical management of ASCUS to be effective, the presence of oncogenic HPV types in an ASCUS smear must be predictive of biopsy-proven high-grade disease.

Initial studies examining the usefulness of HPV testing for colposcopy triage of women with ASCUS used the relatively insensitive HC I (first generation tube test). Nonetheless, the results were promising.[83–85] The sensitivity of HPV-positive results versus repeat abnormal Pap smear (ASCUS or worse) for detecting biopsy proven CIN were similar (46–86 per cent versus 60–86 per cent). When examining the sensitivity for detecting high-grade CIN by HPV testing, there was a range from 50 per cent to 93 per cent. Overall, the combination of HPV testing and repeat Pap smear achieved better detection than either one alone and approached 100 per cent for detection of any CIN without referring for colposcopy all the women with ASCUS on initial Pap smear.

Recent evaluations with new HPV assays have reported higher sensitivities for detection of histological HSIL. In a comparison between the HC I and the newer HC II tests, the sensitivity for detecting high-grade CIN increased from 55.6 per cent to 90 per cent in women with Pap smear showing ASCUS.[86] Accordingly, there was an increase in sensitivity for any CIN from 49 per cent to 80 per cent, but a decrease in specificity from 71 per cent to 45 per cent. A recent study of 265 women with an abnormal Pap smear (ASCUS or LSIL) found that HPV testing with HC II, using cells remaining in a liquid-based cytological fluid collection after preparation of a thin-layer slide, identified 93 per cent of high-grade CIN with a specificity of 30 per cent.[87] Receiver operating characteristic curves demonstrated that HPV DNA testing was more appropriate for women older than 30 years of age and for women with ASCUS as opposed to LSIL.

Finally, a recent study evaluated the performance of HC II HPV testing in identifying women with ASCUS smears who had biopsy-confirmed HSIL.[88] From a cohort of 46 009 women who had routine cervical examinations at a large health maintenance organization (HMO), this study enrolled 995 consenting patients who had ASCUS on conventional cervical smears. A thin-layer slide preparation and HPV testing were done for these 995 women using the residual material left on the collection device for the conventional smear and preserved in liquid cytology medium. All women had colposcopy with repeat conventional Pap smear and at least one histological sample taken. HC II identified 89.2 per cent of women with HSIL or a more serious lesion compared with 76.2 per cent by a repeat Pap diagnosis of ASCUS or worse, but this difference did not reach statistical significance ($P = 0.09$).

Despite these encouraging results, the clinical value of HPV testing in clinical practice remains a matter of debate.[89–91] The biggest concern stems from the fact that in certain populations women with a benign reason for an ASCUS Pap smear have at least the same chance of being HPV-positive as women with normal Pap smears of the same age and recent sexual history.[79] In summary, the usefulness of ancillary HPV testing depends on the analytical sensitivity of the assay, the characteristics of the population tested and the cytology laboratory reporting the equivocal results.

AGUS

Human papillomavirus DNA testing may also be helpful for the clarification of equivocal glandular cervical cytology results. Similar to ASCUS, most cases of AGUS represent an exuberant reactive change. However, either HSIL or, less commonly, adenocarcinoma-*in-situ* (AIS) may be the underlying reason of AGUS. In some series, the percentage of HSIL on follow up biopsies of patients with AGUS is higher than that of ASCUS.[92–94] In the same HMO population as for the recent ASCUS study,[88] 137 women had a diagnosis of AGUS. Hybrid capture II HPV DNA testing identified 92 per cent of the women with biopsy-proven HSIL and 100 per cent of those with AIS.[95] The study also demonstrates the value of careful cytological review in managing these women. A triage approach using a combination of review cytological diagnosis and HPV DNA testing would have produced the best results. Although it is usually possible to distinguish atypical endocervical cells from atypical endometrial cells, it is important to remember that AGUS related to an underlying endometrial carcinoma would not be expected to yield a positive HPV test.

Quality assurance

TO EVALUATE DIAGNOSTIC PERFORMANCE

HPV testing could be used as an independent reference standard for improving the diagnosis of equivocal smears in cytopathology laboratories. In a study examining the relationship between TBS diagnoses and HPV typing, 200 Pap smears that were originally classified as atypical were independently reclassified by five expert cytopathologists and these diagnoses were compared with HPV DNA detection in concurrently obtained lavages.[79] The reviewers classified 38–62 per cent of the smears as negative, 16–39 per cent as ASCUS and 21–28 per cent as SIL. Although interobserver agreement between reviewers was poor and there was not a single smear unanimously classified as ASCUS by the panel, the pattern of HPV DNA detection across TBS diagnostic categories was similar for each reviewer. Specifically, detection of oncogenic types of HPV DNA was lowest in women with negative smears, intermediate in women with ASCUS smears and highest in women with SIL. The detection of low-risk HPV DNA was unrelated to cytological diagnosis; however, cytological diagnosis was strongly related with the detection of oncogenic HPV types. HPV DNA was detected in 100 per cent of cases unanimously diagnosed as SIL by the five panelists. The detection of oncogenic HPV types was extremely rare in cases in which the five pathologists agreed that the smear was negative. Similar results were found in a recent study based on ThinPrep cervical cytology.[96]

The extraordinarily consistent relationship between diagnoses of negative, ASCUS and SIL in TBS and the detection of oncogenic HPV types suggests that pathologists could evaluate their diagnostic performance through determining the rate of oncogenic HPV types for their various diagnostic categories. Failure to detect the highest rate of oncogenic HPV types in SIL, the lowest frequency in negative smears and an intermediate frequency in ASCUS would suggest that TBS criteria had been misapplied. In particular, liberal, non-specific use of the ASCUS category would result in a low rate of HPV DNA detection in these specimens, similar to that found in the negative smears.

TO GUIDE NEGATIVE PAP SMEAR RESCREENING

Current standards of practice in the USA dictate that a cytotechnologist or pathologist rescreen 10 per cent of smears diagnosed as negative/normal by each screener.[97] Whether or not this practice contributes anything to ensuring quality performance is a matter of debate.[98] An interesting question is whether HPV testing can be used to determine which negative smears are more likely to be falsely negative and therefore should be rescreened. An unpublished study by van der Linden et al. found a 7 per cent false negative rate in the rescreening of high-risk HPV-positive smears (PCR-based method), whereas there was a <1 per cent false-negative rate associated with the rescreening of HPV-negative smears.[99]

TO ASSESS ACCURACY OF NEW TECHNOLOGIES

Human papillomavirus testing has been performed in several studies to validate positive results with a new cytological technique.[100,101] For example, in a masked, independent review of split samples, thin-layer slides detected more SIL than conventional smears did and the HPV-positive rate in the cytological diagnoses of SIL was similar for these two techniques. This finding supports the notion that the increased SIL detection rate by the thin-layer technique reflects an increased sensitivity,[101] otherwise, one could have argued that a higher proportion of SIL diagnoses with thin layer slides represented non-specific false-positive diagnoses.

For prediction/prognostication

Prospective studies have shown that women with 'normal' Pap smears and detectable oncogenic HPV DNA are at an increased risk for developing HSIL compared with HPV-negative women.[30,31,102] The probability for a HPV-positive woman with normal smears to develop an abnormal smear within 2 years may be as high as 70 per cent.[103] In a study with a PCR-based HPV test, the estimated risk of developing an HSIL following detection of HPV 16 was less than 10 per cent, but this risk was 100-fold of that for HPV-negative women.[102] These data suggest that women who are positive for an oncogenic type of HPV DNA could be placed under closer surveillance. However, perhaps of more value than an isolated finding of HPV DNA would be the detection of HPV persistence. Viral persistence has been associated with greater age, oncogenic HPV types and infection with multiple types of HPV.[2] Several studies using semiquantitative or quantitative HPV testing have found that a high level of HPV DNA is a possible predictor of prevalent HSIL,[83,104] however the relationship between viral load and persistent HPV infection has not been examined. The clinical utility of viral quantification, while seemingly promising, is currently under investigation. Viral load measurements are affected by the cellularity of the material collected and the sensitivity of the HPV DNA assay, among others, in addition to the number of viral copies per cell.

HPV testing may be useful as a prognostic marker following cervical conization. In one study, women whose cervices remained HPV-positive after conization for HSIL were more likely to develop recurrent disease than those who had no detectable HPV DNA after treatment.[105]

Whether or not the specific HPV type is related to the clinical behavior of cervical carcinomas is under investigation. In several studies of women with invasive cancer, HPV 18 was associated with a poorer prognosis than other HPV types.[106,107] Specifically, the 5-year survival for tumors with HPV 18 was significantly lower compared with those with HPV 16 or other less common HPV types, and HPV 18 was identified as an independent prognostic parameter in multivariate analysis. However, other studies have not confirmed this finding.[108,109] Furthermore, a recent epidemiological study examining risk factors for rapid-onset cervical cancer found no significant association between HPV type 18 and possible rapid-onset disease.[110] Larger studies are necessary to examine the usefulness of HPV typing for prognostic and therapeutic purposes of cervical carcinoma.

Financial implications

The financial impact of HPV testing in cervical cancer screening is difficult to determine. Factors that can influence the cost–benefit analysis include disease prevalence, age of the women tested, interval between tests, and the sensitivity and cost of the HPV DNA test. HPV testing would prove to be cost-effective if colposcopy referrals could be reduced or screening intervals lengthened for HPV-negative women.

Initial cost analysis for the use of HPV testing in the management of patients with ASCUS was promising.[83,111] However, other studies did not show significant cost savings over immediate referral to colposcopy because of the requirement of a second office visit to collect the virological sample.[85] Clearly, the cost-effectiveness of HPV testing is increased if the sample for virological testing is collected concurrently with taking the cytological sample, as was done in a recent study.[88] The results of that study demonstrated that HPV-based triage of ASCUS would provide more sensitive detection of HSIL and a more serious lesion without an increase in the costs of the cervical screening program. The extra costs of the HPV testing and liquid-based Pap tests would be offset by the reduction in colposcopies and repeat Pap tests.

The cost of introducing HPV testing into a cervical screening program has also been evaluated in the UK.[112] It was suggested that the use of HPV testing as part of routine screening in women over the age of 30 years could safely increase the screening interval from 3 to 5 years and would result in an estimated saving of £30 million/year from the currently estimated costs of £130 million/year. The biggest savings occur with increasing the screening interval from 3 to 5 years as there would be 40 per cent fewer smears screened. In addition, as samples are rarely inadequate for HPV testing (about 1 per cent), HPV testing would substantially reduce the number of inadequate smears (about 8 per cent). The increased detection rate associated with a stringent, quality-controlled HPV test would be balanced by the fewer number of women screened each year. To remain cost-effective, referral of women with negative smears must be limited to those with oncogenic HPV types only. Further analysis of the estimated financial impact of HPV testing awaits the results of large-scale clinical trials.

FUTURE DIRECTIONS

ASCUS/LSIL triage study

A large multi-center National Cancer Institute sponsored study has been conducted and has provided additional data on the utility of HPV DNA testing in the triage of women with

ASCUS and LSIL (ALTS).[55,113,114] The baseline data from the study showed that women with an LSIL diagnosis from Pap smears had a very high frequency of oncogenic-type HPV positivity (82.9 per cent),[55] therefore, LSIL was dropped from the study. Subjects with ASCUS were randomized into one of three arms: colposcopy at the initial referral visit, HPV testing with colposcopy performed only on women with oncogenic HPV types, and follow-up by cytology and colposcopy only as indicated by a diagnosis of HSIL. Subjects were followed every 6 months for 2–3 years from the time of enrollment and only persistent low-grade CIN or high-grade CIN were treated. The results demonstrated that HCII testing for oncogenic-type HPV DNA is a viable option in the management of women with ASCUS.[114] It has greater sensitivity (96.3%) to detect CIN III or above than a single repeat Pap smear indicating ASCUS or above (85.3%) with comparable specificity for the two tests.

Elimination of ASCUS

It may be possible to eliminate the ASCUS category based on HPV testing results. It has been suggested that all the early HPV-related diagnoses, ranging from HPV DNA detectable only by sensitive molecular techniques to cytologically confirmed LSIL be 'lumped' together.[115] ASCUS would essentially disappear since HPV-negative ASCUS could safely be called 'benign' and followed routinely, and HPV-positive ASCUS could be called LSIL or 'HPV infection' to reflect what is now known about the natural history of this lesion. The risk of missing significant lesions could be further decreased by referral for immediate colposcopy of the small percentage of ASCUS that are suggestive HSIL, such as atypical metaplastic cells.[116]

HPV testing in other countries

Groups in both The Netherlands and the UK have suggested that HPV testing could be used as an adjunct test in primary cervical cancer screening.[99,112] They recommend that HPV testing for a limited number of oncogenic types be done in conjunction with cytology for women older than 30 years of age and increasing the screening interval from 3 to 5 years in women aged between 30 and 60 years old. In women under the age of 30 years, they suggest primary screening by Pap smear cytology first because of the relatively high prevalence of oncogenic HPV types. HPV testing is performed only if abnormal cells (less serious than HSIL) are identified and patients with HSIL are immediately referred for colposcopy. The appropriate time interval between cervical cancer screenings has not been established. Some suggest that the interval can be at least 6 years or even 8–10 years by combining cytology and HPV testing.[99]

Cervical cancer is the most common cause of cancer in much of Africa, South and Central America, Southeast Asia and other developing countries.[40] While the issue in the developed countries is whether HPV testing should be added to the existing cytology-based screening program, in countries where screening is non-existent, or is ineffective, the current issue is screening by cytology versus by HPV testing.[117] Primary HPV testing has been suggested as a possible primary screening technique because the cost and expertise required to conduct cytological screening is beyond the capacity of most developing countries. The effectiveness and feasibility of this approach has recently been ascertained in South Africa[118] and Costa Rica.[119] HPV testing with self-collected vaginal samples and Papanicolaou smear showed comparable sensitivity in detecting HSIL and invasive cancer (66 per cent versus 68 per cent).[118] However, the false-positive rate dependent on the cut-off point was significantly higher for HPV testing than for cytology. Certain technical issues and the cost-effectiveness of primary screening with HPV DNA testing need to be further evaluated before this approach can be widely applied.

Centralization of laboratories and treatment facilities and the establishment of a countrywide information system could help to optimize the resources already available,[120] regardless of which screening approach is adapted.

HPV vaccine

Immunization of dogs, cattle and rabbits with papillomavirus vaccines has proven effective in preventing the development of PV-related diseases. HPV vaccines for humans are currently in the preliminary stages. The rationale for developing a prophylactic vaccine includes the following: (1) cervical cancer is linked to sexually acquired HPV infection; (2) HPV is etiologically implicated in nearly all cervical cancers; (3) relatively few HPV types account for the majority of cervical cancers; and (4) host immune responses to HPV appear to be important in controlling HPV infection. Prophylactic strategies have focused on the induction of the humoral immune response against virus-like particles that do not contain any viral DNA and are capable of inducing high titers of strongly neutralizing type-specific antibodies to HPV. Treatment of existing HPV infection is targeted on enhancing viral antigen recognition of the oncogenic proteins E6 and E7. For more detail on vaccine development and discussion of the future implications of a prophylactic HPV vaccine, the reader is referred to recent reviews.[121,122]

Potential impact on cervical cancer screening

Human papillomavirus testing would significantly decrease the need for cytology screening by reducing the number of repeat Pap tests and by lengthening the screening intervals. In some countries, HPV DNA testing has the potential to become the primary screening test for cervical cancer. The introduction of effective HPV vaccines directed against the most oncogenic viral types would have a major impact on cervical cancer screening. Cytological abnormalities would become increasingly rare and more often related to less oncogenic viral types that rarely persist and progress to neoplastic lesions. In this setting, automated screening could efficiently classify the great majority of cytological samples as normal and the demand for manual screening of microscopic slides would significantly decrease. Therefore, one might predict that cytotechnologists and cytopathologists of the future will expand their roles as microscopists to include operating automatic screeners, HPV testing and integration of multidisciplinary information.

Acknowledgments: Dr Sherman has received research support from Cytyc Corporation (Boxborough, MA, USA), Digene Corporation (Silver Spring, MD, USA) and Merck (Westpoint, PA, USA) and has pending support from AutoCyte (Burlington, NC, USA).

REFERENCES

1 Koutsky L. Epidemiology of genital human papillomavirus infection. *Am J Med* 1997; **102**: 3–8.

2 Ho GY, Bierman R, Beardsley L, Chang CJ, Burk RD. Natural history of cervicovaginal papillomavirus infection in young women. *N Engl J Med* 1998; **338**: 423–8.

3 Chow LT, Broker TR. Papillomavirus DNA replication. *Intervirology* 1994; **37**: 150–8.

4 Turek LP. The structure, function, and regulation of papillomaviral genes in infection and cervical cancer. *Adv Virus Res* 1994; **44**: 305–56.

5 de Villiers EM. Human pathogenic papillomavirus types: an update. *Curr Top Microbiol Immunol* 1994; **186**: 1–12.

6 Bosch FX, Manos MM, Munoz N, et al. Prevalence of human papillomavirus in cervical cancer: a worldwide perspective. International biological study on cervical cancer (IBSCC) Study Group [see comments]. *J Natl Cancer Inst* 1995; **87**: 796–802.

7 Pecoraro G, Morgan D, Defendi V. Differential effects of human papillomavirus type 6, 16, and 18 DNAs on immortalization and transformation of human cervical epithelial cells. *Proc Natl Acad Sci USA* 1989; **86**: 563–7.

8 Dyson N, Howley PM, Munger K, Harlow E. The human papilloma virus-16 E7 oncoprotein is able to bind to the retinoblastoma gene product. *Science* 1989; **243**: 934–7.

9 Werness BA, Levine AJ, Howley PM. Association of human papillomavirus types 16 and 18 E6 proteins with p53. *Science* 1990; **248**: 76–9.

10 Crook T, Fisher C, Masterson PJ, Vousden KH. Modulation of transcriptional regulatory properties of p53 by HPV *E6*. *Oncogene* 1994; **9**: 1225–30.

11 Munger K, Scheffner M, Huibregtse JM, Howley PM. Interactions of HPV E6 and E7 oncoproteins with tumour suppressor gene products. *Cancer Surv* 1992; **12**: 197–217.

12 Lechner MS, Laimins LA. Inhibition of p53 DNA binding by human papillomavirus E6 proteins. *J Virol* 1994; **68**: 4262–73.

13 Cullen AP, Reid R, Campion M, Lorincz AT. Analysis of the physical state of different human papillomavirus DNAs in intraepithelial and invasive cervical neoplasms. *J Virol* 1991; **65**: 606–12.

14 Durst M, Croce CM, Gissmann L, Schwarz E, Huebner K. Papillomavirus sequences integrate near cellular oncogenes in some cervical carcinomas. *Proc Natl Acad Sci USA* 1987; **84**: 1070–4.

15 Choo KB, Pan CC, Han SH. Integration of human papillomavirus type 16 into cellular DNA of cervical carcinoma: preferential deletion of the *E2* gene and invariable retention of the long control region and the *E6/E7* open reading frames. *Virology* 1987; **161**: 259–61.

16 Jeon S, Lambert PF. Integration of human papillomavirus type 16 DNA into the human genome leads to increased stability of *E6* and *E7* mRNAs: implications for cervical carcinogenesis. *Proc Natl Acad Sci USA* 1995; **92**: 1654–8.

17 Arbeit JM, Howley PM, Hanahan D. Chronic estrogen-induced cervical and vaginal squamous carcinogenesis in human papillomavirus type 16 transgenic mice. *Proc Natl Acad Sci USA* 1996; **93**: 2930–5.

18 Taylor JA, Tewari K, Liao SY, Hughes CC, Villarreal LP. Immunohistochemical analysis, human papillomavirus DNA detection, hormonal manipulation, and exogenous gene expression of normal and dysplastic human cervical epithelium in severe combined immunodeficiency mice. *J Virol* 1999; **73**: 5144–8.

19 Storey A, Thomas M, Kalita A, et al. Role of a p53 polymorphism in the development of human papillomavirus-associated cancer [see comments]. *Nature* 1998; **393**: 229–34.

20 Helland A, Langerod A, Johnsen H, Olsen AO, Skovlund E, Borresen-Dale AL. p53 polymorphism and risk of cervical cancer [letter; comment]. *Nature* 1998; **396**: 530–1; discussion 532.

21 Hildesheim A, Schiffman M, Brinton LA, et al. p53 polymorphism and risk of cervical cancer [letter; comment]. *Nature* 1998; **396**: 531–2.

22 Josefsson AM, Magnusson PK, Ylitalo N, et al. p53 polymorphism and risk of cervical cancer [letter; comment]. *Nature* 1998; **396**: 531; discussion 532.

23 Klaes R, Ridder R, Schaefer U, Benner A, von Knebel Doeberitz M. No evidence of p53 allele-specific predisposition in human papillomavirus-associated cervical cancer. *J Mol Med* 1999; **77**: 299–302.

24 Schiffman MH, Bauer HM, Hoover RN, et al. Epidemiologic evidence showing that human papillomavirus infection causes most cervical intraepithelial neoplasia [see comments]. *J Natl Cancer Inst* 1993; **85**: 958–64.

25 Bosch FX, Castellsague X, Munoz N, et al. Male sexual behavior and human papillomavirus DNA: key risk factors for cervical cancer in Spain. *J Natl Cancer Inst* 1996; **88**: 1060–7.

26 zur Hausen H, Gissmann L, Steiner W, Dippold W, Dreger I. Human papilloma viruses and cancer. *Bibl Haematol* **1975**: 569–71.

27 Franco EL. The sexually transmitted disease model for cervical cancer: incoherent epidemiologic findings and the role of misclassification of human papillomavirus infection. *Epidemiology* 1991; **2**: 98–106.

28 Schiffman MH, Schatzkin A. Test reliability is critically important to molecular epidemiology: an example from studies of human papillomavirus infection and cervical neoplasia [see comments]. *Cancer Res* 1994; **54**: 1944s–7s.

29 Walboomers JM, Meijer CJ. Do HPV-negative cervical carcinomas exist? [editorial]. *J Pathol* 1997; **181**: 253–4.

30 Koutsky LA, Holmes KK, Critchlow CW, et al. A cohort study of the risk of cervical intraepithelial neoplasia grade 2 or 3 in relation to papillomavirus infection. *N Engl J Med* 1992; **327**: 1272–8.

31 Liaw KL, Glass AG, Manos MM, et al. Detection of human papillomavirus DNA in cytologically normal women and subsequent cervical squamous intraepithelial lesions. *J Natl Cancer Inst* 1999; **91**: 954–60.

32 Schiffman MH, Burk RD. Human papillomaviruses. In: Evans AS, Kaslow RA, eds. *Viral infections of humans: epidemiology and control*. New York: Plenum Publishing, 1997: 983–1023.

33 Schiffman MH, Brinton LA. The epidemiology of cervical carcinogenesis. *Cancer* 1995; **76**: 1888–901.

34 Kuhn L, Sun XW, Wright Jr TC. Human immunodeficiency virus infection and female lower genital tract malignancy. *Curr Opin Obstet Gynecol* 1999; **11**: 35–9.

35 Apple RJ, Becker TM, Wheeler CM, Erlich HA. Comparison of human leukocyte antigen DR-DQ disease associations found with cervical dysplasia and invasive cervical carcinoma. *J Natl Cancer Inst* 1995; **87**: 427–36.

36 Apple RJ, Erlich HA, Klitz W, Manos MM, Becker TM, Wheeler CM. HLA DR-DQ associations with cervical carcinoma show papillomavirus-type specificity. *Nat Genet* 1994; **6**: 157–62.

37 Hildesheim A, Schiffman M, Scott DR, et al. Human leukocyte antigen class I/II alleles and development of human papillomavirus-related cervical neoplasia: results from a case-control study conducted in the United States. *Cancer Epidemiol Biomarkers Prev* 1998; **7**: 1035–41.

38 McArdle JP, Muller HK. Quantitative assessment of Langerhans' cells in human cervical intraepithelial neoplasia and wart virus infection. *Am J Obstet Gynecol* 1986; **154**: 509–15.

39 Tsukui T, Hildesheim A, Schiffman MH, et al. Interleukin 2 production *in vitro* by peripheral lymphocytes in response to human papillomavirus-derived peptides: correlation with cervical pathology. *Cancer Res* 1996; **56**: 3967–74.

40 Parker SL, Tong T, Bolden S, Wingo PA. Cancer statistics, 1997 [erratum appears in *CA Cancer J Clin* 1997; **47**(2): 68]. *CA Cancer J Clin* 1997; **47**: 5–27.

41 Jones BA. Rescreening in gynecologic cytology. Rescreening of 3762 previous cases for current high-grade squamous intraepithelial lesions and carcinoma – a College of American Pathologists Q-Probes study of 312 institutions. *Arch Pathol Lab Med* 1995; **119**: 1097–103.

42 Hildesheim A, Schiffman MH, Gravitt PE, et al. Persistence of type-specific human papillomavirus infection among cytologically normal women [see comments]. *J Infect Dis* 1994; **169**: 235–40.

43 Melkert PW, Hopman E, van den Brule AJ, et al. Prevalence of HPV in cytomorphologically normal cervical smears, as determined by the polymerase chain reaction, is age-dependent. *Int J Cancer* 1993; **53**: 919–23.

44 Melnikow J, Nuovo J, Willan AR, Chan BK, Howell LP. Natural history of cervical squamous intraepithelial lesions: a meta-analysis. *Obstet Gynecol* 1998; **92**: 727–35.

45 Ostor AG. Natural history of cervical intraepithelial neoplasia: a critical review. *Int J Gynecol Pathol* 1993; **12**: 186–92.

46 Schiffman MH, Brinton LA, Devesa SS, Fraumeni JF. Cervical cancer. In: Schottenfeld D, Fraumeni JF, eds. *Cancer epidemiology and prevention*, 2nd edn. New York: Oxford University Press, 1996: 1090–116.

47 Kiviat NB, Critchlow CW, Kurman RJ. Reassessment of the morphological continuum of cervical intraepithelial lesions: does it reflect different stages in the progression to cervical carcinoma? In: Munoz N, Bosch FX, Shah KV, Meheus A, eds. *The epidemiology of human papillomavirus and cervical cancer*. Lyon: International Agency for Research on Cancer, 1992: 59–66.

48 Remmink AJ, Walboomers JM, Helmerhorst TJ, et al. The presence of persistent high-risk HPV genotypes in dysplastic cervical lesions is associated with progressive disease: natural history up to 36 months. *Int J Cancer* 1995; **61**: 306–11.

49 Bergeron C, Barrasso R, Beaudenon S, Flamant P, Croissant O, Orth G. Human papillomaviruses associated with cervical intraepithelial neoplasia. Great diversity and distinct distribution in low- and high-grade lesions. *Am J Surg Pathol* 1992; **16**: 641–9.

50 Lorincz AT, Reid R, Jenson AB, Greenberg MD, Lancaster W, Kurman RJ. Human papillomavirus infection of the cervix: relative risk associations of 15 common anogenital types. *Obstet Gynecol* 1992; **79**: 328–37.

51 Lungu O, Sun XW, Felix J, Richart RM, Silverstein S, Wright Jr TC. Relationship of human papillomavirus type to grade of cervical intraepithelial neoplasia. *JAMA* 1992; **267**: 2493–6.

52 Stoler MH, Broker TR. *In situ* hybridization detection of human papillomavirus DNAs and messenger RNAs in genital condylomas and a cervical carcinoma. *Hum Pathol* 1986; **17**: 1250–8.

53 Chang DY, Chen RJ, Lee SC, Huang SC. Prevalence of single and multiple infection with human papillomaviruses in various grades of cervical neoplasia. *J Med Microbiol* 1997; **46**: 54–60.

54 Kalantari M, Karlsen F, Johansson B, Sigurjonsson T, Warleby B, Hagmar B. Human papillomavirus findings in relation to cervical intraepithelial neoplasia grade: a study on 476 Stockholm women, using PCR for detection and typing of HPV. *Hum Pathol* 1997; **28**: 899–904.

55 The Atypical Squamous Cells of Undetermined Significance/Low-Grade Squamous Intraepithelial Lesions Triage Study (ALTS) Group. Human papillomavirus testing for triage of women with cytologic evidence of low-grade squamous intraepithelial lesions: baseline data from a randomized trial [see comments]. *J Natl Cancer Inst* 2000; **92**: 397–402.

56 Sherman ME, Schiffman MH, Erozan YS, Wacholder S, Kurman RJ. The Bethesda System. A proposal for reporting abnormal cervical smears based on the reproducibility of cytopathologic diagnoses. *Arch Pathol Lab Med* 1992; **116**: 1155–8.

57 Duggan MA, McGregor SE, Benoit JL, Inoue M, Nation JG, Stuart GC. The human papillomavirus status of invasive cervical adenocarcinoma: a clinicopathological and outcome analysis. *Hum Pathol* 1995; **26**: 319–25.

58 Stoler MH, Mills SE, Gersell DJ, Walker AN. Small-cell neuroendocrine carcinoma of the cervix. A human papillomavirus type 18-associated cancer. *Am J Surg Pathol* 1991; **15**: 28–32.

59 Tenti P, Romagnoli S, Silini E, et al. Human papillomavirus types 16 and 18 infection in infiltrating adenocarcinoma of the cervix: PCR analysis of 138 cases and correlation with histologic type and grade. *Am J Clin Pathol* 1996; **106**: 52–6.

60 Kurman RJ, Schiffman MH, Lancaster WD, et al. Analysis of individual human papillomavirus types in cervical neoplasia: a possible role for type 18 in rapid progression. *Am J Obstet Gynecol* 1988; **159**: 293–6.

61 Walker J, Bloss JD, Liao SY, Berman M, Bergen S, Wilczynski SP. Human papillomavirus genotype as a prognostic indicator in carcinoma of the uterine cervix. *Obstet Gynecol* 1989; **74**: 781–5.

62 Kleter B, van Doorn LJ, ter Schegget J, et al. Novel short-fragment PCR assay for highly sensitive broad-spectrum detection of anogenital human papillomaviruses [see comments]. *Am J Pathol* 1998; **153**: 1731–9.

63 Zehbe I, Wilander E. Human papillomavirus infection and invasive cervical neoplasia: a study of prevalence and morphology. *J Pathol* 1997; **181**: 270–5.

64 Kurman RJ, Malkasian Jr GD, Sedlis A, Solomon D. From Papanicolaou to Bethesda: the rationale for a new cervical cytologic classification. *Obstet Gynecol* 1991; **77**: 779–82.

65 Nuovo GJ, Darfler MM, Impraim CC, Bromley SE. Occurrence of multiple types of human papillomavirus in genital tract lesions. Analysis by *in situ* hybridization and the polymerase chain reaction. *Am J Pathol* 1991; **138**: 53–8.

66 Pirog EC, Chen YT, Isacson C. Mib-1 immunostaining is a beneficial adjunct test for accurate diagnosis of vulvar condyloma acuminatum. *Am J Surg Pathol* 2000; **24**: 1393–9.

67 Huang CC, Kashima ML, Chen H, Shih IM, Kurman RJ, Wu TC. HPV *in situ* hybridization with catalyzed signal amplification and polymerase chain reaction in establishing cerebellar metastasis of a cervical carcinoma. *Hum Pathol* 1999; **30**: 587–91.

68 Lorincz AT. Methods of DNA hybridization and their clinical applicability to human papillomavirus detection. In: Franco E, Monsonego J, eds. *New developments in cervical cancer screening and prevention*. Oxford: Blackwell Science Ltd, 1997: 325–37.

69 Resnick RM, Cornelissen MT, Wright DK, et al. Detection and typing of human papillomavirus in archival cervical cancer specimens by DNA amplification with consensus primers. *J Natl Cancer Inst* 1990; **82**: 1477–84.

70 Snijders PJ, van den Brule AJ, Schrijnemakers HF, Snow G, Meijer CJ, Walboomers JM. The use of general primers in the polymerase chain reaction permits the detection of a broad spectrum of human papillomavirus genotypes. *J Gen Virol* 1990; **71**: 173–81.

71 Qu W, Jiang G, Cruz Y, et al. PCR detection of human papillomavirus: comparison between MY09/MY11 and GP5+/GP6+ primer systems. *J Clin Microbiol* 1997; **35**: 1304–10.

72 Gregoire L, Arella M, Campione-Piccardo J, Lancaster WD. Amplification of human papillomavirus DNA sequences by using conserved primers. *J Clin Microbiol* 1989; **27**: 2660–5.

73 Shibata DK, Arnheim N, Martin WJ. Detection of human papilloma virus in paraffin-embedded tissue using the polymerase chain reaction. *J Exp Med* 1988; **167**: 225–30.

74 Gravitt PE, Peyton CL, Apple RJ, Wheeler CM. Genotyping of 27 human papillomavirus types by using *L1* consensus PCR products by a single-hybridization, reverse line blot detection method. *J Clin Microbiol* 1998; **36**: 3020–7.

75 Kleter B, van Doorn LJ, Schrauwen L, et al. Development and clinical evaluation of a highly sensitive PCR-reverse hybridization line probe assay for detection and identification of anogenital human papillomavirus. *J Clin Microbiol* 1999; **37**: 2508–17.

76 Harper DM, Hildesheim A, Cobb JL, Greenberg M, Vaught J, Lorincz AT. Collection devices for human papillomavirus. *J Fam Pract* 1999; **48**: 531–5.

77 Ferenczy A, Franco E, Arseneau J, Wright TC, Richart RM. Diagnostic performance of Hybrid Capture human papillomavirus deoxyribonucleic acid assay combined with liquid-based cytologic study. *Am J Obstet Gynecol* 1996; **175**: 651–6.

78 Sherman ME, Schiffman MH, Lorincz AT, et al. Cervical specimens collected in liquid buffer are suitable for both cytologic screening and ancillary human papillomavirus testing. *Cancer* 1997; **81**: 89–97.

79 Sherman ME, Schiffman MH, Lorincz AT, et al. Toward objective quality assurance in cervical cytopathology. Correlation of cytopathologic diagnoses with detection of high-risk human papillomavirus types. *Am J Clin Pathol* 1994; **102**: 182–7.

80 Saminathan T, Lahoti C, Kannan V, Kline TS. Postmenopausal squamous-cell atypias: a diagnostic challenge. *Diagn Cytopathol* 1994; **11**: 226–30.

81 Ferenczy A, Jenson AB. Tissue effects and host response. In: Lorincz A, Reid R, eds. *Obstetrics and gynecology clinics of North America: human papillomavirus II*. Vol. 23. Philadelphia: WB Saunders, 1996: 759–82.

82 Kurman RJ, Henson DE, Herbst AL, Noller KL, Schiffman MH. Interim guidelines for management of abnormal cervical cytology. The 1992 National Cancer Institute Workshop. *JAMA* 1994; **271**: 1866–9.

83 Cox JT, Lorincz AT, Schiffman MH, Sherman ME, Cullen A, Kurman RJ. Human papillomavirus testing by hybrid capture appears to be useful in triaging women with a cytologic diagnosis of atypical squamous cells of undetermined significance. *Am J Obstet Gynecol* 1995; **172**: 946–54.

84 Ferris DG, Wright Jr TC, Litaker MS, et al. Triage of women with ASCUS and LSIL on Pap smear reports: management by repeat Pap smear, HPV DNA testing, or colposcopy? [see comments]. *J Fam Pract* 1998; **46**: 125–34.

85 Wright TC, Sun XW, Koulos J. Comparison of management algorithms for the evaluation of women with low-grade cytologic abnormalities. *Obstet Gynecol* 1995; **85**: 202–10.

86 Ferris DG, Wright Jr TC, Litaker MS, et al. Comparison of two tests for detecting carcinogenic HPV in women with Papanicolaou smear reports of ASCUS and LSIL [see comments]. *J Fam Pract* 1998; **46**: 136–41.

87 Wright Jr TC, Lorincz A, Ferris DG, et al. Reflex human papillomavirus deoxyribonucleic acid testing in women with abnormal Papanicolaou smears. *Am J Obstet Gynecol* 1998; **178**: 962–6.

88 Manos MM, Kinney WK, Hurley LB, et al. Identifying women with cervical neoplasia: using human papillomavirus DNA testing for equivocal Papanicolaou results [see comments]. *JAMA* 1999; **281**: 1605–10.

89 Cox JT. Evaluating the role of HPV testing for women with equivocal Papanicolaou test findings [editorial; comment]. *JAMA* 1999; **281**: 1645–7.

90 Crum CP. Detecting every genital papilloma virus infection: what does it mean? [comment]. *Am J Pathol* 1998; **153**: 1667–71.

91 Kaufman RH, Adam E. Is human papillomavirus testing of value in clinical practice? *Am J Obstet Gynecol* 1999; **180**: 1049–53.

92 Goff BA, Atanasoff P, Brown E, Muntz HG, Bell DA, Rice LW. Endocervical glandular atypia in Papanicolaou smears. *Obstet Gynecol* 1992; **79**: 101–4.

93 Kinney WK, Manos MM, Hurley LB, Ransley JE. Where's the high-grade cervical neoplasia? The importance of minimally abnormal Papanicolaou diagnoses. *Obstet Gynecol* 1998; **91**: 973–6.

94 Raab SS, Isacson C, Layfield LJ, Lenel JC, Slagel DD, Thomas PA. Atypical glandular cells of undetermined significance. Cytologic criteria to separate clinically significant from benign lesions. *Am J Clin Pathol* 1995; **104**: 574–82.

95 Ronnett BM, Manos MM, Ransley JE, et al. Atypical glandular cells of undetermined significance (AGUS): cytopathologic features, histopathologic results, and HPV DNA detection. *Hum Pathol* 1999; **30**: 816–25.

96 Crum CP, Genest DR, Krane JF, et al. Subclassifying atypical squamous cells in Thin-Prep cervical cytology correlates with detection of high-risk human papillomavirus DNA. *Am J Clin Pathol* 1999; **112**: 384–90.

97 Clinical Laboratory Improvement Amendments of 1988. Publ no 100–578. *Congress Rec* 1988; **134**: 3828–63.

98 Sherman ME. Quality assurance in cervical cytopathology. In: Franco E, Monsonego J, eds. *New developments in cervical cancer screening and prevention*. Oxford: Blackwell Science Ltd, 1997: 159–62.

99 Meijer CJLM, Rozendaal L, van der Linden JC, Helmerhorst TJM, Voorhorst FJ, Walboomers JMM. Human papillomavirus testing for primary cervical cancer screening. In: Franco E, Monsonego J, eds. *New developments in cervical cancer screening and prevention*. Oxford: Blackwell Science Ltd, 1997: 338–47.

100 Hutchinson ML, Zahniser DJ, Sherman ME, et al. Utility of liquid-based cytology for cervical carcinoma screening: results of a population-based study conducted in a region of Costa Rica with a high incidence of cervical carcinoma. *Cancer* 1999; **87**: 48–55.

101 Sherman ME, Mendoza M, Lee KR, et al. Performance of liquid-based, thin-layer cervical cytology: correlation with reference diagnoses and human papillomavirus testing. *Mod Pathol* 1998; **11**: 837–43.

102 Rozendaal L, Walboomers JM, van der Linden JC, et al. PCR-based high-risk HPV test in cervical cancer screening gives objective risk assessment of women with cytomorphologically normal cervical smears. *Int J Cancer* 1996; **68**: 766–9.

103 Richart RM, Masood S, Syrjanen KJ, et al. Human papillomavirus. International Academy of Cytology Task Force summary. Diagnostic Cytology Towards the 21st Century: An International Expert Conference and Tutorial. *Acta Cytol* 1998; **42**: 50–8.

104 Cuzick J, Szarewski A, Terry G, et al. Human papillomavirus testing in primary cervical screening [see comments]. *Lancet* 1995; **345**: 1533–6.

105 Chua KL, Hjerpe A. Human papillomavirus analysis as a prognostic marker following conization of the cervix uteri. *Gynecol Oncol* 1997; **66**: 108–13.

106 Lombard I, Vincent-Salomon A, Validire P, et al. Human papillomavirus genotype as a major determinant of the course of cervical cancer. *J Clin Oncol* 1998; **16**: 2613–19.

107 Nakagawa S, Yoshikawa H, Onda T, Kawana T, Iwamoto A, Taketani Y. Type of human papillomavirus is related to clinical features of cervical carcinoma. *Cancer* 1996; **78**: 1935–41.

108 Chen TM, Chen CA, Wu CC, Huang SC, Chang CF, Hsieh CY. The genotypes and prognostic significance of human papillomaviruses in cervical cancer. *Int J Cancer* 1994; **57**: 181–4.

109 van Muyden RC, ter Harmsel BW, Smedts FM, et al. Detection and typing of human papillomavirus in cervical carcinomas in Russian women: a prognostic study. *Cancer* 1999; **85**: 2011–16.

110 Hildesheim A, Hadjimichael O, Schwartz PE, et al. Risk factors for rapid-onset cervical cancer. *Am J Obstet Gynecol* 1999; **180**: 571–7.

111 Cox JT, Schiffman MH, Winzelberg AJ, Patterson JM. An evaluation of human papillomavirus testing as part of referral to colposcopy clinics. *Obstet Gynecol* 1992; **80**: 389–95.

112 Cuzick J, Sasieni P. Estimates of the cost impact of introducing human papillomavirus testing into a cervical screening programme. In: Franco E, Monsonego J, eds. *New Developments in Cervical Cancer Screening and Prevention*. Oxford: Blackwell Science Ltd, 1997: 364–72.

113 Schiffman M, Adrianza ME. ASCUS–LSIL Triage Study. Design, methods and characteristics of trial participants. *Acta Cytol* 2000; **44**: 726–42.

114 Solomon D, Schiffman M, Tarone R for the ALTS Group. Comparison of three management strategies for patients with atypical squamous cells of undetermined significance: baseline results from a randomised trial. *J Natl Cancer Inst* 2001; **93**: 293–9.

115 Schiffman M, Solomon D, Liaw KL, Sherman M. Why, how and when the cytologic diagnosis of ASCUS should be eliminated. *J Lower Tract Dis* 1998; **2**: 165–9.

116 Sherman ME, Tabbara SO, Scott DR, et al. 'ASCUS, rule out HSIL': cytologic features, histologic correlates, and human papillomavirus detection. *Mod Pathol* 1999; **12**: 335–42.

117 Cuzick J. Human papillomavirus testing for primary cervical cancer screening [editorial]. *JAMA* 2000; **283**: 108–9.

118 Wright Jr TC, Denny L, Kuhn L, Pollack A, Lorincz A. HPV DNA testing of self-collected vaginal samples compared with cytologic screening to detect cervical cancer. *JAMA* 2000; **283**: 81–6.

119 Schiffman M, Herrero R, Hildesheim A, et al. HPV DNA testing in cervical cancer screening: results from women in a high-risk province of Costa Rica. *JAMA* 2000; **283**: 87–93.

120 Herrero R, Schiffman MH, Hildesheim A, et al. Is cervical cancer cytological screening valuable in developing countries? In: Franco E, Monsonego J, eds. *New Developments in Cervical Cancer Screening and Prevention.* Oxford: Blackwell Science Ltd, **1997**: 241–9.

121 Murakami M, Gurski KJ, Steller MA. Human papillomavirus vaccines for cervical cancer. *J Immunother* 1999; **22**: 212–18.

122 Sherman ME, Schiffman MH, Strickler H, Hildesheim A. Prospects for a prophylactic HPV vaccine: rationale and future implications for cervical cancer screening. *Diagn Cytopathol* 1998; **18**: 5–9.

7

Benign (squamous) cellular changes

JEFFREY A STEAD

INTRODUCTION

The original and current primary goal of screening with Papanicolaou smears is to detect neoplastic cells, including malignant cells and their precursors. Benign, non-neoplastic cellular changes, however, are important because they can mimic neoplastic changes and may also indicate specific infections or offending agents that can be subject to treatment. The awareness of normal cellular components and benign cellular changes on a Pap smear is a prerequisite for recognizing the neoplastic cells.

WITHIN NORMAL LIMITS

For a slide to be within 'normal limits', no cellular atypicality, including reactive changes or infectious agents other than the normal flora, should be noted. Many types of squamous and glandular cells, including endometrial cells, may be normally seen. The presence of endometrial cells should be consistent with the clinical picture, such as menstrual and hormonal status. The hormonal status should be congruent with the age and history, including menopausal status, post-partum state, and use of hormones.

Squamous cells

For a Pap smear to be considered adequate, at least 10 per cent of the slide should be covered by squamous cells. Superficial, intermediate, and parabasal squamous cells may be present in varying proportions. Superficial squamous cells are the most mature of the squamous cells. They are large and polygonal with small, dark, pyknotic nuclei, and their cytoplasm usually stains pink. They predominate in conditions of estrogen stimulation such as the first half of the menstrual cycle. Intermediate squamous cells are less mature. They are still large and

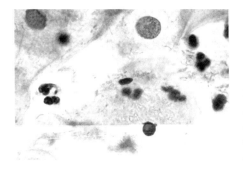

Figure 7.1 *Superficial and intermediate cell. The superficial cell has the smaller, darker nucleus. The intermediate cell has a larger nucleus with a more open chromatin pattern (conventional smear, original magnification ×100).*

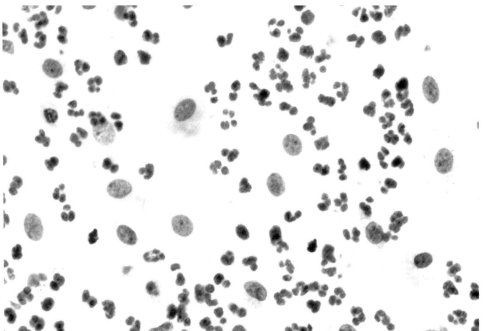

Figure 7.2 *Atrophic Pap smear. The smear is composed entirely of parabasal cells in a background of inflammatory cells (conventional smear, original magnification ×40).*

polygonal, but their nuclei are slightly larger than those of superficial squamous cells, and contain finely dispersed chromatin and inconspicuous nucleoli, and their cytoplasm usually stains green (Fig. 7.1). They predominate in conditions of progesterone stimulation such as the second half of the menstrual cycle. Since the cytoplasmic staining varies according to the pH, among other factors, nuclear features are the most reliable means of distinguishing superficial from intermediate squamous cells. Parabasal cells are the least mature squamous cells. They are round to oval, small, and usually have higher nucleus-to-cytoplasm ratios and larger nuclei than those of intermediate squamous cells. They predominate in low hormonal (atrophic) states such as post-menopausal, post-partum, post-bilateral oophorectomy, and pre-menarche (Fig. 7.2).

Endocervical cells

Cells from the transformation zone, whether endocervical or squamous metaplastic cells, are required, under the Bethesda System, for specimen adequacy in any woman who has a cervix.

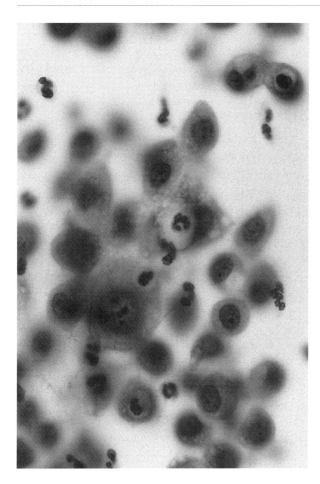

Figure 7.3 *Exodus. This occurs between days 7 and 10 and is composed of endometrial cells, histiocytes, and stromal cells. Better-preserved superficial stromal cells usually resemble histiocytes (conventional smear, original magnification ×100).*

Endocervical cells are mucin-producing columnar cells shed as strips, sheets or individually. In strips (lateral view), the nuclei line up like boards in a picket fence. Sheets (viewed en face) have a honeycomb appearance because of uniform cell size and well-defined cell borders. Whether in strips and sheets or singly, the cells should have abundant clear cytoplasm and round- to oval-shaped nuclei with finely dispersed chromatin and inconspicuous nucleoli. Sheets of endocervical cells may be folded but true stratification should be absent.

Endometrial cells

Endometrial cells may normally be present during the first 12 days of the menstrual cycle. However, their presence later in a cycling woman (out of phase) is usually of little significance, although a polyp or endometritis may be responsible. Their presence in smears from a post-menopausal woman raises the question of endometrial hyperplasia or neoplasia. Spontaneously exfoliated normal endometrial cells are degenerated by nature and, because of their long journey down the endocervical canal, are present as balls of small, dark-blue cells. When degenerated, stromal and glandular epithelial cells appear similar. Better-preserved superficial stromal cells resemble histiocytes and may be seen in 'exodus', which is a discharge of endometrial cells, histiocytes, and stromal cells between days 7 and 10 of a normal cycle (Fig. 7.3). Deep stromal cells are shed during menstruation; they are small, darkly staining, single

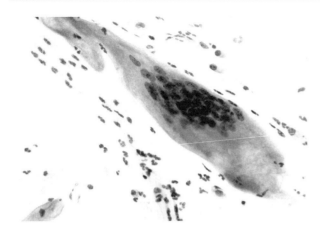

Figure 7.4 *Syncytiotrophoblast. The cell is large with many darkly staining nuclei that lack nuclear irregularity (conventional smear, original magnification ×100).*

rounded or spindly cells. The significance of endometrial cells is often problematic for the laboratory as the date of the last menstrual period and iatrogenic hormonal usage is not always provided in the clinical history. (See Chapter 11 for a detailed discussion of significance of endometrial cells on Pap smears.)

Trophoblastic cells

Rarely, syncytiotrophoblastic cells are seen in smears from pregnant women.[1–3] They are large, multinucleated cells with granular chromatin, and can mimic human papillomavirus (HPV)-infected cells. Their nuclei, however, lack the wrinkled nuclear membranes ('rasinoid' appearance) and the hyperchromasia of dysplastic cells. These nuclei stain more darkly than those of multi-nucleated histiocytes and lack the molding and ground-glass appearance of herpes infection (Fig. 7.4). Cytotrophoblasts are rare and can be difficult to distinguish from severe dysplasia. They are small, single cells with a high nucleus-to-cytoplasm ratio, hyperchromatic nuclei, and occasional prominent nucleoli. The cytoplasm is often basophilic and is either finely vacuolated and blurs with the background, or well outlined and contains few vacuoles that indent the nuclei. Occasionally, the cytotrophoblasts occur in cords or tight clusters and resemble endometrial cells. The presence of trophoblastic cells on Pap smears does not seem to have any clinical significance and is not a reliable indicator of impending abortion.[4]

Decidual cells

Decidualization may occur in the stroma of the cervix of a pregnant woman and may sometimes result in polypoid growths (decidual polyps). Decidual cells may be seen in the Pap smear as individual large, oval to polygonal cells with large nuclei and prominent nucleoli (Fig. 7.5).[2,3] Their cytoplasm stains either basophilic or less commonly eosinophilic. Cytoplasmic extensions between the adjacent cells are common. Abundant cytoplasm often appears degenerated. Atypical cells interpreted as most likely degenerating decidual cells have been reported in 12 per cent of smears from pregnant and post-partum women:[5] it is important not to confuse these with malignant cells. Another potential pitfall is the uncommon presence of cells from Arias–Stella reaction in a cervicovaginal smear during pregnancy.[6] Cells from Arias–Stella reaction have abundant vacuolated cytoplasm and prominent nucleoli (Fig. 7.6). They need to be distinguished from clear cell carcinoma cells, which have much higher nucleus-to-cytoplasm ratios.

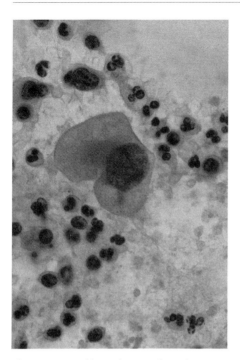

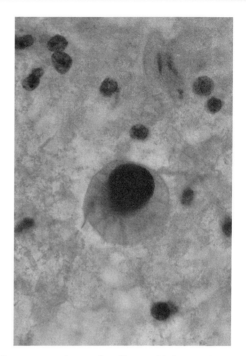

Figure 7.5 *Decidua. The cytoplasm is abundant and granular with a vesicular nucleus and nucleolus (conventional smear, original magnification ×100).*

Figure 7.6 *Arias–Stella effect. Cells from Arias–Stella reaction have abundant vacuolated cytoplasm and prominent nucleoli. In contrast to neoplastic cells, their nucleus to cytoplasm ratio is not increased (conventional smear, original magnification ×100).*

IATROGENIC CHANGES

Radiation

Pap smears are routinely used to follow patients with genital cancer treated with irradiation for the detection of recurrent tumor and post-radiation dysplasia.[7,8] It is essential to be familiar with radiation-induced changes/atypia and to distinguish these changes from neoplastic changes. Irradiated cells are not all killed immediately. The cells and their nuclei may continue to divide. Conversely, the cells may lose the ability to divide while their nuclei continue to do so, leading to multinucleation. If both cytoplasm and nuclei of proliferating cells lose the ability to divide, both may enlarge. In either case, there is cytomegaly, with a normal or near-normal nucleus-to-cytoplasm ratio for affected cells. Cytoplasmic vacuoles are also common. Cellular and nuclear enlargement with a normal or near-normal nucleus-to-cytoplasm ratio, cytoplasmic polychromasia and vacuolization, and slightly hyperchromatic nuclei with smudged chromatin are typical features of radiated cells (Fig. 7.7A). Multinucleation is common (Fig. 7.7B). All or some of these changes may be present, and affected cells occur singly and in groups. When these changes, individually or multiply, are pronounced, the cells affected may appear quite bizarre. Radiation-induced changes have been detected in 28 per cent of the Pap smears taken from 88 women within the first 4 months after radiotherapy.[9] Radiation changes usually subside gradually after 1 year following treatment,[10] however, they may sometimes persist for prolonged periods, perhaps even for the life of the patient.[11]

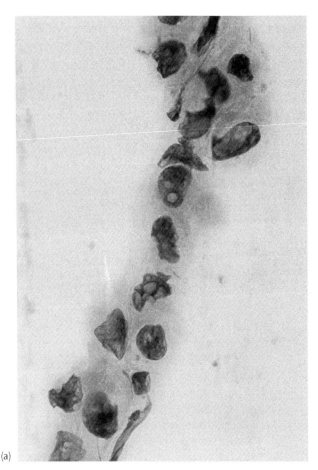

(a)

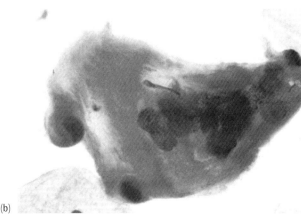

(b)

Figure 7.7 *Radiation changes. (a) The cells are somewhat air-dried and exhibit a smudged nuclear chromatin pattern. Cytoplasmic vacuolization and polychromasia may also be seen (conventional smear, original magnification ×100). (b) Multinucleated cells are common in Pap smears from irradiated women. The nuclear and cytoplasmic changes resulting from radiation are also commonly observed (conventional smear, original magnification ×100).*

Irradiated cancer cells may undergo similar nuclear and cellular enlargement, but have hyperchromatic nuclei and an increased nucleus-to-cytoplasm ratio. Cancer cells showing radiation changes may be seen in the Pap smear for several weeks following therapy. However, they may or may not represent viable tumor.

Radiation changes were studied in 2020 sequential vaginal smears collected from 101 patients with cancer of the uterine cervix at 12–14 days, 15–24 days, and 25 days to 6 weeks following radiotherapy at cumulative doses of 1500 rad, 2000–2500 rad, and 3500 rad or more.[12] According to this study, radiation-induced cell changes are seen in vaginal smears soon after initiation of radiation treatment. The percentage of cells exhibiting these changes can vary from only about 5 per cent in some smears to more than 70 per cent in others. Changes observed at 12–14 days (1500 rad), 15–24 days (2000–2500 rad) and 25 days to 6 weeks (3500 rad or more) were similar. The effects of radiation on benign cells and cancer cells are also similar. However, radiation-induced changes appear in benign cells earlier than in cancer cells. First to be affected are the metabolically active parabasal cells, followed by intermediate cells and superficial cells. Cytoplasmic changes generally precede nuclear changes. Cytoplasmic changes include enlargement, vacuolization, ground-glass appearance and perinuclear halos. Nuclear changes include enlargement of both nuclei and nucleoli, wrinkling of the nuclear membrane, multinucleation, chromatin clumping, pyknosis, karyorrhexis and loss of nuclei. Bizarre cells are not uncommon, and distinguishing bizarre benign cells from cancer cells can be difficult.

The same study also showed that during radiation treatment, neutrophils are almost always present in increased numbers, as are histiocytes, which may exhibit phagocytosis of red blood cells and degenerated cellular material. In this study, mean cancer cell percentage decreased from approximately 42 per cent in pretreatment smears to 19 per cent after 12–14 days, 9 per cent after 15–24 days, and 7 per cent after 25 days to 6 weeks. Complete clearing of cancer cells was seen in approximately 26 per cent of smears after 12–14 days, 63 per cent after 15–24 days and 83 per cent after 25 days to 6 weeks. Smears can be classified as good response (rapid clearing of cancer cells), delayed response and poor response. Cancer cells in the first post-radiation treatment smear were not significant, however, if persisting after 4 months, portended a relatively poor prognosis.[12]

Post-radiation dysplasia is cervical intraepithelial neoplasia (CIN)-like atypia that develops within several months to many years of radiation treatment. If it develops within the first 3 years, there is a significant risk of progression to carcinoma.[13,14]

Radiation changes superimposed on those of repair may result in cells that appear quite bizarre, although these are not usually numerous. A helpful feature is that, as in typical repair, irradiated repair cells are usually seen in cohesive groups.[15]

Chemotherapy

Chemotherapeutic agents may induce changes similar to those caused by radiation. Some of these changes resemble folate/B_{12} deficiency. These changes are reversible and the affected cells are not usually numerous.[16] A more common finding, also reversible, is a hormonal pattern resembling atrophy.[16,17] However, the most common finding is a normal cellular pattern.[18] Malignant and premalignant changes in squamous epithelial cells are probably not related to the effects of chemotherapy.[16,18]

Hormonal therapy (other than estrogen replacement)

Progestational agents in large doses result in an intermediate cell pattern in which 90 per cent or more of squamous epithelial cells in the smear are intermediate cells. Tamoxifen may produce estrogenic changes in Pap smears,[19] but the role of cervical screening in following such women for endometrial pathology remains controversial.[20]

Laser and loop electrocautery excision procedure

When an epithelial abnormality is detected on Pap smear and/or biopsy, the transformation zone may be excised for definitive diagnosis and treatment. A cone biopsy may be done

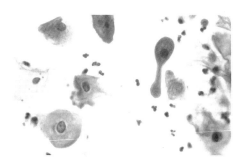

Figure 7.8 *Laser effect. There is a smudgy appearance of both cytoplasm and nucleus (conventional smear, original magnification ×100).*

surgically (cold-knife cone) or by laser. The loop electrocautery excision procedure (LEEP) has become a popular alternative because it can be done on an outpatient basis, even in an office setting, under colposcopic guidance. It has the advantage of being easy to perform. A disadvantage is the electrocautery artifact in tissue removed for histological diagnosis. A follow-up Pap smear should not be taken after a LEEP or laser or cold-knife cone until the surgical site has had ample opportunity to heal, otherwise atypia associated with repair of thermal injury may hamper interpretation. This atypia most frequently manifests as 'taffy-pulled' nuclei in elongated endocervical cells, cell aggregates with coalesced cytoplasm, hockey stick nuclei, notched and enlarged nuclei, and smudgy chromatin; bleeding may also partly obscure cellular details (Fig. 7.8).[21]

Intrauterine contraceptive devices

Inflammation and various reactive and reparative changes are common in women using intrauterine contraceptive devices (IUDs). The IUDs may elicit a foreign body reaction. In addition, two types of reactive glandular atypia involving endometrial and endocervical cells may be observed.[22] One resembles adenocarcinoma. Vacuolated or signet-ring-type cells with enlarged nuclei and prominent nucleoli may occur in small groups. Single cells, however, which are common in adenocarcinoma, are uncommon in this reactive pattern. Another pattern consisting of single non-vacuolated cells with a high nucleus-to-cytoplasm ratio resembles high-grade squamous intraepithelial lesion (HSIL), except that these atypical cells contain conspicuous nucleoli that are usually absent in HSIL. These atypical cells may persist in Pap smears for several months after removal of an IUD. Endometrial cells may be seen in the smear of a woman using an IUD at any time. Squamous metaplastic cells and inflammation are also common.[23] *Actinomyces* infection of endometrium is a well-known complication in women using IUDs,[24] and can be seen on Pap smears.

NUTRITIONAL CHANGES

B$_{12}$/folate deficiency

In vitamin B$_{12}$ or folate deficiency, changes similar to those seen with radiation and chemotherapy may be seen. There may be multinucleation and cytoplasmic polychromasia (Fig. 7.9). The main features are enlargement of both the cells and their nuclei with normal nucleus-to-cytoplasm ratio. These enlarged cells may be mistaken for dysplasia (usually low-grade). Their nuclei do not exhibit the hyperchromasia and irregularities of neoplastic cells. If B$_{12}$/folate deficiency is considered, the number of lobes of polymorphonuclear leukocytes should be counted as increased number of lobes would confirm this diagnosis.[11]

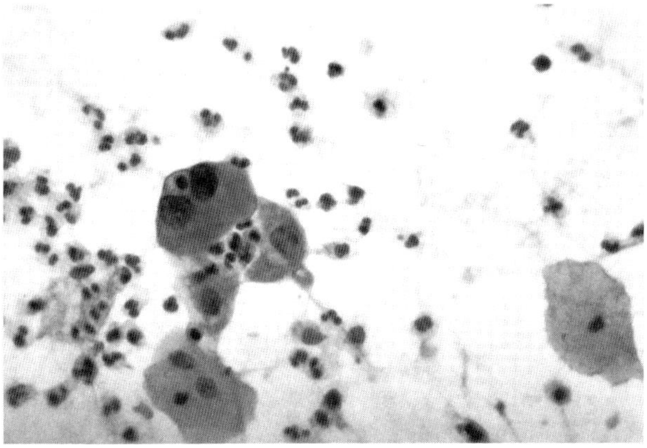

Figure 7.9 *B$_{12}$/folate deficiency. Note the resemblance to radiation changes. Multinucleation and cytoplasmic polychromasia are common. There are often more than seven lobes in polymorphonuclear leukocytes in the background (conventional smear, original magnification ×40).*

INFECTIONS (OTHER THAN HPV)

Inflammation and inflammatory changes

The presence of inflammatory cells does not necessarily imply the presence of active inflammation of the cervix.[25] There may be many inflammatory cells without epithelial cell changes that can be related to the effects of inflammation. The inflammation may be all catarrhal. A variety of non-specific cellular changes due to inflammation may occur. There may be decreased staining intensity, or cytoplasmic polychromasia. Cellular enlargement and cytoplasmic vacuoles, which may contain neutrophils, may be seen. Nuclei may become mildly to moderately enlarged and even slightly hyperchromatic; chromatin clumping may occur, but it is not irregular. Nuclear membranes have uniform thickness, but may become slightly irregular in shape, and perinuclear halos are sometimes present. Nuclei may also accumulate excess water and undergo hydropic degeneration resulting in loss of chromatin pattern.

Normal flora/lactobacilli

The biofilm of the vagina is populated by a community of microorganisms that is normally dominated by rod-shaped lactobacilli. They are Gram positive and stain blue with the Papanicolaou stain. They metabolize glycogen in squamous cells. When there is an overgrowth of lactobacilli, they may destroy many intermediate squamous cells by consuming their glycogen, resulting in cytolysis, which is a profusion of naked nuclei of intermediate squamous cells. Cytolysis may sometimes be mistaken for dysplasia if the observer over-interprets nuclear enlargement caused by air-drying, when in fact dysplastic cells typically lack significant glycogen and therefore seldom undergo cytolysis.[15] Cytolysis may be one cause of a 'ratty' background (cluttered with granular debris) on a liquid-based Pap test. Cocci and coccobacilli may also be present in normal individuals. When conditions change, such that the biofilm of the vagina is no longer composed of lactobacilli, there is said to be a 'shift in flora', which may, or may not, be associated with a clinical disorder such as bacterial vaginosis.

Coccobacilli/*Gardnerella*

If the community in the biofilm of the vagina is altered (shift in flora) such that a 'predominance of coccobacilli' is present, bacterial vaginosis may be present. Bacterial vaginosis is a clinical

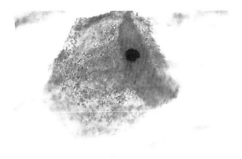

Figure 7.10 *Clue cells. These are squamous cells covered by coccobacillary forms and are indicative of bacterial vaginosis (shift in vaginal flora; conventional smear, original magnification ×100).*

condition associated with itching, burning and a thin, milky, yellow-gray discharge which has a foul fishy smell (positive 'whiff' test) when mixed with 10 per cent potassium hydroxide. *Gardnerella vaginalis* has long been considered the causative agent. Most infections are, however, probably polymicrobial. The term anaerobic pattern has been suggested for patterns of small bacteria seen on Pap smears that lack a predominance of large bacilli (lactobacilli), because the majority of these smears contain a mixture of microorganisms.[26] Also, clue cells (squamous epithelial cells coated by small coccobacilli) should be reported, as they are highly sensitive for detecting a shift in flora from *Lactobacillus*-predominant to a mixed anaerobic/ *G. vaginalis* population likely to be associated with bacterial vaginosis, even though such cells are not particularly sensitive specifically for the presence of *G. vaginalis* (Fig. 7.10).

Gardnerella vaginalis has been cultured from 89 per cent of patients with anaerobic-type smears containing clue cells and 88 per cent of such smears with no clue cells. *Mobiluncus* sp. has been cultured from 83 per cent of patients with anaerobic-type smears containing curved bacilli and from 14 per cent of such smears lacking them.[26] *Gardnerella* may also be cultured from the vaginal biofilm of clinically healthy women.[27] Other bacteria, including *Lactobacillus*, can also coat cells; they are usually also found in large numbers in the background. In contrast, the coccobacilli associated with bacterial vaginosis tend to coat the clue cells only and leave the background clean. Neutrophils are usually scanty, and *Lactobacilli* are absent in cases of bacterial vaginosis. According to the Bethesda System, when a predominance of coccobacilli is present, with or without clue cells, the smear should be reported as 'bacteria morphologically consistent with shift in vaginal flora.' Clinical correlation is essential, as the associated cytological findings are neither sufficient, by themselves, nor necessary for the diagnosis of bacterial vaginosis.

Trichomonas

Trichomonas vaginalis is an 8–30 μm motile, pear-shaped protozoan. Each has a flagellum that may be seen on wet preparations, although it is not seen on Pap smears. To avoid confusion with degenerated cell fragments and other debris, it is necessary for the organism's narrow, elongated nucleus to be identified for diagnosis; identification of red cytoplasmic granules is also very helpful, but they are not always present (Fig. 7.11).

When trichomonads are present in small numbers, patients are usually asymptomatic carriers. When clinical infection is present, it may be manifested by burning, itching, and yellow-green discharge. The Pap smear contains evidence of inflammation, including increased numbers of lymphocytes.[28] Maturation of superficial squamous cells is retarded; some appear metaplastic or almost parakeratotic, and others may have darkly-staining nuclei and indistinct perinuclear halos and mimic a low-grade squamous intraepithelial lesion (LSIL).

Leptothrix is a non-pathogenic, long, filamentous bacterium, which is often seen in the background. It is said to have a spaghetti-like appearance. Small, pear-shaped trichomonads are usually present when *Leptothrix* is, although the reverse does not hold true (with 'spaghetti',

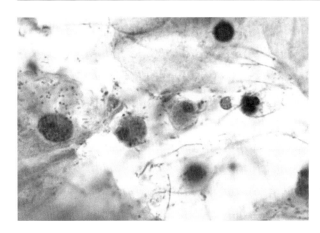

Figure 7.11 Trichomonas. *Note the small forms in the background. A faint nucleus is observed. Trichomonads are often observed in conjunction with* Leptothrix, *seen here, as long, slender, filamentous bacterial forms (conventional smear, original magnification ×100).*

start looking for the 'meatballs'!). *Leptothrix* are thicker, and generally longer, than filamentous forms of *Lactobacilli*.

Candida

Alterations in the community of the vaginal biofilm associated with changes in pH, such as in pregnancy, immune suppression (debilitated states, use of steroids), antibiotic treatment and diabetes mellitus, may be associated with infections by *Candida albicans* or *Candida glabrata* (*Torulopsis*).[15] These infections may be asymptomatic, or may be manifested by burning, itching and a thick, white, cheesy discharge. Yeasts are 3–7 μm and may exhibit budding. When only yeasts are seen, *C. glabrata* is the likely organism. In *C. albicans* infections, hyphae and yeasts are usually both present. *Candida* is eosinophilic on the Papanicolaou stain and the hyphae may appear as tangled masses. The Pap smear detects approximately 80 per cent of *Candida* infections.

Herpes

Infections may be caused by Herpes simplex types I or II, which are morphologically identical. Infected cells characteristically are large and multinucleated. Infected cells with single nuclei may also be found early in the infection and may be confused with HSIL. When multiple, the nuclei may exhibit molding. Nuclei have a pale ground-glass appearance, and a scant amount of chromatin marginated peripherally beneath the nuclear membrane, making it appear thickened (Fig. 7.12). A centrally located eosinophilic (Cowdry Type A) viral inclusion may be present.

Reactive endocervical cells exhibiting nuclear molding or multinucleation that can mimic herpes virus are a potential pitfall in the cytological diagnosis of herpes infection.[29] Ground-glass chromatin has been found to be 95 per cent sensitive and specific; intranuclear inclusions, while pathognomonic, were found to have a sensitivity of only 42 per cent in one study.[29]

Chlamydia

Chlamydia trachomatis is a common sexually transmitted pathogen. It is the most common cause of non-gonococcal cervicitis and urethritis, and accounts for many cases of endometritis and pelvic inflammatory disease. Many infections are asymptomatic. Attempts to diagnose

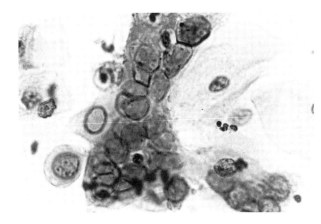

Figure 7.12 *Herpes viral cytopathic effect. Note the multinucleated cells with ground-glass chromatin pattern due to chromatin margination that are molded to each other (conventional smear, original magnification ×100).*

Chlamydia on cytology triggered numerous studies with the following consensus: *Chlamydia* cannot be reliably diagnosed by cytology.[30] Cytological findings can include inflammation, squamous metaplasia, and repair. Inflammation varies from mild to intense and can consist of a mixture of transformed lymphocytes, corresponding to follicular cervicitis on histology, or neutrophils. Cytoplasmic vacuoles or targetoid cytoplasmic inclusions have been described. The cytology findings, however, lack diagnostic sensitivity or specificity,[31,32] and most laboratories employ culture or immunoassay for diagnosis.[33]

Human immunodeficiency virus infection

Human immunodeficiency virus (HIV) has been detected in cervical secretions from HIV-infected women.[34,35] Antigens have been detected in mononuclear cells in the cervical submucosa and mucosa and in endothelial cells of cervical biopsies. No specific changes associated with this infection have been reported on Pap smear.

Actinomyces

Infections with *Actinomyces* are uncommon. Most occur in women that have an IUD. Long, branching filamentous organisms form tangled clumps. Indistinct basophilic masses of bacteria may be present. Granules are larger and consist of colonies of *Actinomyces* with adherent neutrophils. While usually of no clinical significance, approximately 15 per cent of cases are associated with pelvic inflammatory disease.[36] There is no general agreement on how these women should be treated. However, if pelvic inflammatory disease is suspected, the IUD should be removed and antibiotics should be given.[37]

Rare infections

All the following infections are uncommon, but have been reported in the literature.[38] Amebiasis caused by *Entamoeba histolytica* is usually associated with cancers. Amebas may be mistaken for large histiocytes. Cytomegalovirus infection may rarely be seen in the cervical/vaginal smears of ill or apparently healthy individuals. Enlarged nuclei contain characteristic basophilic inclusions surrounded by a pale halo (Fig. 7.13). Multiple smaller cytoplasmic inclusions may also be present. The virus appears to affect glandular cells of the endocervix. Lymphogranuloma

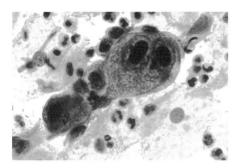

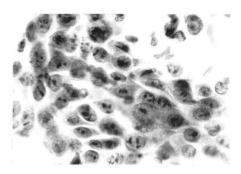

Figure 7.13 *Cytomegalovirus infection. This Pap smear was from a patient infected with human immunodeficiency virus (HIV). There are two large basophilic nuclear inclusions. Cytoplasmic inclusions are also often seen. This infection can be distinguished from Herpes by the lack of molding and the basophilia of the nuclear inclusions (conventional smear, original magnification ×100).*

Figure 7.14 *Reactive/reparative endocervical cells. There is nuclear enlargement and prominent nucleoli, but the cells are arranged in a honeycomb pattern without single cells, nuclear pleomorphism, or a coarsely granular chromatin pattern (conventional smear, original magnification ×100).*

venereum usually involves the labia as an ulcerative condition. Rarely, the cervix is involved. The organisms infect histiocytes and are not seen with the Papanicolaou stain; the Giemsa stain demonstrates them. It is rare to see manifestations of tuberculosis in the Pap smear, but it may be a cause of giant cells. Malakoplakia, a rare disorder, can involve the cervix.[39,40] Characteristic Michaelis–Gutman bodies may be seen on Pap smears of such patients.

REACTIVE AND REPARATIVE CHANGES

Normal or abnormal

Reactive and reparative changes are normal responses by the body to abnormal conditions. Causes may include trauma, infection, radiation or the use of an IUD. Most of the time, reactive squamous epithelial cells exhibit changes that are not striking and the size and shape of the cells and their nuclei exhibit little variability. Nuclei may be slightly enlarged, but not usually more than twice the area of a normal intermediate cell. Nuclear membranes are regular. Hyperchromasia is absent or mild, and chromatin is evenly distributed and fine. However, the responses are sometimes so dramatic, and the cells involved so metabolically active, that distinguishing repair from a significant abnormality, even cancer, is not easy (Fig. 7.14).

Squamous metaplasia

Squamous metaplasia is a common reactive change that occurs at the transformation zone and is particularly common in infection or mechanical irritation. The columnar endocervical cells slough and the reserve cells proliferate to give rise to squamous metaplastic cells. The metaplastic cells resemble parabasal cells and occur in interlocking sheets and as individual cells. Their nuclei may be slightly hyperchromatic and vary slightly in size. Nuclear membranes may become somewhat irregular. When these changes are more pronounced than usual, they may suggest the presence of HSIL and the term 'atypical squamous metaplasia' is sometimes used.[41]

Atypical squamous cells of undetermined significance (ASCUS) is a term used to describe squamous cells that exhibit some, but not all, of the features necessary for diagnosis of SIL. This is discussed in detail in Chapter 8.

Transitional cell metaplasia

Transitional cell metaplasia (TCM) of the uterine cervix and vagina is a newly described entity. It is also a controversial one. The cytological findings in the initial description of TCM were based on observations on histological sections.[42] The cytological findings described included spindled nuclei with tapered ends and frequent longitudinal nuclear grooves, low nucleus-to-cytoplasm ratios, perinuclear halos, and absent to rare mitotic figures. Nuclei were wrinkled, had powdery or smudgy chromatin and nucleoli were inconspicuous. In tissue sections, the nuclei were found to be vertically oriented in the deeper layers and horizontally oriented with a streaming pattern superficially. The diagnosis was an incidental one in all 59 patients. Fifty-seven of the 59 were postmenopausal, and the other two were perimenopausal; ages ranged from 50 to 84 years. Retrospectively, cytological findings considered to represent TCM were found in seven of 127 cervicovaginal smears from 31 patients in whom the diagnosis had been made histologically.

Transitional cell metaplasia of the cervix has been described as a benign condition with the potential to be mistaken for a HSIL.[42–44] Opinions as to the exact nature of TCM vary. One author raises the possibility that it represents the effects of atrophy superimposed upon a squamous intraepithelial lesion, and not simply a benign metaplasia.[45] However, it is argued that TCM is distinguishable from squamous carcinoma *in situ*, as well as tubal metaplasia and atrophy, by the cytological findings of cohesive groups of streaming spindled nuclei with halos, grooves, tapered ends, and wrinkled contours.[46]

Another possibility expressed is that TCM probably represents an uncommon metaplastic reaction to an altered hormonal environment (drop in circulating estrogen and increase in androgen).[43] Distinction of TCM from squamous and glandular areas of the cervix is claimed on the basis of differential cytokeratin staining, with the opinion that it is best called immature transitional metaplasia.[47] This is most likely an uncommon manifestation of cellular atrophy superimposed upon epithelium that has already manifested hyperplastic and/or squamous metaplastic changes.

Papillary immature metaplasia

Papillary immature metaplasia (PIM) is a recently described histological lesion, which involves the upper portion of the transformation zone of the uterine cervix. The metaplasia consists of slender, filiform papillae covered by immature metaplastic cells that are usually positive for HPV 6/11, and is considered to be an exophytic variant of condyloma/LSIL.[48] There is virtual absence of koilocytic atypia often seen in LSIL. Tissue sections lack typical features of HSIL, as the metaplastic cells exhibit uniform nuclear size and staining intensity, multiple chromocenters, and only rare mitoses. Although populations of immature squamous cells may manifest both HSIL and LSIL, PIM has been described as the only well-defined immature LSIL.[49] Areas resembling condyloma or coexisting HSIL may be seen in a minority of cases. PIM is often treated by cone biopsy, but may extend far into the endocervical canal and persist after conization.[50]

Cervicovaginal smears from affected patients reveal atypical metaplastic cells (ASCUS) or LSIL.[51] PIM is a variant of condyloma and some cytological/histological discrepancies may be resolved if PIM is diagnosed histologically.

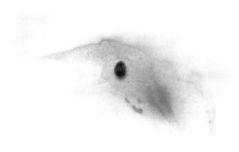

Figure 7.15 *Parakeratosis. Note the orangeophilic, keratinized squamous cell with a pyknotic, darkly staining nucleus (conventional smear, original magnification ×100).*

Hyperkeratosis

Hyperkeratosis is a response of stratified squamous epithelium to chronic irritation and is of no clinical significance by itself.[52,53] Anucleated mature polygonal squamous cells are seen, and may sometimes be numerous. If such cells are isolated, they probably represent nothing serious. Similarly, plaques of such cells usually represent nothing serious. However, jagged keratin plaques are associated with HSIL or squamous carcinoma. In addition, abnormal keratinization associated with abnormal nuclei is indicative of dysplasia.[54] Contamination from skin of the vulva or the hands of a person handling the slide may mimic hyperkeratosis.

Parakeratosis

Parakeratosis without atypia is also a response of stratified squamous epithelium to chronic irritation and is of no clinical significance by itself.[52,53] Parakeratotic squames are small with dense, almost refractile-appearing heavily keratinized orangeophilic cytoplasm and small, pyknotic nuclei (Fig. 7.15). When nuclear atypia is present in parakeratotic cells, they should be classified as an epithelial cell abnormality and may be called 'atypical parakeratotic cells' or 'dyskeratocytes.' Atypical parabasal cells of dyskeratotic appearance are not infrequently encountered in inflamed atrophic smears and may raise the possibility of a keratinizing dysplasia or squamous carcinoma; these cells disappear after a short course of topical estrogen if dysplasia or cancer are not present.

Repair

When injury causes a defect in the epithelium of the cervix, reserve cells at the margin of the defect proliferate to restore the integrity of the epithelium. Usually, this is a fairly orderly process. Repair cells are quite cohesive. They resist being pulled apart, and often have prominent cytoplasmic processes where pulling apart has been attempted or taken place ('taffy-pull'). They form sheets of cells aligned in the same direction (like a school of fish). Single cells are uncommon in repair and, when seen, are usually near a cohesive cluster of repair cells. Conversely, single cells are usually easy to find in cancer. Since they are part of an attempt to rapidly repair damage, repair cells are metabolically active. Such cells may exhibit prominent nuclear and nucleolar enlargement. Nucleoli are often multiple. However, chromatin is usually finely granular and regularly dispersed. Mitotic figures are often seen. Tumor diathesis is absent. Repair cells tend to look more worrisome in bloody smears, but blood alone is not a tumor diathesis.

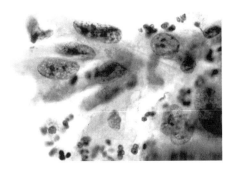

Figure 7.16 *Atypical repair. There is pronounced nuclear atypicality with a coarsely granular chromatin pattern and large irregular nucleoli. However, there is still a stretched-out appearance, and this smear lacked single atypical cells (conventional smear, original magnification ×100).*

Atypical repair

Some repair reactions are difficult to differentiate from carcinoma. Nuclei may be crowded and contain coarsely granular chromatin and large nucleoli (Fig. 7.16). Single cells are more frequent – they tend to be most numerous in the most atypical repair reactions. It is best to diagnose it as an epithelial cell abnormality and make some disclaimer concerning its significance such as 'ASCUS.'

FUTURE DIRECTIONS

Technology is offering us different ways to perform cervical/vaginal (and other) cytological examinations. There is a growing body of literature that suggests that liquid-based thin-layer preparations, such as ThinPrep™ (see Chapter 3), provide consistently better cytological preparations. Cytologists need to become familiar with a new set of artifacts inherent in such preparations. Cells are generally better preserved than in conventional smears. Some patterns, such as streaks of atypical cells, are eliminated and tumor diathesis, for example, appears different. However, for the most part, those familiar with the conventional Pap smear should have no difficulty adapting to liquid-based techniques. These new technologies will probably not completely replace conventional smears in the immediate future. In time, however, everyone who is engaged in the examination of cervical/vaginal cytology specimens will be called upon to examine some liquid-based preparations.

The new technologies also provide new opportunities for diagnosis with ancillary studies. Molecular markers can be applied to the residual materials in the vial to identify specific infections and even to separate atypical repair from a neoplastic process when such markers become available.

REFERENCES

1 Frank TS, Bhat N, Noumoff JS, Yeh IT. Residual trophoblastic tissue as a source of highly atypical cells in the postpartum cervicovaginal smear. *Acta Cytol* 1991; **35**: 105–8.

2 Michael CW, Esfahani FM. Pregnancy-related changes: a retrospective review of 278 cervical smears. *Diagn Cytopathol* 1997; **17**: 99–107.

3 Pisharodi LR, Jovanoska S. Spectrum of cytologic changes in pregnancy. A review of 100 abnormal cervicovaginal smears, with emphasis on diagnostic pitfalls. *Acta Cytol* 1995; **39**: 905–8.

4 Fiorella RM, Cheng J, Kragel PJ. Papanicolaou smears in pregnancy. Positivity of exfoliated cells for human chorionic gonadotropin and human placental lactogen. *Acta Cytol* 1993; **37**: 451–6.

5 Murad TM, Terhart K, Flint A. Atypical cells in pregnancy and postpartum smears. *Acta Cytol* 1981; **25**: 623–30.

6 Mulvany NJ, Khan A, Ostor A. Arias-Stella reaction associated with cervical pregnancy. Report of a case with a cytologic presentation. *Acta Cytol* 1994; **38**: 218–22.

7 McLennan MT, McLennan CE. Significance of cervicovaginal cytology after radiation therapy for cervical carcinoma. *Am J Obstet Gynecol* 1975; **121**: 96–100.

8 Shield PW, Daunter B, Wright RG. Post-irradiation cytology of cervical cancer patients. *Cytopathology* 1992; **3**: 167–82.

9 Rintala MA, Rantanen VT, Salmi TA, Klemi PJ, Grenman SE. PAP smear after radiation therapy for cervical carcinoma. *Anticancer Res* 1997; **17**: 3747–50.

10 Gupta S, Gupta YN, Sanyal B. Radiation changes in vaginal and cervical cytology in carcinoma of the cervix uteri. *J Surg Oncol* 1982; **19**: 71–3.

11 Naib ZM. *Exfoliative Cytopathology*, 3rd edn. Boston/Toronto: Little, Brown and Connoly, 1985.

12 Gupta S, Mukherjee K, Gupta YN, Kumar M. Sequential radiation changes in cytology of vaginal smears in carcinoma of cervix uteri during radiotherapy. *Int J Gynaecol Obstet* 1987; **25**: 303–8.

13 Murad TM, August C. Radiation-induced atypia. A review. *Diagn Cytopathol* 1985; **1**: 137–52.

14 Wentz WB, Reagan JW. Clinical significance of postirradiation dysplasia of the uterine cervix. *Am J Obstet Gynecol* 1970; **106**: 812–17.

15 DeMay R. *The art and science of cytopathology*. Chicago: ASCP Press, 1996.

16 Schachter A, Kopmar A, Avram E, Gorodeski IG, Segal A. Hormonal and cytopathological changes in vaginal and cervical smears from women undergoing chemotherapy for extragenital malignant diseases. *Acta Obstet Gynecol Scand* 1983; **62**: 621–4.

17 Kraus H, Schuhmann R, Ganal M, Geier G. Cytologic findings in vaginal smears from patients under treatment with cyclophosphamide. *Acta Cytol* 1977; **21**: 726–30.

18 Liu K, Marshall J, Shaw HS, Dodge RK, Layfield LJ. Effects of chemotherapy and tamoxifen on cervical and vaginal smears in bone marrow transplant recipients. *Acta Cytol* 1999; **43**: 1027–33.

19 Eells TP, Alpern HD, Grzywacz C, MacMillan RW, Olson JE. The effect of tamoxifen on cervical squamous maturation in Papanicolaou stained cervical smears of post-menopausal women. *Cytopathology* 1990; **1**: 263–8.

20 Seoud M, Shamseddine A, Khalil A, et al. Tamoxifen and endometrial pathologies: a prospective study. *Gynecol Oncol* 1999; **75**: 15–19.

21 Thomas PA. Postprocedural Pap Smears: a LEEP of faith? *Diagn Cytopathol* 1997; **17**: 440–6.

22 Fornari ML. Cellular changes in the glandular epithelium of patients using IUCD – a source of cytologic error. *Acta Cytol* 1974; **18**: 341–3.

23 Kaplan B, Orvieto R, Hirsch M, et al. The impact of intrauterine contraceptive devices on cytological findings from routine Pap smear testing. *Eur J Contracep Reprod Health Care* 1998; **3**: 75–7.

24 Gupta PK, Hollander DH, Frost JK. Actinomycetes in cervico-vaginal smears: an association with IUD usage. *Acta Cytol* 1976; **20**: 295–7.

25 Bertolino JG, Rangel JE, Blake Jr RL, Silverstein D, Ingram E. Inflammation on the cervical Papanicolaou smear: the predictive value for infection in asymptomatic women. *Fam Med* 1992; **24**: 447–52.

26 Schnadig VJ, Davie KD, Shafer SK, Yandell RB, Islam MZ, Hannigan EV. The cytologist and bacterioses of the vaginal–ectocervical area. Clues, commas and confusion. *Acta Cytol* 1989; **33**: 287–97.

27 Hammann R, Kronibus A, Lang N, Werner H. Quantitative studies on the vaginal flora of asymptomatic women and patients with vaginitis and vaginosis. *Zentralbl Bakteriol Mikrobiol Hyg [A]* 1987; **265**: 451–61.

28 Kiviat NB, Paavonen JA, Brockway J, et al. Cytologic manifestations of cervical and vaginal infections. I. Epithelial and inflammatory cellular changes. *JAMA* 1985; **253**: 989–96.

29 Stowell SB, Wiley CM, Powers CN. Herpesvirus mimics. A potential pitfall in endocervical brush specimens. *Acta Cytol* 1994; **38**: 43–50.

30 Bernal JN, Martinez MA, Dabancens A. Evaluation of proposed cytomorphologic criteria for the diagnosis of *Chlamydia trachomatis* in Papanicolaou smears. *Acta Cytol* 1989; **33**: 309–13.

31 Arroyo G, Linnemann C, Wesseler T. Role of the Papanicolaou smear in diagnosis of chlamydial infections. *Sex Transm Dis* 1989; **16**: 11–14.

32 Vinette-Leduc D, Yazdi HM, Jessamine P, Peeling RW. Reliability of cytology to detect chlamydial infection in asymptomatic women. *Diagn Cytopathol* 1997; **17**: 258–61.

33 Addiss DG, Vaughn ML, Golubjatnikov R, Pfister J, Kurtycz DF, Davis JP. Chlamydia trachomatis infection in women attending urban midwestern family planning and community health clinics: risk factors, selective screening, and evaluation of non-culture techniques. *Sex Transm Dis* 1990; **17**: 138–46.

34 Pomerantz RJ, de la Monte SM, Donegan SP, et al. Human immunodeficiency virus (HIV) infection of the uterine cervix. *Ann Intern Med* 1988; **108**: 321–7.

35 Wofsy CB, Cohen JB, Hauer LB, et al. Isolation of AIDS-associated retrovirus from genital secretions of women with antibodies to the virus. *Lancet* 1986; **i**: 527–9.

36 Spence MR, Gupta PK, Frost JK, King TM. Cytologic detection and clinical significance of *Actinomyces israelii* in women using intrauterine contraceptive devices. *Am J Obstet Gynecol* 1978; **131**: 295–8.

37 Dybdahl H, Hastrup J, Baandrup U. The clinical significance of *Actinomyces* colonization as seen in cervical smears. *Acta Cytol* 1991; **35**: 142–3.

38 Cibas ES, Ducatman BS, eds. *Cytology. Diagnostic Principles and Clinical Correlates.* Philadelphia: WB Saunders, 1996.

39 Falcon-Escobedo R, Mora-Tiscareno A, Pueblitz-Peredo S. Malacoplakia of the uterine cervix. Histologic, cytologic and ultrastructural study of a case. *Acta Cytol* 1986; **30**: 281–4.

40 Stewart CJ, Thomas MA. Malacoplakia of the uterine cervix and endometrium. *Cytopathology* 1991; **2**: 271–5.

41 Duggan MA. Cytologic and histologic diagnosis and significance of controversial squamous lesions of the uterine cervix [In Process Citation]. *Mod Pathol* 2000; **13**: 252–60.

42 Weir MM, Bell DA, Young RH. Transitional cell metaplasia of the uterine cervix and vagina: an underrecognized lesion that may be confused with high-grade dysplasia. A report of 59 cases [see comments]. *Am J Surg Pathol* 1997; **21**: 510–17.

43 Egan AJ, Russell P. Transitional (urothelial) cell metaplasia of the uterine cervix: morphological assessment of 31 cases [see comments]. *Int J Gynecol Pathol* 1997; **16**: 89–98.

44 Jones MA. Transitional cell metaplasia and neoplasia in the female genital tract: an update [see comments]. *Adv Anat Pathol* 1998; **5**: 106–13.

45 Koss LG. Transitional metaplasia of cervix: a misnomer [letter; comment]. *Am J Surg Pathol* 1998; **22**: 774–6.

46 Weir MM, Bell DA. Transitional cell metaplasia of the cervix: a newly described entity in cervicovaginal smears. *Diagn Cytopathol* 1998; **18**: 222–6.

47 Harnden P, Kennedy W, Andrew AC, Southgate J. Immunophenotype of transitional metaplasia of the uterine cervix. *Int J Gynecol Pathol* 1999; **18**: 125–9.

48 Ward BE, Saleh AM, Williams JV, Zitz JC, Crum CP. Papillary immature metaplasia of the cervix: a distinct subset of exophytic cervical condyloma associated with HPV-6/11 nucleic acids. *Mod Pathol* 1992; **5**: 391–5.

49 Park JJ, Genest DR, Sun D, Crum CP. Atypical immature metaplastic-like proliferations of the cervix: diagnostic reproducibility and viral (HPV) correlates. *Hum Pathol* 1999; **30**: 1161–5.

50 Trivijitsilp P, Mosher R, Sheets EE, Sun D, Crum CP. Papillary immature metaplasia (immature condyloma) of the cervix: a clinicopathologic analysis and comparison with papillary squamous carcinoma. *Hum Pathol* 1998; **29**: 641–8.

51 Mosher RE, Lee KR, Trivijitsilp P, Crum CP. Cytologic correlates of papillary immature metaplasia (immature condyloma) of the cervix. *Diagn Cytopathol* 1998; **18**: 416–21.

52 Andrews S, Miyazawa K. The significance of a negative Papanicolaou smear with hyperkeratosis or parakeratosis. *Obstet Gynecol* 1989; **73**: 751–3.

53 Nuovo GJ, Nuovo MA, Cottral S, Gordon S, Silverstein SJ, Crum CP. Histological correlates of clinically occult human papillomavirus infection of the uterine cervix. *Am J Surg Pathol* 1988; **12**: 198–204.

54 Navarro M, Furlani B, Songco L, Alfieri ML, Nuovo GJ. Cytologic correlates of benign versus dysplastic abnormal keratinization. *Diagn Cytopathol* 1997; **17**: 447–51.

8

ASCUS (atypical squamous cells of undetermined significance)

AN INCREASING PROBLEM

Atypical squamous cells of undetermined significance (ASCUS) are defined according to the Bethesda System (TBS) as 'squamous cellular abnormalities that are more marked than those attributable to reactive changes but that quantitatively or qualitatively fall short of a definite diagnosis of squamous intraepithelial lesion (SIL). Because the cellular changes in the ASCUS category may reflect an exuberant benign change or a potentially serious lesion, which cannot be classified unequivocally, they are interpreted as being of 'undetermined significance'.[1-3] This diagnostic category was introduced in 1988 by the Bethesda System[1] with the following aims: (1) to provide a uniform standardized terminology for reporting equivocal Pap smears, thus facilitating the communication between cytopathologist and clinician; and (2) to eliminate the ambiguity associated with the vague term 'atypia' which was used to designate anything from benign reactive change to preinvasive cellular change.

The designation of ASCUS under the Bethesda System was not intended to be equivalent to previously used terms such as 'inflammatory atypia', 'reactive atypia', 'koilocytic atypia' or 'Class II Papanicolaou', but rather restricted to squamous abnormalities that are of uncertain significance. Borderline changes cannot always be classified accurately; these should be considered ASCUS. However, clearly reactive cellular or pre-neoplastic/neoplastic changes should not be included in the ASCUS category.

The National Cancer Institute published interim guidelines to suggest that the reporting rate of ASCUS should not exceed 5 per cent, and that a greater frequency may represent overuse of that diagnosis.[4] However, in high-risk populations (e.g. sexually transmitted disease clinics or colposcopy referral centers) with a higher prevalence of SIL, the rate of ASCUS may be correspondingly higher. Therefore, the ASCUS–SIL ratio is a better indicator of its proper use and should be 2–3.[3] The College of American Pathologists (CAP) inter-laboratory comparison program data showed that although ASCUS rates varied widely, the ASCUS–SIL ratio was more constant. The median ASCUS rate was 2.9 per cent with 10 per cent of the laboratories reporting rates greater than 9 per cent. The median ASCUS–SIL ratio was 1.3 and 90 per cent of the laboratories had ratios less than 4.[5]

While most laboratories appear to use the ASCUS category appropriately, ASCUS remains an increasing problem for several reasons, including poor inter-observer reproducibility, variable follow up results and the overwhelming number of women with ASCUS that need to be managed. Minor cytological alterations are most subject to interpretative variability. This difficulty may reflect an attempt to minimize liability, particularly among less experienced cytopathologists, but results in inconsistent diagnoses and subsequent controversy in management. The quandary is further compounded by the clinician's response in the current litigious atmosphere. Therefore, the health-care finance system shoulders the burden of coping with the large number of women needing further evaluation – undoubtedly a problem that will receive further scrutiny as the prevalence of capitated health care reimbursement increases.

CYTOLOGICAL CRITERIA

Atypical squamous cells of undetermined significance encompasses a spectrum of borderline cellular changes. The Bethesda System for reporting cervical/vaginal cytological diagnoses have recently published specific criteria for what constitutes ASCUS.[3] A summary of these features, modified from the Bethesda System Atlas, is listed in Table 8.1 and examples of ASCUS are illustrated in Figs 8.1–8.4.

The nuclear abnormalities of ASCUS are essentially similar to, but of lesser degree than those of low-grade squamous intraepithelial lesions (LSIL). Compared with LSIL, the nuclei of ASCUS are slightly smaller and less hyperchromatic, with generally either mildly coarse, evenly distributed chromatin or smudged and dark chromatin. Mildly coarse, as opposed to smudged chromatin, may be the cytological feature in ASCUS most predictive of SIL on histology.[6] Artifacts, such as degenerative changes or air-drying, often contribute to the nuclear abnormalities and thus to the diagnostic difficulty. Any limitations in smear quality should be reported. Included in the ASCUS category are cells with some but not all of the features suggestive of human papillomavirus (HPV). However, cytoplasmic vacuolization alone without nuclear abnormality should be considered a benign cellular change and not a feature of ASCUS. This can be seen in normal glycogenated squamous epithelium or in association with inflammatory conditions such as those caused by *Trichomonas* or *Candida*.[7] Similarly, binucleation alone without significant nuclear abnormalities may be seen in reactive conditions and should not be considered a feature of ASCUS. Most often, ASCUS involves cells with mature superficial or intermediate-type cytoplasm. In such cases the differential diagnosis is between a reactive process and LSIL. In a small minority of ASCUS cases the cellular changes involve small or metaplastic type cells where the differential diagnosis is between a benign process and high-grade squamous intraepithelial lesions (HSIL). Other specific settings or cellular changes included in the ASCUS category in the Bethesda System are also described in Table 8.1.

The terminology for reporting equivocal diagnoses and the morphological criteria of ASCUS are ongoing subjects of debate in cytology. These issues were addressed by the International Academy of Cytology Task Force at a recent international expert conference and

Table 8.1 *Atypical squamous cells of undetermined significance (ASCUS): The Bethesda System (TBS) criteria*

ASCUS – general features

Nuclear enlargement to 2.5–3 times the size of a normal intermediate squamous cell nucleus

Slight increase in the nuclear/cytoplasmic ratio

Variation in nuclear size and shape

Binucleation may be observed

Mild hyperchromasia may be present, but the chromatin remains evenly distributed without granularity

Nuclear outlines usually are smooth and regular; very limited irregularity may be observed

Cells with some but not all features suggestive of human papillomavirus (HPV) cytopathic effect

1. ASCUS involving squamous metaplastic cells (atypical metaplasia)

    Nuclear enlargement to 1.5–2 times the area of a normal squamous metaplastic nucleus or 3 times the size of a normal intermediate size nucleus

    Increased nuclear/cytoplasmic ratio

    Remaining nuclear features as in 'ASCUS – general features' above

    Nucleoli may be present

The differential diagnosis of ASCUS involving metaplastic cells is high-grade squamous intraepithelial lesion (HSIL).

2. ASCUS involving tissue fragments (atypical repair)

    Marked cellular changes (exceeding those seen in typical repair) involving tissue fragments or syncytial sheets of immature squamous cells with:

        Nuclear piling

        Significant nuclear pleomorphism

        Irregular chromatin distribution

        Nucleoli may be present

The differential diagnosis is HSIL involving glands versus carcinoma versus exuberant reparative process; however, the dyshesion, tumor diathesis and other nuclear criteria diagnostic of carcinoma are absent.

3. ASCUS associated with atrophy

    Should be considered in the setting of atrophy if cells demonstrate:

        Both nuclear enlargement (at least 2 times normal) and hyperchromasia

        Irregularities in nuclear contour or chromatin distribution

        Marked pleomorphism with tadpole or spindle cells

A course of estrogen therapy with repeat smear may be useful to establish a definitive diagnosis and exclude HSIL or squamous carcinoma. Benign reactive changes are expected to resolve after estrogen, whereas significant pre-neoplastic or neoplastic lesions will persist and will be easier to diagnose. Minor cytological abnormalities are more likely to be reactive in the setting of atrophy since the prevalence of HPV infection is low in older women.

4. ASCUS in parakeratotic-type cells (atypical parakeratosis)

    Miniature polygonal squamous cells with dense orangeophilic cytoplasm shed singly or in three-dimensional clusters that demonstrate any or all of the following:

        Cellular pleomorphism with caudate or elongate shapes

        Increased nuclear size

        Hyperchromasia

Atypical parakeratosis is a known cause of diagnostic difficulty on Pap smears and may be associated with a HSIL or even carcinoma. However, hyperkeratosis and parakeratosis without nuclear atypia are not included in TBS.

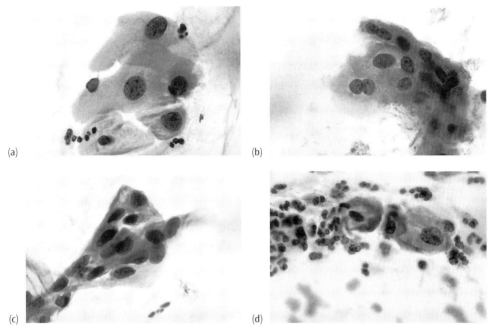

Figure 8.1 *Pap smears with atypical squamous cells of undetermined significance (ASCUS) involving superficial and/or intermediate type squamous cells. (a) Single cells with nuclear enlargement, mild hyperchromasia and slight nuclear membrane irregularity. (b) Sheet of superficial squamous cells with nuclear enlargement and binucleation. (c) Sheet of squamous cells with hyperchromatic smudged chromatin (ASCUS favor reactive). Biopsy showed cervicitis with squamous metaplasia. (d) Few cells with some features suggestive of human papillomavirus (HPV) cytopathic effect [ASCUS favor LSIL (low-grade squamous intraepithelial lesions)]. (All conventional smears, original magnification ×100.)*

tutorial.[8] While conference participants agreed that a term reflecting diagnostic uncertainty is necessary to communicate cytological findings that are equivocal, their opinions differed as to the terminology (atypical or abnormal morphologic changes) and to the value of defining morphological criteria for this diagnosis.[8]

REPRODUCIBILITY AND CONSISTENCY

The major problem with ASCUS is perhaps its poor inter-observer reproducibility. Among 13 cases of ASCUS reviewed by 17 CAP pathologists only 62 per cent of the diagnoses rendered by the panel was ASCUS, while the remaining diagnoses were normal, reactive and SIL.[9] Furthermore, no reviewed case received a unanimous ASCUS diagnosis. Of 31 35-mm color Kodachromes of 'ASCUS' presented to a group of 17 CAP members, only 23 per cent were confirmed as ASCUS by more than 70 per cent of the participants, while the remaining cases were interpreted as benign, LSIL and HSIL.[9] Similarly, in a study of 200 smears originally classified as 'atypical' and reviewed by five expert cytopathologists,[10] not a single smear received a unanimous diagnosis of ASCUS from all five cytopathologists. Exact two-way agreement was generally less than 66 per cent. Moreover, about 50 per cent of the cases were downgraded to negative.[10]

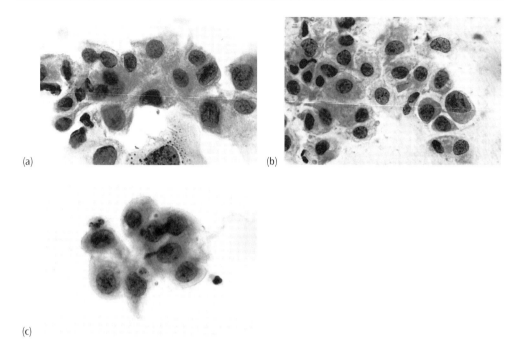

(a)

(b)

(c)

Figure 8.2 *Pap smears with atypical squamous cells of undetermined significance (ASCUS) involving squamous metaplastic type cells. (a and b) Sheets of small metaplastic cells showing increased nuclear–cytoplasmic ratio, variation in nuclear size and shape and slight nuclear membrane irregularity [ASCUS favor HSIL (high-grade squamous intraepithelial lesion) or cannot exclude HSIL]. Biopsy on case a showed HSIL, while follow up Pap smear on case b shows ASCUS (both conventional smears, original magnification ×100). (c) An aggregate of cells showing increased nuclear–cytoplasmic ratio and mild hyperchromasia; follow-up Pap smear showed ASCUS (ThinPrep, original magnification ×100).*

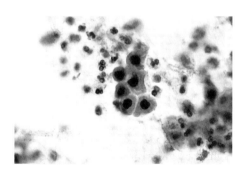

Figure 8.3 *Pap smear with atypical squamous cells of undetermined significance (ASCUS) involving parakeratotic-type cells [ASCUS favor HSIL (high-grade squamous intraepithelial lesion)]. Small, polygonal squamous cells showing hyperchromasia and increased nuclear size; biopsy showed HSIL (conventional smear, original magnification × 100).*

This poor reproducibility, along with the specter of malpractice litigation contributes to the clinician's dilemma in managing ASCUS patients. Since the Pap smear is a screening rather than a diagnostic test, intra-laboratory consistency over time may be the most essential parameter to determine and validate the recommendations for patient management.

Various quality assurance/improvement programs can be used to improve and monitor the intra-laboratory reproducibility and consistency in the use of ASCUS. First, criteria should be evaluated and established among various cytotechnologists and cytopathologists. However, it should be kept in mind that even the 'objective' criteria (e.g. nuclear enlargement and chromatin

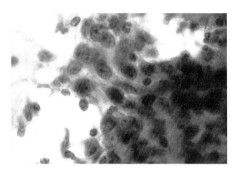

Figure 8.4 *Pap smear with atypical squamous cells of undetermined significance (ASCUS) involving tissue fragments 'atypical repair' [ASCUS favor HSIL (high-grade squamous intraepithelial lesion)]. Irregularly shaped thick tissue fragment showing enlarged crowded nuclei and nucleoli; biopsy showed squamous cell carcinoma (conventional smear, original magnification ×100).*

pattern) are largely subjective. Periodic review of selected cases over a multi-headed microscope may help refine and standardize those criteria. Histocytological correlation of ASCUS cases may also be used for intra-laboratory standardization over time. For example, similar prevalence rates of SIL on follow-up biopsies in women with ASCUS over different periods would indicate that there is consistency in the application of ASCUS criteria within a laboratory. As was stressed previously, the ASCUS rate and the ASCUS–SIL ratio are very useful for monitoring the consistency of ASCUS over time and for comparison of data between laboratories.[11]

Human papillomavirus testing is another objective tool that may be used to ensure that the diagnosis of ASCUS is being used appropriately.[10] In view of the substantial data linking SIL and carcinoma to HPV infection, 'ASCUS' diagnoses should correlate with a higher rate of HPV infection than 'negative' smears and less than smears showing 'SIL'. In a review by five cytopathologists of 200 Pap smears originally diagnosed as 'atypical', there was a consistent correlation between the rate of detection of high-risk HPV types and the revised diagnoses. The rate of detection of high-risk HPV types was greater for smears reclassified as ASCUS (30 per cent) compared with those interpreted as negative (10 per cent) but lower than that of SIL (60 per cent).[10] These data indicate that correlating HPV detection with cytological/histological diagnosis may be a useful and objective quality assurance measure, particularly in laboratories with high rates of ASCUS.

HISTOLOGICAL CORRELATES

Based on the more restricted use of the term 'atypia', a diagnosis of ASCUS was expected to be more predictive of SIL on biopsy than the previously used diagnoses of 'inflammatory atypia' and 'benign or reactive atypia'. When cases of 'inflammatory atypia' were reclassified using a set of predefined morphological criteria similar to TBS criteria as either reactive/reparative change (RC) or ASCUS, the incidence of SIL on biopsy in the ASCUS group was significantly greater than that of the RC group (61.3 per cent versus 5.2 per cent).[12]

An inter-laboratory comparison and evaluation study concluded that the ASCUS–SIL ratio is an important laboratory monitor that can be predictive of the rate of SIL on follow-up in women with ASCUS on Pap smear.[11] An inverse relationship was noted between the ASCUS–SIL ratio (range = 0.8:1–2.7:1) and the rate of SIL on follow-up (range = 10–45 per cent). The laboratory rates of ASCUS will be determined by the patient population being screened, by the cytological criteria used, and by the experience of the cytopathologists.

A review of 17 published studies shows that the prevalence of biopsy-proven SIL (both low grade and high grade) in women with a Pap smear showing 'squamous atypia' varies between 18.7 per cent and 84.4 per cent (Table 8.2).[6,12–27] The rate of biopsy-proven HSIL ranges

Table 8.2 *Prevalence rate of squamous intraepithelial lesions (SIL) on follow up biopsies in women with Pap smear showing 'squamous atypia' [atypical squamous cells of undetermined significance (ASCUS)]*

Author	Year	Number of cases	Laboratory ASCUS rate (%)	ASCUS–SIL ratio	% Biopsy-proven SIL	% Biopsy-proven HSIL[a]
Abu-Jawdeh et al.[6]	1994	97	8	1.5	31	13
Andrews et al.[13]	1989	353			15.6	5.4
Collins et al.[14]	1996	304	7	1.9	30	9
Davis et al.[15]	1987	406			18.7	7.6
Dvorak et al.[16]	1999	249	3.8	1.76	72	18
Genest et al.[17]	1998	452		3.2	24	13
Gonzalez et al.[18]	1996	118	11	2.2	24.5	1.7
Jones et al.[19]	1987	236			25	4.2
Kaminski et al.[20]	1989	1074			18.8	6.8
Lindheim and Smith-Nguyen[21]	1990	101			29.7	16.8[b]
Noumoff[22]	1987	375			29	10
Paavonen et al.[39]	1989	124			41.1	13.7
Sidawy et al.[12]	1993	31			61.3	3.2
Slawson et al.[23]	1993	96			84.4	15.6
Soutter et al.[25]	1986	44			40.9	38.6[b]
Tay et al.[26]	1987	44	1.27		75	40.9
Williams et al.[27]	1997	284	4.5	0.5	56	8

[a]HSIL, high-grade squamous intraepithelial lesion.
[b]Includes one case of invasive carcinoma.

between 1.7 per cent and 40.9 per cent, including only rare cases of invasive carcinoma.[21,25] This wide variability results, at least in part, from the differing criteria used between laboratories in the definition of 'squamous atypia'. Furthermore, some studies were based on the pre-Bethesda definition of 'squamous atypia'. Among those reports including the ASCUS–SIL ratio, the prevalence of biopsy-proven SIL correlated inversely with the ASCUS–SIL ratio (Table 8.2). This observation confirms the findings of the CAP inter-laboratory comparison data,[11] and further underscores the importance of the ASCUS–SIL ratio as a useful quality assurance monitor.

Other factors that may correlate with the presence of SIL in those patients with ASCUS include age and previous history. One study found that following a diagnosis of ASCUS, women aged 40 years or less are significantly more likely to have SIL on biopsy than older women.[20] Similarly, Rader et al.[28] reported that the incidence of ASCUS and the frequency of an underlying SIL are lower in women over the age of 55 years than in the general population. In pregnant women, ASCUS may be associated with an underlying biopsy-proven SIL in 21 per cent of cases.[29] It should be pointed out that the prevalence rates of underlying SIL reported in histological/cytological correlation studies are probably not representative of all women with ASCUS on Pap smears. The cases included in these studies may represent a selected group of women with ASCUS since not all women with such a diagnosis have biopsy follow-up. It is possible that the selection of patients for biopsy is biased by clinical findings or past history, as suggested by Ghoussoub et al.[30] They report that in women with ASCUS who have biopsy follow-up, the prevalence rate of SIL is about twice that in those women followed with Pap smears.[30]

In contrast to SIL, the natural history of ASCUS has not been extensively documented. Hirschowitz et al.[31] reported that 98 out of 437 (22.4 per cent) women with smears showing borderline changes had subsequent smears showing high-grade lesions within 13–106 months. Fifty per cent of the cases that progressed did so within the first 3 years; the risk of progression was greater in women aged 20 to 39 years.[31] In another study, progression to SIL in 29.1 per cent of women with ASCUS was observed on biopsy and/or follow-up cytology within 12–18 months.[32] It is possible, however, that some of these women had underlying SIL instead of developing SIL during the follow-up period. Similar findings on follow-up cytology and biopsy were observed in the inter-laboratory comparison study.[11] In a recent study on 651 women with a diagnosis of ASCUS followed regularly for 6 years, HSIL developed in 9 per cent of the women but none had invasive cancer.[33] In a review of 123 cervical smears on 18 patients with HSIL and three with squamous cell carcinoma (each with at least three prior negative results), 30 per cent of the original negatives were reclassified as ASCUS.[34]

Two conclusions may be drawn. (1) The majority of women with ASCUS on Pap smear do not have evidence of a significant lesion; nevertheless, about one-third are at high risk of either having or developing SIL including HSIL. (2) ASCUS may be the only abnormality preceding a diagnosis of HSIL. Moreover, ASCUS smears represent the largest source of HSIL in the population. In a prospective study of more than 46 000 women, Kinney et al.,[35] reported that of all cases of biopsy-proven HSIL, ASCUS was the most frequent associated cytological diagnosis, accounting for 38 per cent of the cases. This underscores the need for cost-effective triage for the management of ASCUS. A comparison of methods of triaging women with ASCUS smears is presented in Chapter 2.

QUALIFICATION OF ASCUS

Since ASCUS represents a heterogeneous category, TBS recommends attempts to morphologically subclassify or qualify the diagnosis into 'favor reactive' or 'favor SIL'. However, given our understanding of the biology of HPV in the pathogenesis of cervical neoplasia and the current management options for SIL, a more rational approach to ASCUS qualification would be to further separate the 'favor-SIL' cases into 'favor LSIL' or 'favor HSIL' categories. Thus, the diagnostic terminology includes: (1) 'ASCUS-favor LSIL', (2) 'ASCUS-favor HSIL or cannot exclude HSIL', and (3) 'ASCUS-favor reactive'.

'ASCUS-favor LSIL' is used predominantly in cases with minor cytopathic effects suggestive of HPV. Since the diagnosis of HPV implies both the presence of a potential cancer precursor and a sexually transmitted disease, this should not be rendered lightly. For cases with minimal cellular changes, i.e. subtle nuclear abnormalities that fall short of a definitive diagnosis of LSIL, one may use a diagnosis such as 'ASCUS, probably representing HPV'. Often the scarcity of abnormal cells precludes a more definitive diagnosis. Smears containing rare cells diagnostic of LSIL have been shown to have confirmatory histology in only 29 per cent of women, compared with 82 per cent of those who display numerous abnormal cells.[36] Thus, TBS recommends that ASCUS include those smears that 'quantitatively' fall short of a definitive diagnosis of LSIL.

'ASCUS-favor HSIL' is used for smears containing syncytial sheets or tissue fragments with nuclear crowding (atypical repair), atypical metaplasia, atypical parakeratosis, atrophy and when a few small atypical cells are present but degeneration or technical artifacts render interpretation difficult. Syncytial sheets or tissue fragments with crowded nuclei are a feature of exuberant reactive processes, atrophy, HSIL involving glands and adenocarcinoma *in situ*. Their interpretation is often challenging as well as subjective, particularly when nuclear crowding precludes adequate evaluation of chromatin pattern and when single cells diagnostic of HSIL are not present. Sherman et al.[37] found that thick tissue fragments were frequent cytological findings in cases interpreted as 'ASCUS rule out HSIL', and that these smears are often reclassified as HSIL on review. 'Atypical metaplasia' or ASCUS involving metaplastic cells has been more highly correlated with HSIL on follow-up or biopsy than other types of ASCUS by up to sevenfold (21 per cent versus 3 per cent).[38–40] Atypical immature metaplasia was found on review in 11 of 17 smears originally reported as negative and immediately preceding smears showing HSIL.[38] These studies underscore the difficulty in differentiating reactive changes from neoplastic processes in immature squamous metaplasia, and the importance of recognizing 'atypical metaplasia' as a potential marker of a more serious lesion. Atrophy may, in some instances, produce changes that mimic HSIL or even carcinoma.[41]

'ASCUS-favor reactive' is used when there is minimal nuclear atypia, smudged chromatin, occasional nucleoli and an inflammatory background.

Qualification of ASCUS may be used to guide patient management. This seems justified based on the results of several studies that demonstrate the stratification of patients into distinct risk groups for SIL, particularly HSIL, by the qualification of ASCUS.[14,17,37,42,43] Collins et al.[14] reported that a significant proportion of biopsy specimens associated with Pap smear diagnosis of 'ASCUS-favor SIL' were HSIL (15 per cent); in contrast, an underlying HSIL was much less likely in patients with ASCUS (unqualified) (3 per cent) and 'ASCUS-favor reactive' (3 per cent). Furthermore, in seven of the 27 ASCUS smears associated with HSIL a HG lesion was favored in the report. Similarly, two other studies have reported that smears classified as 'ASCUS favor dysplasia' were associated with an underlying HSIL on biopsy in 9.6 per cent and 27.3 per cent of cases, whereas smears classified as ASCUS favor reactive were associated with HSIL in 2.6 per cent and 5 per cent of cases.[42,43] Other investigators have found a significantly lower rate of HSIL at biopsy in women whose smears were qualified as ASCUS–NOS compared with those with ASCUS–suggestive of HSIL (11 and 1.2 per cent versus 53 and 23.9 per cent, respectively).[17,37] Schooland et al.[44] reported that Pap smears diagnosed as 'Inconclusive–Possible high-grade epithelial abnormality' (using the Australian Terminology for Cervical Cytology Reporting) were associated with HSIL on biopsy in 55.9 per cent of cases.

Limited data available from studies correlating HPV DNA detection and ASCUS seem to further validate the qualification of ASCUS. Crum et al.[45] found a significantly higher rate of detection of high-risk HPV DNA in Thin-Prep cervical smears classified as ASCUS–favor SIL compared with ASCUS–NOS or ASCUS–favor reactive (47.8 per cent, 17.4 per cent, and 8.8 per cent, respectively).

While most studies seem to suggest that there is consistency in the associated SIL rate between laboratories for different categories of ASCUS, some studies have indicated otherwise.[18,46] In a study by Gonzalez et al.,[18] a diagnosis of ASCUS favoring either a reactive process or LSIL was associated with a relatively low rate of SIL on biopsy (8.6 per cent and 15 per cent, respectively). However, much higher rates of underlying SIL were reported by Malik et al. for all ASCUS categories.[46] Smears classified as 'ASCUS favor reactive', 'favor LSIL' and 'favor HSIL' were associated with SIL on biopsy in 48 per cent, 78 per cent, and 100 per cent of cases, respectively.[46]

In conclusion, since a major goal of Pap smear screening is to identify those patients requiring immediate treatment, particularly those with suspected HSIL, the qualification of ASCUS appears useful. It at least stratifies those patients with a diagnosis of ASCUS into different risk groups. Each laboratory then needs to communicate to their clinicians what the risk for SIL associated with each category of ASCUS actually is.

MANAGEMENT OF ASCUS

There is no consensus regarding the management of women with ASCUS: 'At present, aggressive follow-up is thought to be the norm in the United States'.[47] While the main concern of the clinicians is a missed diagnosis in those patients who have HSIL or invasive cancer, overtreatment and cost are serious problems for the health-care system. Interim guidelines[4] have been proposed by the 1992 National Cancer Institute-sponsored workshop and include several management options, such as: (1) repeat Pap smear without colposcopy for women with ASCUS unqualified or when the diagnosis favors a reactive process, (2) repeat Pap smear after treatment for inflammation or with topical estrogen in the setting of atrophy, and (3) colposcopy and biopsy for high-risk women, or when a neoplastic process is favored. Although ASCUS in postmenopausal women most commonly represents a benign reactive change,[28] there is still a substantial risk that women with such findings on Pap smear may have a cervical or even a vaginal lesion.[48] Repeat Pap smear after estrogen treatment may be advised to clarify the nature of these abnormalities. Testing for HPV and cervicography[49,50] may be used by physicians who understand their limitations.

FUTURE TRENDS

The use of ASCUS as a diagnostic category remains a source of debate and controversy. It has been argued that the use of ASCUS is an incomplete evaluation of the Pap smear and should be replaced by a more definitive diagnosis.[51] Uncertainty in the ASCUS category eventually may be resolved by the use of intermediate triage tests. An ideal triage test is expected to be cost effective and to have both high sensitivity and high specificity in identifying those women at high risk for high-grade lesions and carcinoma. Studies evaluating the usefulness of new modalities in the clarification of ASCUS are ongoing. These new modalities include HPV testing, cervicography and ancillary new technologies for Pap smear collection and screening.

Studies have shown that HPV testing may be useful in identifying women with ASCUS who require immediate colposcopy[52–54] (see Chapters 2 and 6 for details). To eliminate the extra cost and delay associated with a second triage office visit, the feasibility of collecting samples for HPV testing on the first visit is currently being addressed. Samples collected in a preservative for liquid-based preparation can be stored until the Pap smear results are available. The PreservCyt buffer (the collection medium used with the ThinPrep technique) has been shown to be an appropriate medium for HPV testing.[55,56] Fluorescence-based *in situ* hybridization is another modality that has been reported to be sensitive in the detection of high-risk HPV subtypes in cervicovaginal samples[57] and could have potential applications in the evaluation of ASCUS smears.

Other methods with potential use in the clarification of ASCUS include new automated technologies for cervicovaginal slide preparation and screening (these are described in detail in Chapter 3). An initial trial comparing matched pairs of conventional and ThinPrep slide preparation indicates that the ASCUS rate in ThinPrep slides is less than that in conventional smears.[56,58] The use of the PAPNET computerized system to re-evaluate and reclassify ASCUS smears has been investigated in a recent study.[59] The main questions that this study addressed were: (1) whether cells diagnostic of SIL were present but missed in ASCUS smears, and (2) whether the PAPNET could detect the presence of such cells. The results indicated that PAPNET-directed rescreening of Pap smears interpreted as ASCUS uncovered SIL in a significant number of cases.[59] However, from a public health perspective, the use of PAPNET to rescreen all slides for quality control does not appear to be cost-effective.[60] Whether the same limitations would apply to ASCUS smears has yet to be determined.

A large prospective multicenter randomized clinical trial to study management of ASCUS, as well as LSIL, on Pap smear has been funded by the National Cancer Institute and is currently underway.[47,61–63] The main objective of this trial, also known as the ASCUS/LSIL Triage Study (ALTS), is to determine effective colposcopy triage strategies to identify women with ASCUS or LSIL on Pap smear who have significant disease and need immediate treatment and those that can be managed more conservatively. The trial compares two colposcopy triage strategies with respect to their sensitivity and specificity of detecting HSIL: (1) triage based on the results of Hypbrid Capture 2™ (HC 2) HPV testing and ThinPrep cytology; and (2) triage based on cytology results alone; the results of immediate colposcopy are used as reference standard. Baseline results from the ALTS trial, summarizing the cross-sectional enrollment results for women with ASCUS, have been recently published.[63] As further discussed in Chapter 6, the preliminary data indicate that HC 2 testing for high-risk HPV DNA may be a potentially viable strategy in the management of women with ASCUS.[63]

REFERENCES

1 National Cancer Institute Workshop. The 1988 Bethesda System for reporting cervical/vaginal cytological diagnoses. *JAMA* 1989; **262**: 931–4.

2 Kurman RJ, Malkasian GD, Sedlis A, Solomon D. From Papanicolaou to Bethesda: the rationale for a new cervical cytologic classification. *Obstet Gynecol* 1991; **77**: 779–82.

3 Kurman RJ, Solomon D. *The Bethesda System for reporting cervical/vaginal cytologic diagnoses: definitions, criteria, and explanatory notes for terminology and specimen adequacy.* New York: Springer-Verlag, 1994: 30–43.

4 Kurman RJ, Henson DE, Herbst AL, Noller KL, Schiffman MH. Interim guidelines for management of abnormal cervical cytology. *J Am Med Assoc* 1994; **271**: 1866–9.

5 Davey DD, Nielsen ML, Naryshkin S, Robb JA, Cohen T, Kline TS. Atypical squamous cells of undetermined significance: current laboratory practices of participants in the College of American Pathologists interlaboratory comparison program in cervicovaginal cytology. *Arch Pathol Lab Med* 1996; **120**: 440–4.

6 Abu-Jawdeh GM, Trawinski G, Wang HH. Histocytological study of squamous atypia on Pap smears. *Mod Pathol* 1994; **7**: 920–4.

7 Miguel Jr NL, Lachowicz CM, Kline TS. *Candida*-related changes and ASCUS: a potential trap! *Diagn Cytopathol* 1997; **16**: 83–6.

8 Solomon D, Frable WJ, Vooijs GP, et al. ASCUS and AGUS criteria. International Academy of Cytology Task Force summary. Diagnostic Cytology Towards the 21st Century: An International Expert Conference and Tutorial. *Acta Cytol* 1998; **42**: 16–24.

9 Robb JA. The 'ASCUS' swamp [editorial] [published erratum appears in *Diagn Cytopathol* 1995; **12**(2): 198] [see comments]. *Diagn Cytopathol* 1994; **11**: 319–20.

10 Sherman ME, Schiffman MH, Lorincz AT. Toward objective quality assurance in cervical cytopathology. Correlation of cytopathologic diagnoses with detection of high-risk human papillomavirus types. *Am J Clin Pathol* 1994; **102**: 182–7.

11 Davey DD, Naryshkin S, Nielsen ML, Kline TS. Atypical squamous cells of undetermined significance: interlaboratory comparison and quality assurance monitors. *Diagn Cytopathol* 1994; **11**: 390–6.

12 Sidawy MK, Tabbara SO. Reactive change and atypical squamous cells of undetermined significance in Papanicolaou smears: a cytohistologic correlation. *Diagn Cytopathol* 1993; **9**: 423–9.

13 Andrews S, Hernandez E, Miyazawa K. Paired Papanicolaou smears in the evaluation of atypical squamous cells. *Obstet Gynecol* 1989; **73**: 747–50.

14 Collins LC, Wang HH, Abu-Jawdeh GM. Qualifiers of atypical squamous cells of undetermined significance help in patient management. *Mod Pathol* 1996; **9**: 677–81.

15 Davis GL, Hernandez E, Davis JL, Miyazawa K. Atypical squamous cells in Papanicolaou smears. *Obstet Gynecol* 1987; **69**: 43–6.

16 Dvorak KA, Finnemore M, Maksem JA. Histology correlation with atypical squamous cells of undetermined significance (ASCUS) and low-grade squamous intraepithelial lesion (LSIL) cytology diagnoses: an argument to ensure ASCUS follow-up that is as aggressive as that for LSIL. *Diagn Cytopathol* 1999; **21**: 292–5.

17 Genest DR, Dean B, Lee KR, Sheets E, Crum CP, Cibas ES. Qualifying the cytologic diagnosis of 'atypical squamous cells of undetermined significance' affects the predictive value of a squamous intraepithelial lesion on subsequent biopsy. *Arch Pathol Lab Med* 1998; **122**: 338–41.

18 Gonzalez D, Hernandez E, Anderson L, Heller P, Atkinson B. Clinical significance of a cervical cytologic diagnosis of atypical squamous cells of undetermined significance. Favoring a reactive process or low grade squamous intraepithelial lesion. *J Reprod Med* 1996; **41**: 719–23.

19 Jones DED, Creasman WT, Dombroski RA, Lentz SS, Waeltz JL. Evaluation of the atypical Pap smear. *Am J Obstet Gynecol* 1987; **157**: 544–9.

20 Kaminski PF, Stevens CWJ, Wheelock JB. Squamous atypia on cytology. The influence of age. *J Reprod Med* 1989; **34**: 617–20.

21 Lindheim SR, Smith-Nguyen G. Aggressive evaluation for atypical squamous cells in Papanicolaou smears. *J Reprod Med* 1990; **35**: 971–3.

22 Noumoff JS. Atypia in cervical cytology as a risk factor for intraepithelial neoplasia. *Am J Obstet Gynecol* 1987; **156**: 628–31.

23 Slawson DC, Bennett JH, Herman JM. Follow-up Papanicolaou smear for cervical atypia: are we missing significant disease? A HARNET Study. *J Fam Pract* 1993; **36**: 289–93.

24 Slevaggi SM, Haefner HK. Reporting atypical squamous cells of undetermined significance on cervical smears: is it significant? *Diagn Cytopathol* 1995; **13**: 352–6.

25 Soutter WP, Wisdom S, Brough AK, Monoghan JM. Should patients with mild atypia in a cervical smear be referred for colposcopy? *Br J Obstet Gynecol* 1986; **93**: 70–4.

26 Tay SK, Jenkins D, Singer A. Management of squamous atypia (borderline nuclear abnormalities): repeat cytology or colposcopy? *Aust NZ J Obstet Gynaecol* 1987; **27**: 140–1.

27 Williams GM, Rimm DL, Pedigo MA, Frable WJ. Atypical squamous cells of undetermined significance: correlative histologic and follow-up studies from an academic medical center. *Diagn Cytopathol* 1997; **16**: 1–7.

28 Rader AE, Rose PG, Rodriguez M, Mansbacher S, Pitlik D, Abdul-Karim FW. Atypical squamous cells of undetermined significance in women over 55. Comparison with the general population and implications for management. *Acta Cytol* 1999; **43**: 357–62.

29 Kaminski PF, Lyon DS, Sorosky JI, Wheelock JB, Podczaski ES. Significance of atypical cervical cytology in pregnancy. *Am J Perinatol* 1992; **9**: 340–3.

30 Ghoussoub RA, Rimm DL. Degree of dysplasia following diagnosis of atypical squamous cells of undetermined significance is influenced by patient history and type of follow-up. *Diagn Cytopathol* 1997; **17**: 14–19.

31 Hirschowitz L, Raffle AE, Mackenzie EF, Hughes AO. Long term follow up of women with borderline cervical smear test results: effects of age and viral infection on progression to high grade dyskaryosis. *BMJ* 1992; **304**: 1209–12.

32 Howell LP, Davis RL. Follow-up of Papanicolaou smears diagnosed as atypical squamous cells of undetermined significance. *Diagn Cytopathol* 1996; **14**: 20–4.

33 Raab SS, Bishop NS, Zaleski MS. Long-term outcome and relative risk in women with atypical squamous cells of undetermined significance. *Am J Clin Pathol* 1999; **112**: 57–62.

34 Sherman ME, Kelly D. High-grade squamous intraepithelial lesions and invasive carcinoma following the report of three negative Papnicolaou smears: screening failures or rapid progression? *Mod Pathol* 1992; **5**: 337–42.

35 Kinney WK, Manos MM, Hurley LB, Ransley JE. Where's the high-grade cervical neoplasia? The importance of minimally abnormal Papanicolaou diagnoses. *Obstet Gynecol* 1998; **91**: 973–6.

36 Hall S, Wu TC, Soudi N. Low-grade squamous intraepithelial lesions: cytologic predictors of biopsy confirmation. *Diagn Cytopathol* 1994; **10**: 3–9.

37 Sherman ME, Tabbara SO, Scott DR, et al. 'ASCUS, rule out HSIL': cytologic features, histologic correlates, and human papillomavirus detection. *Mod Pathol* 1999; **12**: 335–42.

38 Hatem F, Wilbur DC. High grade squamous cervical lesions following negative Papanicolaou smears: false negative cervical cytology or rapid progression? *Diagn Cytopathol* 1995; **12**: 135–41.

39 Paavonen J, Kiviat NB, Wolner-Hanssen P, Stevens CE, Vontver LA. Significance of mild cervical cytologic atypia in a sexually transmitted disease clinic population. *Acta Cytol* 1989; **33**: 831–8.

40 Sheils LA, Wilbur DC. Atypical squamous cells of undetermined significance. Stratification of the risk of association with, or progression to, squamous intraepithelial lesions based on morphologic subcategorization [see comments]. *Acta Cytol* 1997; **41**: 1065–72.

41 Weintraub NT, Violi E, Freedman ML. Cervical cancer screening in women aged 65 and over. *J Am Geriatr Soc* 1987; **35**: 870–5.

42 Kline MJ, Davey DD. Atypical squamous cells of undetermined significance qualified: a follow-up study. *Diagn Cytopathol* 1996; **14**: 380–4.

43 Lachman MF, Cavallo-Calvanese C. Qualification of atypical squamous cells of undetermined significance in an independent laboratory: is it useful or significant? *Am J Obstet Gynecol* 1998; **179**: 421–9.

44 Schoolland M, Sterrett GF, Knowles SA, Mitchell KM, Kurinczuk JJ. The 'Inconclusive–possible high grade epithelial abnormality' category in Papanicolaou smear reporting. *Cancer* 1998; **84**: 208–17.

45 Crum CP, Genest DR, Krane JF, et al. Subclassifying atypical squamous cells in Thin-Prep cervical cytology correlates with detection of high-risk human papillomavirus DNA. *Am J Clin Pathol* 1999; **112**: 384–90.

46 Malik SN, Wilkinson EJ, Drew PA, Bennett BB, Hardt NS. Do qualifiers of ASCUS distinguish between low- and high-risk patients? *Acta Cytol* 1999; **43**: 376–80.

47 McNeil C. Getting a handle on ASCUS: a new clinical trial could show how [news]. *J Natl Cancer Inst* 1995; **87**: 787–90.

48 Saminathan T, Lahoti C, Kannan V, Kline TS. Postmenopausal squamous-cell atypias: a diagnostic challenge. *Diagn Cytopathol* 1994; **11**: 226–30.

49 August N. Cervicography for evaluating the 'atypical' Papanicolaou smear. *J Reprod Med* 1991; **36**: 89–94.

50 Ferris DG. Cervicography – an adjunct to Papanicolaou screening. *Am Fam Physician* 1994; **85**: 337–42.

51 Gupta PK. Cytopathology today: challenges and opportunities. *Acta Cytol* 1997; **41**: 1–10.

52 Cox JT, Lorincz AT, Schiffman MH, Sherman ME, Cullen A, Kurman RJ. Human papillomavirus testing by hybrid capture appears to be useful in triaging women with a cytologic diagnosis of atypical squamous cells of undetermined significance. *Am J Obstet Gynecol* 1995; **172**: 946–54.

53 Manos MM, Kinney WK, Hurley LB, et al. Identifying women with cervical neoplasia: using human papillomavirus DNA testing for equivocal Papanicolaou results [see comments]. *JAMA* 1999; **281**: 1605–10.

54 Wright TC, Sun XW, Koulos J. Comparison of management algorithms for the evaluation of women with low-grade cytologic abnormalities. *Obstet Gynecol* 1995; **85**: 202–10.

55 Linder J, Zahniser D. The ThinPrep Pap test. A review of clinical studies. *Acta Cytol* 1997; **41**: 30–8.

56 Zahniser DJ, Sullivan PJ. CYTYC Corporation. *Acta Cytol* 1996; **40**: 37–44.

57 Siadat-Pajouh M, Periasamy A, Ayscue AH, et al. Detection of human papillomavirus type 16/18 DNA in cervicovaginal cells by fluorescence based *in situ* hybridization and automated image cytometry. *Cytometry* 1994; **15**: 245–57.

58 Wilbur DC, Cibas ES, Merritt S. ThinPrep processor. Clinical trials demonstrate an increased detection rate of abnormal cervical cytologic specimens. *Am J Clin Pathol* 1994; **101**: 209–14.

59 Ryan MR, Stastny JF, Remmers R, Pedigo MA, Cahill LA, Frable WJ. PAPNET-directed rescreening of cervicovaginal smears. A study of 101 cases of atypical squamous cells of undetermined significance. *Am J Clin Pathol* 1996; **105**: 711–18.

60 Hutchinson ML. Assessing the costs and benefits of alternative rescreening strategies. *Acta Cytol* 1996; **40**: 4–8.

61 Ferris DG. ASCUS and LSIL Pap smear. Results: triage considerations [editorial]. *Am Fam Physician* 1996; **53**: 1057–8, 60, 64 passim.

62 Titus K. Abnormal Pap smears, ASCUS still ob/gyn puzzle [news]. *JAMA* 1996; **276**: 1014–16.

63 Solomon D, Schiffman M, Tarone R. Comparison of three management strategies for patients with atypical squamous cells of undetermined significance: baseline results from a randomized trial. *J Natl Cancer Inst* 2001; **93**: 293–9.

9

Squamous lesions

LINNEA W GARCIA, ROBERT A GOULART

HISTORICAL OVERVIEW

Historically, there were three widely used classification systems before the introduction of the Bethesda System in the late 1980s: Papanicolaou's numeric classification, the dysplasia/carcinoma in situ scheme (CIS) and the cervical intraepithelial neoplasia (CIN) classification.

Prior to Papanicolaou's own diagnostic terminology for exfoliative cytology, advanced in 1954, no widely accepted reporting scheme for cervical cytology existed.[1] It is important to remember that the use of the Papanicolaou's classification system was not limited to cervico-vaginal cytology and did not incorporate any understanding of the concept of progression from precursor to invasive cancer. The terminology was designed for use with any exfoliated cytological preparation to convey the degree of suspicion that the patient had cancer (Table 9.1). The design of his classification into five groups of cytological findings or classes (I–V) was meant to demonstrate the difficulty of unequivocal cytological diagnosis and to reflect graded suspicion to conclusive malignancy.[2]

As the scientific understanding of the evolution of cervical carcinogenesis from precursor lesions expanded, dissatisfaction with reporting by Papanicolaou's classification also increased. Histological and corresponding cytological classification schemes that better reflected this new knowledge emerged. In the early 1960s, the first widely accepted descriptive terms were dysplasia and carcinoma in situ. They were defined by the International Congress of Cytology in 1961 as disturbances of differentiation in the squamous epithelium of the cervix involving less than (dysplasia) or the full thickness (carcinoma in situ).[3] Dysplasia could be further subdivided into grades ranging from very mild to severe, with varying degrees of diagnostic reproducibility and an undefined risk of progression. The clinical significance of these terms was poorly understood, the gynecological approach to treatment was surgical and the extent of that surgery was generally based on whether the lesion was considered dysplasia (conization) or carcinoma in situ (radical hysterectomy). While the terminology changed very little over

Table 9.1 *Papanicolaou classification system (1954)*

Class I	Absence of atypical or abnormal cells
Class II	Atypical cytology but no evidence of malignancy
Class III	Cytology suggestive of, but not conclusive for, malignancy
Class IV	Cytology strongly suggestive of malignancy
Class V	Cytology conclusive for malignancy

a decade, there was a trend towards upgrading lesions previously considered dysplasia to carcinoma *in situ*, resulting in an increase in the number of hysterectomies.[4]

The next decade (1960–70) saw the introduction of scientific and technological advances that permitted visualization of cervical lesions (colposcopy) and treatment limited to conservative ablation (electrocautery, cryotherapy and laser ablation) of precursor lesions. In addition, clinical and experimental studies led to a greater understanding of the biology of cervical cancer, which concluded that all intraepithelial neoplasia was a continuum that began as mild dysplasia and ended (although not inevitably) as carcinoma *in situ*.[4] Therefore, cervical intraepithelial neoplasia (CIN) was proposed as a generic term to designate the spectrum of intraepithelial disease that antedates invasive cervical cancer. It has been shown that, on average, women with invasive squamous cell carcinoma of the cervix are 10 years older than those with high-grade dysplasia,[5] although there is preliminary evidence of a possible subgroup of women with an apparently shorter preinvasive disease phase, of the order of 1–2 years, often without an intervening diagnosis of low-grade dysplasia.[6] Other studies have demonstrated a progression rate of severe dysplasia/carcinoma *in situ* to invasive disease to range from 30 to 80 per cent.[7–9] Once the severity of the initial diagnosis has been taken into account, age has not proven to be a strong independent predictor of progression to high-grade cervical dysplasia.[10]

Initially, CIN was a five-grade classification (very mild, mild, moderate, severe dysplasia and carcinoma *in situ*) but was later modified to a three-grade system (mild dysplasia, moderate dysplasia and severe dysplasia/carcinoma *in situ* corresponding to CIN I, CIN II and CIN III, respectively). However, Richart[4] believed that the critical decision was whether a lesion was present and, if so, whether it was intraepithelial or invasive. Because the behavior of precancerous lesions could not be predicted by morphology, treatment of all neoplasia was required, but all intraepithelial disease, including carcinoma *in situ*, could potentially be managed with local eradication.

Two seminal events led to another evaluation of the national and international reporting systems for cervical/vaginal cytological diagnoses in the late 1980's – the establishment of the link between human papillomavirus (HPV) infection and cervical neoplasia and the intense media and subsequent government scrutiny of cytology laboratories.[11,12] (Please also see Chapter 6.) A new classification system was sought to improve quality assurance by providing unambiguous and clinically relevant communication between cytologists and clinicians, to incorporate what was known about the association between HPV and cervical neoplasia, to facilitate cytological–histological correlation and research, and to provide reproducible data for national and international analyses. The 1988 Bethesda System for Reporting Cervical/Vaginal Cytologic Diagnoses was a response to this call.[13]

THE BETHESDA SYSTEM

The Bethesda System for Reporting Cervical/Vaginal Cytologic Diagnoses was first recommended under the auspices of the National Cancer Institute (NCI) in 1988. Its format included three elements: a statement of specimen adequacy for diagnostic evaluation, a general diagnostic categorization, and a descriptive diagnosis. In addition, specific terminology was recommended for use with each of the three elements of the cervical/vaginal cytology report (Table 9.2). However, no specific criteria were provided for determining specimen adequacy or for descriptive diagnoses. Similarly, although the Workshop participants unanimously affirmed that the cytopathology report be considered a medical consultation and that 'the diagnostic

Table 9.2 *The 1988 Bethesda System for reporting cervical/vaginal cytological diagnoses*

Statement of specimen adequacy
  Satisfactory for interpretation
  Less than optimal
  Unsatisfactory
Explanation for less than optimal/unsatisfactory specimen:
  Scant cellularity
  Poor fixation or preservation
  Presence of foreign material (e.g. lubricant)
  Partially or completely obscuring inflammation
  Partially or completely obscuring blood
  Excessive cytolysis
  No endocervical component in a premenopausal woman who has a cervix
  Not representative of the anatomic site
  Other

General categorization
  Within normal limits
  Other:
    See descriptive diagnosis
    Further action recommended

Descriptive diagnoses
Infection
  Fungal
    Fungal organisms morphologically consistent with *Candida* species
    Other
  Bacterial
    Microorganisms morphologically consistent with *Gardnerella* species
    Microorganisms morphologically consistent with *Actinomyces* species
    Cellular changes suggestive of *Chlamydia* species infection, subject to confirmatory studies
  Other
  Protozoan
    Trichomonas vaginalis
    Other
  Viral
    Cellular changes associated with cytomegalovirus
    Cellular changes associated with herpesvirus simplex
    Other
  Note: for human papillomavirus (HPV), refer to 'Epithelial Cell Abnormalities, Squamous Cell'
Reactive and reparative changes
  Inflammation
    Associated cellular changes
    Follicular cervicitis
  Miscellaneous (as related to patient history)

Table 9.2 *Continued*

Effects of therapy
  Ionizing radiation
  Chemotherapy
  Effects of mechanical devices (e.g. intrauterine contraceptive device)
  Effects of non-steroidal estrogen exposure (e.g. diethylstilbestrol)
Epithelial cell abnormalities
Squamous cell
  Atypical squamous cells of undetermined significance (recommended follow-up and/or
    type of further investigation: specify)
  Squamous intraepithelial lesion (SIL) (comment on presence of cellular changes associated
    with HPV if applicable)
    Low-grade squamous intraepithelial lesion, encompassing:
      Cellular changes associated with HPV
      Mild (slight) dysplasia/cervical intraepithelial neoplasia grade 1 (CIN I)
    High-grade squamous intraepithelial lesion, encompassing:
      Moderate dysplasia/CIN II
      Severe dysplasia/CIN III
      Carcinoma *in situ*/CIN III
  Squamous cell carcinoma
Glandular cell
  Presence of endometrial cells in one of the following circumstances:
    Out of phase in a menstruating woman
    In a postmenopausal woman
    No menstrual history available
    Atypical glandular cells of undetermined significance (recommended follow-up
      and/or type of further investigation: specify)
    Endometrial
    Endocervical
    Not otherwise specified
  Adenocarcinoma
    Specify probable site of origin: endocervical, endometrial, extrauterine
    Not otherwise specified
  Other epithelial malignant neoplasm: specify
Non-epithelial malignant neoplasm: specify
Hormonal evaluation (applies to vaginal smears only)
  Hormonal pattern compatible with age and history
  Hormonal pattern incompatible with age and history: specify
  Hormonal evaluation not possible
    Cervical specimen
    Inflammation
    Insufficient patient history
Other

report should include a recommendation for further patient evaluation when appropriate', no specific guidelines for such a recommendation were provided. To address these issues and other issues raised by clinicians, NCI sponsored a second workshop in 1991 to assess the use of the Bethesda System in actual practice and to consider modifications (Table 9.3).

The 1991 workshop resulted in the first revision of the Bethesda System that was significantly simpler and more streamlined than its predecessor. The general reporting format was retained, but minor modifications were made to each of the three elements. The issues of specific adequacy and diagnostic criteria were addressed by the publication of a monograph

Table 9.3 *The 1991 Bethesda System*

Adequacy of the specimen
Satisfactory for evaluation
Satisfactory for evaluation but limited by … (specify reason)
Unsatisfactory for evaluation … (specify reason)
General categorization (optional)
Within normal limits
Benign cellular changes: see descriptive diagnosis
Epithelial cell abnormality: see descriptive diagnosis
Descriptive diagnoses
Benign cellular changes
Infection
Trichomonas vaginalis
Fungal organisms morphologically consistent with *Candida* sp.
Predominance of coccobacilli consistent with shift in vaginal flora
Bacteria morphologically consistent with *Actinomyces* sp.
Cellular changes associated with herpes simplex virus
Other
Reactive changes
Reactive cellular changes associated with:
Inflammation (includes typical repair)
Atrophy with inflammation ('atrophic vaginitis')
Radiation
Intrauterine contraceptive device (IUD)
Other
Epithelial cell abnormalities
Squamous cell
Atypical squamous cells of undetermined significance: qualify[a]
Low-grade squamous intraepithelial lesion encompassing HPV[b] mild
dysplasia/cervical intraepithelial neoplasia (CIN) I
High-grade squamous intraepithelial lesion encompassing moderate and severe
dysplasia, carcinoma *in situ* (CIS)/CIN II and CIN III
Squamous cell carcinoma
Glandular cell
Endometrial cells, cytologically benign, in a postmenopausal woman
Atypical glandular cells of undetermined significance: qualify[a]
Endocervical adenocarcinoma
Endometrial adenocarcinoma
Extrauterine adenocarcinoma
Adenocarcinoma, not otherwise specified
Other malignant neoplasms: specify
Hormonal evaluation (applies to vaginal smears only)
Hormonal pattern compatible with age and history
Hormonal pattern incompatible with age and history: specify
Hormonal evaluation not possible due to … (specify)

[a]Atypical squamous or glandular cells of undetermined significance should be further qualified, if possible, as to whether a reactive or a premalignant process is favored.
[b]Cellular changes of HPV previously termed koilocytosis, koilocytotic atypia or condylomatous atypia are included in the category of low-grade squamous intraepithelial lesion.

with color photomicrographs to illustrate the definition of various entities.[14] The issue of recommendations for management in the report was addressed along with other issues raised by clinicians as described below.

While leaders in the field of obstetrics and gynecology had applauded a uniform reporting system that included clear definition of terminology, they remained skeptical about several aspects of the System according to their own perspectives.[15–18] Specifically, three aspects of the initial proposal were identified as problematic: the affirmation of the cytopathology report as a medical consultation, the language used to describe specimen adequacy ('Unsatisfactory' or 'Less than Optimal') and the terminology to describe squamous epithelial abnormalities. These issues were raised because of concern about how the language of the cytology report might affect patient care.

To label the cytopathology report as a medical consultation seemed to imply that recommendations for patient evaluation and follow-up would be made by those who had never examined the patient. The 1991 Bethesda Workshop concluded that recommendations, if given by cytopathologists in the cytology report, should focus on the need for additional steps to clarify pathological issues in order to reach a more definitive diagnosis. Examples of such recommendations include requesting a repeat smear after topical estrogen therapy to resolve the diagnostic dilemma of atypical squamous cells of undetermined significance (ASCUS) versus atrophy, and suggesting tissue confirmation of high-grade squamous intraepithelial lesion (HSIL). Furthermore, a qualifying phrase, such as 'as clinically indicated', should be included with all recommendations to avoid any impressions of directing patient management. Finally, recommendations in the cytology report are entirely optional.

The other two problem areas were associated with introducing new terms without knowledge of their clinical or scientific significance. While there were no data to either affirm or refute the validity of diagnosis in specimens deemed anything other than satisfactory, up to 20 per cent of patients with otherwise normal smears would be recalled and possibly retested unnecessarily because a specimen was labeled as 'less than optimal'.[17] Similarly, some clinicians felt that the new terminology to describe squamous epithelial abnormalities (ASCUS and SIL) created ambiguities, since no information existed concerning the clinical/biological significance of these terms. Consequently, this would again lead to costly, and perhaps unnecessary, testing and therapy.[19] Many felt that the 'classic terminology of dysplasia' (either CIN terminology or dysplasia/CIS) better represented their understanding of the biology and, therefore, better served the purpose of guiding the treatment of pre-cancerous squamous lesions of the cervix. The most controversial aspect of the new terminology involved including koilocytosis or cellular changes associated with HPV in the category of low-grade squamous intraepithelial lesions (LSIL), along with mild dysplasia (CIN I). It has been estimated that including HPV changes into the category of LSIL would cause an increase of 2–6 per cent in the number of women requiring additional evaluation and possibly treatment, which could result in additional health-care expenditures of over a billion dollars.[18,20]

To alleviate the clinicians' concern, the term 'less than optimal' was changed to 'satisfactory but limited by' in the revision. In an attempt to provide guidance to clinicians on appropriate management of patients with abnormalities of either specimen adequacy or epithelial cells, as defined by the Bethesda System, the Early Detection Branch of the National Cancer Institute convened a workshop in 1992. The participants included representatives from the fields of medicine, gynecology, pathology, family practice and epidemiology. Although interim guidelines for the management of abnormal cervical cytology were published in 1994,[21] it was recognized that final guidelines await more experience with the Bethesda System and data from clinical trials to determine the biological behavior of LSIL and the efficacy of adjunctive screening techniques, such as HPV typing. A revision of the 1991 Bethesda system guidelines has been scheduled by the National Institutes of Health (NIH) for 2001.

By 1992, The Bethesda System or a modification thereof were in widespread use in laboratories in the USA for reporting cervical cytology results, although the international adoption has been slow.[20,22] It therefore appears that the Bethesda System has achieved its first and foremost goal of improving communication by providing uniformity in reporting Pap smear results. This does not mean, however, that the System needs no improvement, as some critics of the Bethesda System would be quick to remind us.[23] For example, the debate on the determination of a satisfactory specimen by the presence of transformation zone cells continues.[24,25] (This topic is covered in detail in Chapter 2.) As proposed, the Bethesda System is a 'work in progress', having already undergone modifications to meet the needs of cytopathologists and clinicians. A current issue is the estimated 2–3 per cent increase in the number of women with abnormal Pap smears (due to changes in terminology for ASCUS and LSIL) that is translated to an increase in health-care cost and possibly morbidity. Can the blame for this be attributed solely to the adoption of The Bethesda System? Unlikely – the call for an improved reporting system came with the awareness of the fact that Pap smears are providing an important health service to women. Cytopathologists and cytotechnologists have become victims of their own success, which has resulted in unrealistic expectations of the Pap smear. A trend toward practicing 'defensive medicine' is the underlying cause of an increasing number of 'atypical' Pap smears, whether they be called 'ASCUS', 'squamous atypia' or any other term. The Bethesda System has at least provided a uniform term, if not definition, to convey the findings. Additional refinements of the Bethesda System are expected to follow more than a decade of experience with the reporting system as well as an increasing body of evidence derived from clinical studies. Most agree that the Bethesda System is a good beginning.

DIAGNOSTIC CRITERIA

Squamous intraepithelial lesion reflects the current concept of cervical carcinogenesis as defined by 'a spectrum of non-invasive cervical epithelial abnormalities traditionally classified as flat condyloma, dysplasia/CIS and CIN',[14] and incorporates the central role of HPV in its pathogenesis. The Bethesda System adopted a binary system for SIL, dividing all cervical precursor lesions into two categories, low and high grade, as opposed to three or more categories employed in previous classifications. The rationale for this choice included: (1) to improve inter- and intra-observer grading reproducibility; (2) to correspond to the increasing scientific data that support the separation of intraepithelial squamous lesions into two categories (low and high grade) based upon the risk of progression to squamous cell carcinoma; (3) to eliminate categories for which biological behavior or treatment does not significantly differ from the next higher grade. An obvious goal of the binary system is to determine patient care according to the grade. Epidemiological data suggest that high-grade lesions are much more likely to progress to carcinoma than low-grade lesions. However, the biological behavior of each individual lesion is still unpredictable based solely on current cytomorphological criteria.

Low-grade squamous intraepithelial lesion

A diagnosis of LSIL is given when the cellular changes associated with HPV cytopathic effect (koilocytosis and koilocytic atypia) or mild dysplasia/CIN I are present. These two previously separate categories share nearly identical HPV types (most often 'low risk' HPV types 6 and 11) and biological significance (more likely to regress without treatment and less likely to progress to carcinoma).[5] Other investigators have shown that a majority (>70 per cent) of cases diagnosed as 'mild dysplasia' have, on review, associated HPV cytopathic effect.[26]

Specific diagnostic criteria for LSIL include anisokaryosis, nuclear enlargement and hyper-chromasia, which are generally confined to cells with superficial-type cytoplasm. Other features, including binucleation or multinucleation and nuclear membrane abnormalities, are variably present. In order to be considered LSIL, cells with the cytoplasmic features of HPV effect (well-defined, optically clear perinuclear cavities or 'halos' with a peripheral dense cyto-plasmic rim) must also show the described nuclear abnormalities.[14] This last requirement appears to make the morphologic features of mild dysplasia/CIN I and koilocytic atypia indi-visible, a conclusion supported by investigators using strict criteria to define koilocytosis ver-sus CIN I.[27,28] Others have argued that diagnostic discrimination between these two lesions is possible and prognostically important in order to prevent overtreatment of non-progressive (koilocytic only) lesions.[19,29]

High-grade squamous intraepithelial lesion

A high-grade squamous intraepithelial lesion is defined by Bethesda terminology as squamous cells with enlarged, hyperchromatic nuclei showing irregular nuclear outlines and immature cytoplasm. The combination of nuclear enlargement in smaller, more immature cells leads to a pronounced increase in the nuclear/cytoplasmic ratio. The presence of syncytial-like aggre-gates of dysplastic cells – hyperchromatic crowded groups (HCGs) – is characteristic of CIS. No attempt is made to subdivide this category into levels of dysplasia. As with LSIL, this merg-ing of diagnostic categories (CIN II/moderate dysplasia and CIN III/severe dysplasia/CIS) has created the impression of biological homogeneity for the lesions. Questions about the validity of this assumption have been raised, based upon studies of the natural history of CIN, which suggest that CIN II has a greater tendency to regress than CIN III and that CIN III has a sig-nificantly higher rate of progression to invasive carcinoma than CIN II.[30,31] At present, these lesions are managed similarly in the USA.

Squamous cell carcinoma

It is generally accepted that lesions categorized as HSIL have a greater likelihood of progression to squamous cell carcinoma than those designated as LSIL. Left untreated, a significant num-ber of cases of HSIL progress to invasive squamous cell carcinoma.[4,30] There are no known cytological characteristics that predict which HSIL lesions will progress to invasion and the cytological features that correspond to histological microinvasion are non-specific and vari-ably represented.

As in CIS, the presence of highly dysplastic cells in syncytial groups is common in microin-vasive squamous cell carcinoma. The appearance of nucleoli (present in up to 25 per cent of the abnormal cells) and a tumor diathesis (which increases in frequency as the depth of inva-sion increases) favors the diagnosis of microinvasion.

Frankly invasive squamous cell carcinoma is characterized by more pronounced malignant features, including marked nuclear irregularity and cell-to-cell variability, the presence of even greater numbers of large and irregular nucleoli as well as the association in many cases with a tumor diathesis. Squamous cell carcinoma has traditionally been divided into three major types (non-keratinizing, keratinizing and small cell) that encompass the vast majority of inva-sive squamous cell carcinoma of the cervix. Other less common variants include verrucous squamous cell carcinoma, papillary squamous cell carcinoma, lymphoepithelial-like squa-mous cell carcinoma and spindle-cell squamous cell carcinoma. These variants may be virtu-ally indistinguishable from the major types of squamous cell carcinoma or other malignancies (sarcoma or melanoma) on cytological preparations.

LSIL versus HSIL

It is still debatable whether it is important or valid to differentiate between LSIL and HSIL on a Pap smear, since the first step in the management of either diagnosis may be histological confirmation.[32,33] If one assumes that the distinction is important, then the difficulty is in determining the 'cut-off' between the two diagnoses. Features that favor a diagnosis of HSIL include a greater number of abnormal cells on the smear, more pronounced nuclear outline and chromatin irregularities and less mature (lacy, delicate or dense/metaplastic) cytoplasm with rounded cell borders (Fig. 9.1a). In contrast, LSIL usually involves cells of the mature (superficial or intermediate) type with well-defined polygonal cell borders (Fig. 9.1b).

Diagnostic challenges

The use of the Bethesda System terminology has led to improved reporting uniformity, but has not eliminated the diagnostic uncertainty of Pap smear interpretations. Squamous lesions that have presented interpretive challenges in the past remain difficult. An entire chapter of this book is devoted to ASCUS. Further examples include non-specific cellular changes that mimic HPV effect versus true koilocytosis, keratinizing HSIL versus invasive squamous cell carcinoma, immature squamous metaplasia versus HSIL, atrophic changes versus HSIL or squamous cell carcinoma, HSIL involving endocervical glands, and repair versus squamous cell carcinoma. We will address these challenges in this section.

The differential diagnosis for koilocytosis includes changes caused by inflammation and infection, the presence of intracytoplasmic glycogen, differential staining of endoplasm and ectoplasm, and even the postmenopausal cervical milieu.[34] Strict adherence to diagnostic criteria may be helpful in excluding those mimics of HPV infection, although studies of reproducibility in making this diagnosis are cautionary.[28]

It is of paramount importance to remember that the nucleus of a true koilocyte must have dysplastic features. It must be enlarged and show nuclear chromatin and contour irregularities. The perinuclear halos that define koilocytes must also be held to strict criteria: the halo should be larger than the width of a typical intermediate cell nucleus ($>8\,\mu m$) and its edges must be sharply defined by a surrounding rim of dense cytoplasm. Reactive perinuclear halos

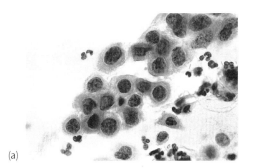
(a)

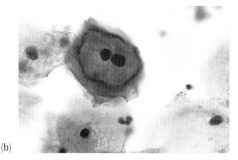
(b)

Figure 9.1 *(a) High-grade squamous intraepithelial lesion (HSIL) in parabasal-sized squamous cells. Note marked increase in nucleus–cytoplasm ratio (conventional smear, original magnification ×100). (b) Superficial squamous cell demonstrating classic features of a low-grade squamous intraepithelial lesion (LSIL) – binucleation with nuclear enlargement and hyperchromasia surrounded by a well-defined nuclear halo (conventional smear, original magnification ×100).*

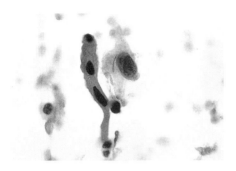

Figure 9.2 *Prominent tumor diathesis (granular material in the background composed of lysed red blood cells and cellular debris) in a smear of squamous cell carcinoma with round to spindle-shaped tumor cells and pyknotic nuclei (conventional smear, original magnification ×100).*

or other types of 'pseudo-koilocytosis' tend to be smaller and more indistinct than true koilocytic perinuclear halos.

The differentiation of keratinizing SIL from invasive squamous cell carcinoma may be aided by the identification of a tumor diathesis (Fig. 9.2). As already stated, the likelihood that bleeding and necrosis will become apparent on Pap smear increases with the increasing depth of invasion. The corollary to this is that microinvasive lesions, such as keratinizing SIL, will not usually demonstrate diathesis and will therefore be indistinguishable from SIL.

Squamous metaplasia of the endocervix is a normal physiological process which is thought to proceed along a maturation continuum from reserve cell hyperplasia to immature and, finally, to mature squamous metaplasia. The cytological features of each phase of this maturation process can be confused with SIL, in particular HSIL. Reserve cell hyperplasia is rarely identified on Pap smears, but can be mistaken for CIS because of its tendency to appear as syncytial sheets of very small cells with a high nucleus–cytoplasm (N/C) ratio. The key to appropriate diagnosis rests on the absence of chromatin or nuclear contour abnormalities and the uniform cell-to-cell appearance.

As reserve cells mature, they acquire the dense cytoplasm and distinct cell borders of immature squamous metaplasia. Immature squamous metaplasia is characterized by parabasal-sized squamous cells with dense cytoplasm and rounded cell borders. In conventional Pap smears, these cells tend to occur in groups often described as 'cobblestone' in appearance. The nucleus is round to oval with smooth contour, and nucleoli can be present as in reactive change. These cells are often admixed with more mature squamous metaplastic cells, contributing to an increase in pleomorphism. Dysplastic change in squamous metaplasia remains extremely difficult and has resulted in problems classifying these lesions using the Bethesda System terminology.[35] The diagnosis of dysplasia in metaplasia relies on very subtle differences in nuclear size, nuclear chromatin and nuclear membrane contour. Increased size and irregularity of the nucleus will favor a dysplastic process.

The search for cytological features of SIL or squamous cell carcinoma in a background of atrophy-related epithelial changes is daunting. While women older than 50 years have a low prevalence of SIL, the prevalence of squamous cell carcinoma increases after the age of 50 years, reflecting the natural history of cervical carcinogenesis. Atrophic smears can be filled with small and very degenerated parabasal cells in an inflammatory background. Diagnostic accuracy may be improved by applying reproducible cytological criteria.[36] Atrophic squamous cells demonstrate nuclear enlargement, mild nuclear hyperchromasia and often prominent degenerative changes. However, in contrast to dysplastic or neoplastic cells, their nuclear chromatin remains homogeneous and the nuclear borders are smooth (Fig. 9.3).

HSIL involving endocervical glands is a well-known diagnostic pitfall both in screening and interpretation. They can be mistaken for either reactive endocervical cells on the one hand or glandular neoplasia on the other.[37] Both architectural arrangements and nuclear features provide clues to the correct diagnosis.[38] Unlike true glandular cells that show peripheral

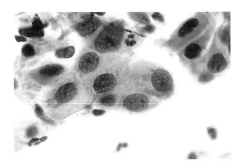

Figure 9.3 *Atropic changes as shown in this figure include nuclear enlargement, mild hyperchromasia and inflammatory background (conventional smear, original magnification ×100).*

palisading, HSIL involving endocervical glands has flattened cells at the periphery of cell clusters without evidence of polarization. The cells within a cluster often show overlapping and crowding but without nuclear molding. In contrast to either reactive or neoplastic glandular cells, neoplastic squamous cells have hyperchromatic nuclei with coarse chromatin and no nucleoli.

Like atrophy, reparative changes in squamous epithelium are notorious mimics of epithelial cell abnormalities. Reparative change can result in the under- or over-diagnosis of squamous lesions by Pap smear examination.[39] A key architectural feature of repair that can be seen in cytological smears is a tendency of these cells to occur in flat, mono-layered sheets with uniform nuclear orientation. Despite worrisome nuclear features (nucleomegaly, prominent nucleoli and even mitoses), other features of malignancy (numerous single cells, hyperchromasia and tumor diathesis) are not present.

Squamous lesions and liquid-based, thin-layer cervical cytology

The use of liquid-based thin-layer technology for cervical cytology in routine gynecological practice is increasing nationally and internationally. The first, and currently most widely used preparation, the ThinPrep Pap test (see Chapter 3), was approved for use by the Food and Drug Administration (FDA) in 1996 as an alternative to the conventional Pap smear. There is a growing body of evidence that points to an improvement in both specimen adequacy and diagnostic yield for this methodology.[40–45]

The cytological features of SIL in liquid-based, thin-layer preparations vary depending on the grade of the lesion. In general, the cytological features of LSIL in liquid-based, thin-layer preparations are not significantly different from those of the conventional Pap smear. Its detection is facilitated in thin-layer preparation and koilocytes are particularly easy to identify at low magnification. It is HSIL, squamous cell carcinoma and their mimics that show significant differences on liquid-based, thin-layer cytological preparations. Cells are generally smaller in liquid-based preparations due to immediate immersion fixation. Nuclear chromaticity can be altered, resulting in (usually) a lesser degree of hyperchromasia or even hypochromasia. The absence of this important diagnostic 'clue', as well as other features peculiar to conventional smears (streaming of dysplastic cells due to smear preparation, etc.) makes attention to nuclear contour abnormalities critical. While variations in thin-layer preparations exist (ThinPrep and AutoCyte), the technique generally results in disaggregation of cell groups, leading to an increased dispersion of similar cell types. Isolated single cells are the rule and cell-to-cell comparison can be difficult. A particular challenge, which many feel has been aggravated by the thin-layer technology, is the problem relating to small immature metaplastic cells. Differentiating between immature metaplasia, atypical immature metaplasia and HSIL is often impossible and may be responsible for false-positive results (Fig. 9.4). As has been shown for the conventional

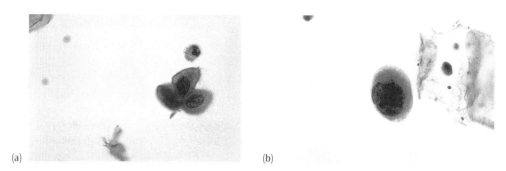

(a)   (b)

Figure 9.4 *(a) Atypical/immature squamous metaplastic cells that proved to be high-grade squamous intraepithelial lesions (HSIL) on biopsy. These cells have features of HSIL that are unique to ThinPrep, namely hypochromasia and irregular nuclear contour (ThinPrep, original magnification ×100). (b) Another example of HSIL in liquid-based, thin-layer preparation that is similar to those seen on conventional smears. The cell is isolated with a prominent hyperchromatic nucleus and irregular contour (ThinPrep, original magnification ×100).*

Pap smear, attention to the nuclear features of the cell in question is critical. Ancillary studies, such as HPV typing, which have been facilitated by the liquid-based technology, can help to make the distinction.

EPIDEMIOLOGICAL REVIEW

As in many types of human carcinogenesis, cervical neoplasia is currently postulated to most likely occur through a multi-step process, with increasing risk of progression to invasive squamous cell carcinoma at points further along the neoplastic progression of pre-invasive precursor lesions. As described in Chapter 6, HPV has been shown to play a pivotal role, and now stands as the primary risk factor in the development of cervical cancer. However, many other cofactors have been identified in the past two to three decades, reinforcing the complex and multifactorial nature of this neoplastic progression. More recent studies of these previously established risk factors have presented supporting evidence of interaction with HPV at a molecular or immunological level. A review of the major epidemiological cofactors and how they relate to the molecular biology of cervical carcinogenesis and (in concert with Chapter 6) the role of HPV follow.

Socioeconomic and marital/sexual factors and non-HPV genital infections

It has been well established that lower socioeconomic status (as measured by both income and education levels), young age at marriage and/or first sexual intercourse, and increasing lifetime number of sexual partners are associated with an increased relative risk of cervical HPV DNA detection.[5,46–52] As Brinton et al.[53] have emphasized, many social factors, such as sexual behavior, are closely related to each other as well as with HPV infection, which must be taken into consideration in the statistical documentation of an independent risk factor. However, these factors remain as persistent, although reduced, risk factors, after correction for HPV infection.

Anti-herpes simplex virus-2 antibodies and *Chlamydia trachomatis* seropositivity have been shown to be associated with cervical dysplasia/neoplasia,[5,51,54–57] but this association is either weakened or becomes inconsistent once the concomitant HPV infection is taken into consideration.[5,55]

Immunosuppression and human immunodeficiency virus infection

The immune responses of the host may function as a cofactor in the progression versus regression of HPV-associated CIN. Certainly, the risk of cervical neoplasia increases dramatically with systemic immunosuppression.[58] However, it is reasonable to postulate that individuals infected with human immunodeficiency virus (HIV) through sexual contact are also at increased risk for exposure to genital HPV infection. In addition to being a marker for exposure, de Sanjose et al.[59] reported a higher prevalence of CIN in HIV-positive prostitutes compared with HIV-negative prostitutes and further suggests that HIV-infection, irrespective of the route of exposure, represents an independent risk factor for the development of HPV-related cervical dysplasia.

Human immunodeficiency virus has also been shown to be associated with a high prevalence of HPV DNA detection, especially in women with low CD4 counts,[60–62] and rapid progression of HPV-induced squamous neoplasia.[63–65] However, as pointed out by Schiffman and Brinton,[5] it is not clear whether the immunosuppression caused by HIV infection increases the rate of progression of SIL to invasive disease and/or affects the prevalence/persistence of SIL.

The cellular immune response to HPV infection is postulated to involve Langerhans' (antigen presenting) cells and cytotoxic T lymphocytes.[66] A decrease in Langerhans' cells has been noted in CIN,[67] although this finding has not been consistently reproduced.[68,69] When present, the decrease has been correlated with increasing severity of CIN.[70] Langerhans' cells and CD4+ (helper) T lymphocytes are also reduced in the cervical transformation zone of smokers, potentially accounting for, in part, the correlation between smoking and cervical dysplasia (see section on Tobacco use).

Oral contraception use

In 1958, Woodruff and Peterson[71] in a review of papillary lesions of the uterine cervix noted that many of the condylomata reported to that date were in pregnant women, with the majority of these lesions spontaneously regressing in the post-partum period. In the 1960s, animal models demonstrated the capability of hormonal steroids to promote cervical cancer,[72,73] with the presence of high-affinity hormonal receptors noted in both normal and pathological cervical tissues,[74–76] particularly in endocervical adenocarcinomas.[75] Steroid hormones were then documented to increase HPV transcription both *in vitro* and *in vivo*, with upstream transcriptional hormonal-sensitive regulatory regions demonstrated.[77–80]

Although the association of oral contraceptive pill (OCP) use with HPV infection has not been consistently documented,[5] a significant association of invasive cervical carcinoma and long-term OCP use in HPV-positive women has been demonstrated in at least some studies.[46,48] It therefore has been suggested that OCP use is likely an important cofactor (with HPV) and may have a promoting role for progression of chronic HPV infection to cervical cancer. After adjustment for confounding factors, such as sexual and social histories, it is generally felt that long-term use of oral contraception (greater than 5 years) confers an increased, albeit a weakly increased, risk of cervical cancer,[5,81] particularly of cervical adenocarcinoma.[82–84] In studying specific types of non-barrier forms of contraception (oral, intrauterine devices and depot-medroxyprogesterone acetate), the New Zealand Contraception and Health Study Group found no difference in the rates of cervical dysplasia in multivariate analyses, with correction for confounding variables such as smoking and sexual history.[85] In contrast, barrier forms of contraception (diaphragm/condom) are associated with a lower risk of cervical cancer, possibly secondary to protection from sexually transmitted diseases, including HPV. However, the studies of these contraception modalities were limited by the short duration of use with the median duration only 2–3 years.

Gynecological/obstetric events

Multiparity appears to be consistently associated with an increased risk. Possible mechanisms include nutritional effects and demands of reproduction as well as the cervical trauma associated with vaginal delivery, as a reduced risk has been identified in individuals with Cesarean section deliveries.[46,86]

Age at menarche/menopause, characteristics of menses, and personal hygiene have been found to be associated with slight or no increased risk of cervical dysplasia/neoplasia.[5]

Tobacco use

Winkelstein[87] was the first to suggest that cigarette smoking may increase the risk of cervical cancer, having found a correlation between the geographic distribution of cervical cancer and that of other smoking-related cancers. This risk appears to be independent of age at first intercourse, number of sexual partners and socioeconomic class. No relationship, however, was noted with the less common cervical adenocarcinoma and/or adenosquamous carcinoma.

The evidence of a relationship between smoking and altered immune function/immunosurveillance has been mounting since the late 1970s.[88–90] In addition, numerous tobacco constituents and metabolites have been identified in cervical mucus at relatively high concentrations when compared with serum levels.[91] Holly et al.[92] also found cervical fluids of smokers to show mutagenic activity at higher rates than non-smokers. More recently Simons et al.[93] have found that smokers have a significantly increased median percentage of DNA adducts (modified or 'damaged' DNA, the formation of which is a critical step in carcinogenesis)[94] as measured by ^{32}P post-labeling, in their ectocervical epithelium, with a similar increase also seen in women with abnormal cervical smears. Furthermore, smoking has been shown to influence the local cervical immunosurveillance in current smokers by significantly decreasing the density of human leukocyte antigen (HLA)-DR-positive and CD1a+ Langerhans' cells.[95] Peripheral blood analysis of T lymphocyte subsets of heavy smokers has also revealed a reversible and relative decrease in CD4+ T lymphocytes.[95] All grades of CIN have been shown to have a significant reduction in the CD4+ T lymphocytes in the transformation zone and a reversed CD4/CD8 lymphocyte ratio has been documented in cervical condyloma. This alteration in intraepithelial lymphocyte populations in smokers may have a similar effect in patients to that of the HIV-related immunodeficiency on HPV progression (see Immunosuppression and human immunodeficiency virus infection).

Population-based age-adjusted incidence rates of cervical cancer (in Norway) have revealed a statistically significant positive association with number of cigarettes smoked per day, cumulative years of smoking and young age at which smoking began,[96] although the associations with duration of smoking and early age of onset of smoking have not been reproduced in other studies.[97] The ex-smoker risk has been shown to be intermediate between that of current smokers and non-smokers, with a lower risk among those with cessation greater than 10 years than for more recent quitters.[97]

Although a positive association of smoking with cervical dysplasia has not been demonstrated after controlling for confounding factors,[51] dysplasia grade-specific analysis has demonstrated an increased risk of high-grade dysplasia in HPV-positive smokers when compared with HPV-positive non-smokers.[98] There appears to be a dose–response relationship between the number of cigarettes smoked daily and the presence of high-risk HPV types (16, 18 and 33) in all grades of CIN, which persists after adjustment for age at first intercourse and lifetime number of sexual partners.[99] In summary, the cumulative evidence suggests a causal relationship between smoking and cervical neoplasia.[100]

The possibility of a synergistic relationship has been raised for smoking and diet/nutritional factors on cervical neoplasia[101] and this will be discussed next.

Dietary/nutritional factors

The evidence supporting a relationship between diet and cancer development has been growing for the past few decades.[102,103] Large international differences in cancer rates are felt to be partly explained by variation in nutritional intake. Epidemiological studies of cancer and dietary micronutrients have specifically suggested that dietary deficiencies of the retinoids, beta-carotene, ascorbate, and folic acid increase risk of cervical neoplasia.[104–115]

The retinoid group includes vitamin A and its natural and synthetic analogues, which are necessary for growth and differentiation of epithelial tissues. Its dietary deficiency increases the risk of squamous pre-neoplastic and neoplastic lesions. In the cervix, they may act by suppressing the expression of the HPV E6 and E7 proteins,[116,117] possibly by increasing secretion of transforming growth factor (TGF)-β[118,119] (see also Cytokines below). Beta-carotene is the most common and active carotenoid found in the diet.[117] Its conversion to vitamin A, with subsequent regulation of epithelial cell differentiation and free radical scavenging, may form the basis of its protective effects for cervical cancer risk.[114] Folate (or folic acid) is a coenzyme of DNA synthesis, necessary for normal cell growth, proliferation and differentiation.[117] Low erythrocytic folate levels appear to enhance patient susceptibility to HPV infection,[120] and *in vitro* studies have demonstrated decreased oncogene expression, including HPV E6, in folate-treated cell lines.[121]

MOLECULAR BIOLOGY REVIEW (EXCLUDING HPV)

A cursory review of the current knowledge of molecular biology and possible tumorigenesis in cervical dysplasia/neoplasia is given below.

Oncogenes

Altered oncogene activity has been described in numerous malignancies,[122] with increasing literature relating the overexpression of oncogenes to premalignant (dysplastic) states, including the uterine cervix. HPV DNA has been found to be integrated near cellular oncogenes in invasive cervical carcinoma.[123] In preinvasive and microinvasive disease, c-*myc* protein expression appears to increase as the lesions progress to high-grade dysplasia and microinvasive carcinomas,[124–127] with similar results described for h-*ras* and c-*erb-2*.[128–132]

Cytokines (growth factors/growth factor receptors/interleukin expression)

Keratinocytes transfected with HPV have been demonstrated to secrete interleukin-6 (IL-6),[133] a multifunctional cytokine that has been shown to act as an *in vitro* growth factor in a number of tumor types and may function in a similar role in cervical carcinoma.[134] Tartour et al.[135] have further described significantly increased expression of the IL-6 gene in invasive cervical carcinoma *in vivo* compared with CIN and normal cervical tissue. Transforming growth factor-β is an additional multifunctional cytokine of interest in cervical carcinogenesis research. It inhibits *in vitro* proliferation of normal genital squamous epithelial cells through apparent autocrine regulation,[136–138] downregulates HPV 16 and 18 E6 and E7 transcription, and inhibits *in vitro* non-tumorigenic HPV DNA-containing genital epithelial cell lines.[139,140] Decreasing expression of cervical epithelial intracellular TGF-β1, one of three homologous isoforms of TGF-β, has been associated with the progression of intraepithelial neoplasia, with concomitant increasing stromal extracellular expression. Thus, the loss of growth-inhibitory effects of epithelial TGF-β1 with tumor growth promotion, via paracrine effects of extracellular stromal TGF-β1[141] and its stromal angiogenesis promotion,[142] may play a role in cervical tumorigenesis.[140]

Interleukin-1, also an autocrine epidermal growth factor,[143] and epidermal growth factor receptor, which may interact with HPV E5 to enhance transformation,[144–146] have been demonstrated by flow cytometry and immunohistochemistry to be increased in high-grade CIN and cervical squamous cell carcinomas.[129]

Integrin expression

Alterations in epithelial cell–basement membrane interaction also represent an area of active research in cervical neoplasia and progression to malignant tumor transformation. Integrins, a family of heterodimeric transmembrane glycoproteins that mediate cell–cell and cell–matrix adhesion, have been shown to vary in epithelial staining distribution patterns from normal to neoplastic cervical epithelium,[70,147,148] with loss or reduction of integrin chain expression in high-grade dysplasia (CIN III)[70] – a finding similar to that observed in dysplastic and invasive squamous cell carcinomas of the skin.[149]

The expression of certain integrin chains has been suggested to possess diagnostic and potentially prognostic capability in cervical neoplasia,[70] however, variability of immunohistochemical integrin expression for given degrees of dysplasia and within individual cases[147] currently limits diagnostic specificity.

Genetics/human leukocyte antigen expression

Histocompatibility-related leukocyte antigens (HLA) class I and II of the major histocompatibility complex (MHC) play a pivotal role in antigen immunorecognition within the cellular immune response. Alterations in this expression may lead to a lack of immune recognition and an escape from cytotoxic T lymphocytes, which are felt to play a major role in the cellular immune response to HPV infection (see Immunosuppression and human immunodeficiency virus infection).[66] Studies have demonstrated a reduced expression of class I MHC antigens,[150,151] with *de novo* expression of class II MHC antigens, primarily HLA-DR, in cervical carcinoma.[151,152] Such alterations are less commonly seen in premalignant (dysplastic) squamous epithelium, particularly that of low grade. This HLA-DR expression in high-grade dysplasia and invasive carcinomas may be related to local influences of cytokines that are possibly derived from increased intraepithelial lymphocytes.[153,154] Epidemiological genetic studies have also linked HLA class II allele expression, particularly HLA-DQ, to the risk of cervical neoplasia.[155,156]

Tumor markers

The study of molecular markers of neoplasia (biomarkers or tumor-associated antigen markers) has become an active area of basic research and clinico-pathological study. Examples of potential markers in cervical carcinogenesis include the membrane antigen designated as MN and the squamous cell carcinoma antigen SCC-Ag.

The MN antigen is associated with the tumorigenic phenotype of HeLa cells (a cervical carcinoma-derived cell line) and HeLa×fibroblast hybrids.[157] Significant levels of its expression over that seen in normal cervical epithelium have been described in CIN, squamous cervical carcinomas and adenocarcinomas,[158] although the original suggestions that this antigen is a marker of high-risk groups and that it reflects neoplastic progression were not corroborated by a subsequent study.[159]

The squamous cell carcinoma antigen SCC-Ag, first described by Kato and Torigoe in 1977,[160] is a subfraction of TA-4, a cervical squamous cell carcinoma-derived tumor antigen. It has been suggested as a marker of response to treatment and post-treatment tumor recurrence, with use in choosing therapeutic modalities in patients with higher than expected values for their clinical stage.[161,162]

Cell cycle proteins

Cell cycle proteins are involved in the regulation of cell proliferation and are postulated to interact with HPV viral oncoproteins, particularly HPV-E6 and HPV-E7. This interaction appears to be coupled to inactivation of the tumor suppressor proteins TP53 and pRB, which are functionally inactivated upon binding with the viral oncoproteins.[163] This inactivation results in the loss of normal cell cycle regulation, which may be manifested by increased transcription of certain cell cycle genes. Thus, it follows that the identification of the corresponding cell cycle proteins or protein complexes in patient material may be helpful as an adjunct marker for HPV infection and related dysplastic and neoplastic lesions.

One of the cell cycle proteins, cyclin E, has been studied with immunohistochemistry in archival cervical biopsies and found to be overexpressed in CIN, particularly within low-grade lesions, and squamous cell carcinoma (SCC), and was rarely seen in normal/reactive cervical epithelium or non-diagnostic squamous atypias.[164] Cyclin E has been further studied in monolayer (ThinPrep) gynecological specimens, and was found strongly correlate with the morphological features of HPV and anti-HPV antibody positivity, although in this study by Weaver et al.[165] histological correlation data were not available. Protein complexes formed by cyclin proteins and cyclin-dependent kinases, most notably p21, are also overexpressed in both high-grade CIN[166] and cervical carcinomas.[167]

Although these proteins and cell cycle protein complexes have potential as surrogate markers for HPV infection and HPV-related gynecological lesions, further large corroborating studies with cytological–histological correlation and cost-effectiveness are needed.

FUTURE TRENDS

At the time of writing, morphology is still the gold standard to triage patient management. High-risk HPV DNA type has shown some promise to aid in this regard (see Chapter 6). With the advancement of molecular biology, a highly sensitive and specific marker to indicate high risk or actual neoplastic progression may replace morphology. MN antigen appeared to hold such a promise at one point. However, it seems that much more work will be needed to verify the initial findings and to extend the research findings to clinical application. The cost of such a marker may be another prohibiting factor for it to completely replace morphology.

REFERENCES

1 Kline TS. The Papanicolaou smear: a brief historical perspective and where we are today. *Arch Pathol Lab Med* 1997; **121**: 205–9.

2 Papanicolaou GN. *Atlas of exfoliative cytology*. Cambridge, MA: Harvard University Press, 1954.

3 Wied GL, ed. Proceedings of First International Congress Exfoliative Cytology. Philadelphia: Lippincott, 1961: 283.

4 Richart RM. Cervical intraepithelial neoplasia. *Pathol Annu* 1973; **8**: 301–28.

5 Schiffman MH, Brinton LA. The epidemiology of cervical carcinogenesis. *Cancer* 1995; **76**: 1888–901.

6 Paterson ME, Peel KR, Joslin CA. Cervical smear histories of 500 women with invasive cervical cancer in Yorkshire. *BMJ (Clin Res Edn)* 1984; **289**: 896–8.

7 Eddy D. ACS report on the cancer-related health checkup. *CA Cancer J Clin* 1980; **30**: 193–240.

8 Kottmeier HL. *Carcinoma of the female genitalia*. Baltimore: Williams & Wilkins, 1953.

9 Petersen O. Spontaneous course of cervical precancerous conditions. *Am J Obstet Gynecol* 1956; **72**: 1063–71.

10 Nasiell K, Roger V, Nasiell M. Behavior of mild cervical dysplasia during long-term follow-up. *Obstet Gynecol* 1986; **67**: 665–9.

11 Bogdanich W. Lax Laboratories: the Pap test misses much cervical cancer through lab's errors. *Wall Street J* 1987; Nov 2: 1.

12 Bogdanich W. Physicians carelessness with Pap tests is cited in procedure's high failure rate. *Wall Street J* 1987; Dec 29: 17.

13 National Cancer Institute Workshop. The 1988 Bethesda System for reporting cervical/vaginal cytological diagnoses. *JAMA* 1989; **262**: 931–4.

14 Kurman RJ, Soloman D. *The Bethesda system for reporting cervical/vaginal cytologic diagnosis: definitions, criteria and explanatory notes for terminology and specimen adequacy*. New York: Springer-Verlag, 1994.

15 Bottles K, Reiter RC, Steiner AL, Zaleski S, Bedrossian CW, Johnson SR. Problems encountered with the Bethesda System: the University of Iowa experience. *Obstet Gynecol* 1991; **78**: 410–14.

16 Greer BE. The gynecologist's perspective of liability and quality issues with the Papanicolaou smear. *Arch Pathol Lab Med* 1997; **121**: 246–9.

17 Herbst AL. The Bethesda System for cervical/vaginal cytologic diagnoses: a note of caution [editorial]. *Obstet Gynecol* 1990; **76**: 449–50.

18 Herbst AL. The Bethesda system for cervical/vaginal cytologic diagnoses. *Clin Obstet Gynecol* 1992; **35**: 22–7.

19 Lonky NM, Navarre GL, Saunders S, Sadeghi M, Wolde-Tsadik G. Low-grade Papanicolaou smears and the Bethesda system: a prospective cytohistopathologic analysis. *Obstet Gynecol* 1995; **85**: 716–20.

20 Jones 3rd HW. Impact of the Bethesda System. *Cancer* 1995; **76**: 1914–18.

21 Kurman RJ, Henson DE, Herbst AL, Noller KL, Schiffman MH. Interim guidelines for management of abnormal cervical cytology. The 1992 National Cancer Institute Workshop. *JAMA* 1994; **271**: 1866–9.

22 Davey DD, Nielsen ML, Rosenstock W, Kline TS. Terminology and specimen adequacy in cervicovaginal cytology. The College of American Pathologists Interlaboratory Comparison Program experience. *Arch Pathol Lab Med* 1992; **116**: 903–7.

23 Koss LG. The new Bethesda System for reporting results of smears of the uterine cervix. *J Natl Cancer Inst* 1990; **82**: 988–91.

24 Mitchell H, Medley G. Influence of endocervical status on the cytologic prediction of cervical intraepithelial neoplasia. *Acta Cytol* 1992; **36**: 875–80.

25 Sherman ME, Weinstein M, Sughayer M, et al. The Bethesda System. Impact on reporting cervicovaginal specimens and reproducibility of criteria for assessing endocervical sampling. *Acta Cytol* 1993; **37**: 55–60.

26 Meisels A, Morin C. Human papillomavirus and cancer of the uterine cervix. *Gynecol Oncol* 1981; **12**: S111–23.

27 Hall S, Wu TC, Soudi N, Sherman ME. Low-grade squamous intraepithelial lesions: cytologic predictors of biopsy confirmation. *Diagn Cytopathol* 1994; **10**: 3–9.

28 Lee KR, Minter LJ, Crum CP. Koilocytotic atypia in Papanicolaou smears. Reproducibility and biopsy correlations. *Cancer* 1997; **81**: 10–15.

29 Syrjanen K, Kataja V, Yliskoski M, Chang F, Syrjanen S, Saarikoski S. Natural history of cervical human papillomavirus lesions does not substantiate the biologic relevance of the Bethesda System. *Obstet Gynecol* 1992; **79**: 675–82.

30 Ostor AG. Natural history of cervical intraepithelial neoplasia: a critical review. *Int J Gynecol Pathol* 1993; **12**: 186–92.

31 Sherman ME, Kurman RJ. The role of exfoliative cytology and histopathology in screening and triage. *Obstet Gynecol Clin North Am* 1996; **23**: 641–55.

32 Joste NE, Rushing L, Granados R, et al. Bethesda classification of cervicovaginal smears: reproducibility and viral correlates. *Hum Pathol* 1996; **27**: 581–5.

33 McGrath CM, Kurtis JD, Yu GH. Evaluation of mild-to-moderate dysplasia on cervical-endocervical (Pap) smear: a subgroup of patients who bridge LSIL and HSIL. *Diagn Cytopathol* 2000; **23**: 245–8.

34 Jovanovic AS, McLachlin CM, Shen L, Welch WR, Crum CP. Postmenopausal squamous atypia: a spectrum including 'pseudo-koilocytosis' [see comments]. *Mod Pathol* 1995; **8**: 408–12.

35 Sherman ME, Tabbara SO, Scott DR, et al. 'ASCUS, rule out HSIL': cytologic features, histologic correlates, and human papillomavirus detection. *Mod Pathol* 1999; **12**: 335–42.

36 Acs G, Gupta PK, Baloch ZW. Glandular and squamous atypia and intraepithelial lesions in atrophic cervicovaginal smears. One institution's experience. *Acta Cytol* 2000; **44**: 611–17.

37 Selvaggi SM. Cytologic features of squamous cell carcinoma *in situ* involving endocervical glands in endocervical cytobrush specimens. *Acta Cytol* 1994; **38**: 687–92.

38 Siziopikou KP, Wang HH, Abu-Jawdeh G. Cytologic features of neoplastic lesions in endocervical glands. *Diagn Cytopathol* 1997; **17**: 1–7.

39 Colgan TJ, Woodhouse SL, Styer PE, Kennedy M, Davey DD. Reparative changes and the false-positive/false-negative Papanicolaou test. *Arch Pathol Lab Med* 2001; **125**: 134–40.

40 Bishop JW, Bigner SH, Colgan TJ, et al. Multicenter masked evaluation of AutoCyte PREP thin layers with matched conventional smears. Including initial biopsy results. *Acta Cytol* 1998; **42**: 189–97.

41 Carpenter AB, Davey DD. ThinPrep Pap Test: performance and biopsy follow-up in a university hospital. *Cancer* 1999; **87**: 105–12.

42 Guidos BJ, Selvaggi SM. Use of the ThinPrep Pap Test in clinical practice. *Diagn Cytopathol* 1999; **20**: 70–3.

43 Papillo JL, Zarka MA, St John TL. Evaluation of the ThinPrep Pap test in clinical practice. A seven-month, 16,314-case experience in northern Vermont. *Acta Cytol* 1998; **42**: 203–8.

44 Vassilakos P, Griffin S, Megevand E, Campana A. CytoRich liquid-based cervical cytologic test. Screening results in a routine cytopathology service. *Acta Cytol* 1998; **42**: 198–202.

45 Wilbur DC, Cibas ES, Merritt S, James LP, Berger BM, Bonfiglio TA. ThinPrep Processor. Clinical trials demonstrate an increased detection rate of abnormal cervical cytologic specimens [see comments]. *Am J Clin Pathol* 1994; **101**: 209–14.

46 Bosch FX, Munoz N, de Sanjose S, et al. Risk factors for cervical cancer in Colombia and Spain. *Int J Cancer* 1992; **52**: 750–8.

47 Brinton LA, Hamman RF, Huggins GR, et al. Sexual and reproductive risk factors for invasive squamous cell cervical cancer. *J Natl Cancer Inst* 1987; **79**: 23–30.

48 Eluf-Neto J, Booth M, Munoz N, Bosch FX, Meijer CJ, Walboomers JM. Human papillomavirus and invasive cervical cancer in Brazil. *Br J Cancer* 1994; **69**: 114–19.

49 Fasal E, Simmons ME, Kampert JB. Factors associated wih high and low risk of cervical neoplasia. *J Natl Cancer Inst* 1981; **66**: 631–6.

50 Hildesheim A, Gravitt P, Schiffman MH, et al. Determinants of genital human papillomavirus infection in low-income women in Washington, DC. *Sex Transm Dis* 1993; **20**: 279–85.

51 Koutsky LA, Holmes KK, Critchlow CW, et al. A cohort study of the risk of cervical intraepithelial neoplasia grade 2 or 3 in relation to papillomavirus infection. *N Engl J Med* 1992; **327**: 1272–8.

52 West DW, Schuman KL, Lyon JL, Robison LM, Allred R. Differences in risk estimations from a hospital and a population-based case-control study. *Int J Epidemiol* 1984; **13**: 235–9.

53 Brinton LA, Schairer C, Haenszel W, et al. Cigarette smoking and invasive cervical cancer. *JAMA* 1986; **255**: 3265–9.

54 Coleman DV, Morse AR, Beckwith P, et al. Prognostic significance of herpes simplex virus antibody status in women with cervical intraepithelial neoplasia (CIN). *Br J Obstet Gynaecol* 1983; **90**: 421–7.

55 de Sanjose S, Munoz N, Bosch FX, et al. Sexually transmitted agents and cervical neoplasia in Colombia and Spain. *Int J Cancer* 1994; **56**: 358–63.

56 Hildesheim A, Mann V, Brinton LA, Szklo M, Reeves WC, Rawls WE. Herpes simplex virus type 2: a possible interaction with human papillomavirus types 16/18 in the development of invasive cervical cancer. *Int J Cancer* 1991; **49**: 335–40.

57 Jha PK, Beral V, Peto J, et al. Antibodies to human papillomavirus and to other genital infectious agents and invasive cervical cancer risk [see comments]. *Lancet* 1993; **341**: 1116–18.

58 Porreco R, Penn I, Droegemueller W, Greer B, Makowski E. Gynecologic malignancies in immunosuppressed organ homograft recipients. *Obstet Gynecol* 1975; **45**: 359–64.

59 de Sanjose S, Palacio V, Tafur L, et al. Prostitution, HIV, and cervical neoplasia: a survey in Spain and Colombia. *Cancer Epidemiol Biomarkers Prev* 1993; **2**: 531–5.

60 Ho GY, Burk RD, Fleming I, Klein RS. Risk of genital human papillomavirus infection in women with human immunodeficiency virus-induced immunosuppression. *Int J Cancer* 1994; **56**: 788–92.

61 Maiman M, Tarricone N, Vieira J, Suarez J, Serur E, Boyce JG. Colposcopic evaluation of human immunodeficiency virus-seropositive women. *Obstet Gynecol* 1991; **78**: 84–8.

62 Vermund SH, Kelley KF, Klein RS, et al. High risk of human papillomavirus infection and cervical squamous intraepithelial lesions among women with symptomatic human immunodeficiency virus infection. *Am J Obstet Gynecol* 1991; **165**: 392–400.

63 Johnson JC, Burnett AF, Willet GD, Young MA, Doniger J. High frequency of latent and clinical human papillomavirus cervical infections in immunocompromised human immunodeficiency virus-infected women. *Obstet Gynecol* 1992; **79**: 321–7.

64 Maiman M, Fruchter RG, Serur E, Remy JC, Feuer G, Boyce J. Human immunodeficiency virus infection and cervical neoplasia. *Gynecol Oncol* 1990; **38**: 377–82.

65 ter Meulen J, Eberhardt HC, Luande J, et al. Human papillomavirus (HPV) infection, HIV infection and cervical cancer in Tanzania, east Africa. *Int J Cancer* 1992; **51**: 515–21.

66 Crawford L. Prospects for cervical cancer vaccines. *Cancer Surv* 1993; **16**: 215–29.

67 Tay SK, Jenkins D, Maddox P, Campion M, Singer A. Subpopulations of Langerhans' cells in cervical neoplasia. *Br J Obstet Gynaecol* 1987; **94**: 10–15.

68 McArdle JP, Muller HK. Quantitative assessment of Langerhans' cells in human cervical intraepithelial neoplasia and wart virus infection. *Am J Obstet Gynecol* 1986; **154**: 509–15.

69 Morris HH, Gatter KC, Sykes G, Casemore V, Mason DY. Langerhans' cells in human cervical epithelium: effects of wart virus infection and intraepithelial neoplasia. *Br J Obstet Gynaecol* 1983; **90**: 412–20.

70 Cristoforoni P, Favre A, Cennamo V, Giunta M, Corte G, Grossi CE. Expression of a novel beta 1 integrin in the dysplastic progression of the cervical epithelium. *Gynecol Oncol* 1995; **58**: 319–26.

71 Woodruff JD, Peterson WF. Condyloma acuminata of the cervix. *Am J Obstet Gynecol* 1958; **75**: 1354–62.

72 Dunn TB. Cancer of the uterine cervix in mice fed a liquid diet containing an antifertility drug. *J Natl Cancer Inst* 1969; **43**: 671–92.

73 Kaminetzky HA. Methylcholanthrene-induced cervical dysplasia and the sex steroids. *Obstet Gynecol* 1966; **27**: 489–93.

74 Cao ZY, Eppenberger U, Roos W, Torhorst J, Almendral A. Cytosol estrogen and progesterone receptor levels measured in normal and pathological tissue of endometrium, endocervical mucosa and cervical vaginal portion. *Arch Gynecol* 1983; **233**: 109–19.

75 Ford LC, Berek JS, Lagasse LD, Hacker NF, Heins YL, DeLange RJ. Estrogen and progesterone receptor sites in malignancies of the uterine cervix, vagina, and vulva. *Gynecol Oncol* 1983; **15**: 27–31.

76 Sanborn BM, Kuo HS, Held B. Estrogen and progestogen binding site concentrations in human endometrium and cervix throughout the menstrual cycle and in tissue from women taking oral contraceptives. *J Steroid Biochem* 1978; **9**: 951–5.

77 Auborn KJ, Woodworth C, DiPaolo JA, Bradlow HL. The interaction between HPV infection and estrogen metabolism in cervical carcinogenesis. *Int J Cancer* 1991; **49**: 867–9.

78 Monsonego J, Magdelenat H, Catalan F, Coscas Y, Zerat L, Sastre X. Estrogen and progesterone receptors in cervical human papillomavirus related lesions. *Int J Cancer* 1991; **48**: 533–9.

79 Pater A, Bayatpour M, Pater MM. Oncogenic transformation by human papillomavirus type 16 deoxyribonucleic acid in the presence of progesterone or progestins from oral contraceptives. *Am J Obstet Gynecol* 1990; **162**: 1099–103.

80 Pater MM, Hughes GA, Hyslop DE, Nakshatri H, Pater A. Glucocorticoid-dependent oncogenic transformation by type 16 but not type 11 human papilloma virus DNA. *Nature* 1988; **335**: 832–5.

81 WHO Collaborative Study of Neoplasia and Steroid Contraceptives. Invasive squamous-cell cervical carcinoma and combined oral contraceptives: results from a multinational study. *Int J Cancer* 1993; **55**: 228–36.

82 Brinton LA, Huggins GR, Lehman HF, et al. Long-term use of oral contraceptives and risk of invasive cervical cancer. *Int J Cancer* 1986; **38**: 399–44.

83 Dallenbach-Hellweg G. On the origin and histological structure of adenocarcinoma of the endocervix in women under 50 years of age. *Pathol Res Pract* 1984; **179**: 38–50.

84 Ursin G, Peters RK, Henderson BE, d'Ablaing 3rd G, Monroe KR, Pike MC. Oral contraceptive use and adenocarcinoma of cervix [see comments]. *Lancet* 1994; **344**: 1390–4.

85 The New Zealand Contraception and Health Study Group. Risk of cervical dysplasia in users of oral contraceptives, intrauterine devices or depot-medroxyprogesterone acetate. *Contraception* 1994; **50**: 431–41.

86 Brinton LA, Reeves WC, Brenes MM, et al. Parity as a risk factor for cervical cancer. *Am J Epidemiol* 1989; **130**: 486–96.

87 Winkelstein Jr W. Smoking and cancer of the uterine cervix: hypothesis. *Am J Epidemiol* 1977; **106**: 257–9.

88 Corberand J, Nguyen F, Do AH, et al. Effect of tobacco smoking on the functions of polymorphonuclear leukocytes. *Infect Immun* 1979; **23**: 577–81.

89 Miller LG, Goldstein G, Murphy M, Ginns LC. Reversible alterations in immunoregulatory T cells in smoking. Analysis by monoclonal antibodies and flow cytometry. *Chest* 1982; **82**: 526–9.

90 White Jr KL, Holsapple MP. Direct suppression of *in vitro* antibody production by mouse spleen cells by the carcinogen benzo(a)pyrene but not by the noncarcinogenic congener benzo(e)pyrene. *Cancer Res* 1984; **44**: 3388–93.

91 Sasson IM, Haley NJ, Hoffmann D, Wynder EL, Hellberg D, Nilsson S. Cigarette smoking and neoplasia of the uterine cervix: smoke constituents in cervical mucus [letter]. *N Engl J Med* 1985; **312**: 315–16.

92 Holly EA, Petrakis NL, Friend NF, Sarles DL, Lee RE, Flander LB. Mutagenic mucus in the cervix of smokers. *J Natl Cancer Inst* 1986; **76**: 983–6.

93 Simons AM, Phillips DH, Coleman DV. Damage to DNA in cervical epithelium related to smoking tobacco [see comments]. *BMJ* 1993; **306**: 1444–8.

94 Miller EC, Miller JA. Searches for ultimate chemical carcinogens and their reactions with cellular macromolecules. *Cancer* 1981; **47**: 2327–45.

95 Poppe WA, Ide PS, Drijkoningen MP, Lauweryns JM, van Assche FA. Tobacco smoking impairs the local immunosurveillance in the uterine cervix. An immunohistochemical study. *Gynecol Obstet Invest* 1995; **39**: 34–8.

96 Gram IT, Austin H, Stalsberg H. Cigarette smoking and the incidence of cervical intraepithelial neoplasia, grade III, and cancer of the cervix uteri. *Am J Epidemiol* 1992; **135**: 341–6.

97 de Vet HC, Sturmans F, Knipschild PG. The role of cigarette smoking in the etiology of cervical dysplasia. *Epidemiology* 1994; **5**: 631–3.

98 Schiffman MH, Bauer HM, Hoover RN, et al. Epidemiologic evidence showing that human papillomavirus infection causes most cervical intraepithelial neoplasia [see comments]. *J Natl Cancer Inst* 1993; **85**: 958–64.

99 Burger MP, Hollema H, Gouw AS, Pieters WJ, Quint WG. Cigarette smoking and human papillomavirus in patients with reported cervical cytological abnormality [see comments]. *BMJ* 1993; **306**: 749–52.

100 Winkelstein Jr W. Smoking and cervical cancer – current status: a review. *Am J Epidemiol* 1990; **131**: 945–57; discussion 58–60.

101 Butterworth Jr CE. Effect of folate on cervical cancer. Synergism among risk factors. *Ann NY Acad Sci* 1992; **669**: 293–9.

102 Willett WC, MacMahon B. Diet and cancer – an overview. *N Engl J Med* 1984; **310:** 633–8.

103 Willett WC, MacMahon B. Diet and cancer – an overview (second of two parts). *N Engl J Med* 1984; **310**: 697–703.

104 Correa P. Vitamins and cancer prevention. *Cancer Epidemiol Biomarkers Prev* 1992; **1**: 241–3.

105 Herrero R, Potischman N, Brinton LA, et al. A case-control study of nutrient status and invasive cervical cancer. I. Dietary indicators. *Am J Epidemiol* 1991; **134**: 1335–46.

106 La Vecchia C, Franceschi S, Decarli A, et al. Dietary vitamin A and the risk of invasive cervical cancer. *Int J Cancer* 1984; **34**: 319–22.

107 Liu T, Soong SJ, Wilson NP, et al. A case control study of nutritional factors and cervical dysplasia. *Cancer Epidemiol Biomarkers Prev* 1993; **2**: 525–30.

108 Marshall JR, Graham S, Byers T, Swanson M, Brasure J. Diet and smoking in the epidemiology of cancer of the cervix. *J Natl Cancer Inst* 1983; **70**: 847–51.

109 Palan PR, Mikhail MS, Basu J, Romney SL. Plasma levels of antioxidant beta-carotene and alpha-tocopherol in uterine cervix dysplasias and cancer. *Nutr Cancer* 1991; **15**: 13–20.

110 Parazzini F, La Vecchia C, Negri E, Fedele L, Franceschi S, Gallotta L. Risk factors for cervical intraepithelial neoplasia. *Cancer* 1992; **69**: 2276–82.

111 Potischman N. Nutritional epidemiology of cervical neoplasia. *J Nutr* 1993; **123**: 424–9.

112 Potischman N, Herrero R, Brinton LA, et al. A case-control study of nutrient status and invasive cervical cancer. II. Serologic indicators. *Am J Epidemiol* 1991; **134**: 1347–55.

113 Romney SL, Palan PR, Duttagupta C, et al. Retinoids and the prevention of cervical dysplasias. *Am J Obstet Gynecol* 1981; **141**: 890–4.

114 Steinmetz KA, Potter JD. Vegetables, fruit, and cancer. I. Epidemiology. *Cancer Causes Control* 1991; **2**: 325–57.

115 VanEenwyk J, Davis FG, Colman N. Folate, vitamin C, and cervical intraepithelial neoplasia [see comments]. *Cancer Epidemiol Biomarkers Prev* 1992; **1**: 119–24.

116 Bartsch D, Boye B, Baust C, zur Hausen H, Schwarz E. Retinoic acid-mediated repression of human papillomavirus 18 transcription and different ligand regulation of the retinoic acid receptor beta gene in non-tumorigenic and tumorigenic HeLa hybrid cells. *EMBO J* 1992; **11**: 2283–91.

117 Mitchell MF, Hittelman WK, Lotan R, et al. Chemoprevention trials and surrogate end point biomarkers in the cervix. *Cancer* 1995; **76**: 1956–77.

118 Batova A, Danielpour D, Pirisi L, Creek KE. Retinoic acid induces secretion of latent transforming growth factor beta 1 and beta 2 in normal and human papillomavirus type 16-immortalized human keratinocytes. *Cell Growth Differ* 1992; **3**: 763–72.

119 Woodworth CD, Notario V, DiPaolo JA. Transforming growth factors beta 1 and 2 transcriptionally regulate human papillomavirus (HPV) type 16 early gene expression in HPV-immortalized human genital epithelial cells. *J Virol* 1990; **64**: 4767–75.

120 Butterworth Jr CE, Hatch KD, Macaluso M, et al. Folate deficiency and cervical dysplasia. *JAMA* 1992; **267**: 528–33.

121 Pietrantoni M, Taylor DD, Gercel-Taylor C, Bosscher J, Doering D, Gall SA. The regulation of HPV oncogene expression by folic acid in cultured human cervical cancer cells. *J Soc Gynecol Invest* 1995; **2**: 228 (Abstr).

122 Slamon DJ, deKernion JB, Verma IM, Cline MJ. Expression of cellular oncogenes in human malignancies. *Science* 1984; **224**: 256–62.

123 Couturier J, Sastre-Garau X, Schneider-Maunoury S, Labib A, Orth G. Integration of papillomavirus DNA near myc genes in genital carcinomas and its consequences for proto-oncogene expression. *J Virol* 1991; **65**: 4534–8.

124 Devictor B, Bonnier P, Piana L, et al. *c-myc* protein and Ki-67 antigen immunodetection in patients with uterine cervix neoplasia: correlation of microcytophotometric analysis and histological data. *Gynecol Oncol* 1993; **49**: 284–90.

125 Di Luca D, Costa S, Monini P, et al. Search for human papillomavirus, herpes simplex virus and *c-myc* oncogene in human genital tumors. *Int J Cancer* 1989; **43**: 570–7.

126 Iwasaka T, Yokoyama M, Oh-uchida M, et al. Detection of human papillomavirus genome and analysis of expression of *c-myc* and *Ha-ras* oncogenes in invasive cervical carcinomas. *Gynecol Oncol* 1992; **46**: 298–303.

127 Kohler M, Janz I, Wintzer HO, Wagner E, Bauknecht T. The expression of EGF receptors, EGF-like factors and *c-myc* in ovarian and cervical carcinomas and their potential clinical significance. *Anticancer Res* 1989; **9**: 1537–47.

128 Bernard C, Mougin C, Laurent R, Lab M. Oncogene activation: an informative marker for the human papillomavirus- lesions severity. *Cancer Detect Prev* 1994; **18**: 273–82.

129 McGlennen RC, Ostrow RS, Carson LF, Stanley MS, Faras AJ. Expression of cytokine receptors and markers of differentiation in human papillomavirus-infected cervical tissues [see comments]. *Am J Obstet Gynecol* 1991; **165**: 696–705.

130 Pinion SB, Kennedy JH, Miller RW, MacLean AB. Oncogene expression in cervical intraepithelial neoplasia and invasive cancer of cervix. *Lancet* 1991; **337**: 819–20.

131 Sagae S, Kudo R, Kuzumaki N, et al. *Ras* oncogene expression and progression in intraepithelial neoplasia of the uterine cervix. *Cancer* 1990; **66**: 295–301.

132 van Dam PA, Lowe DG, Watson JV, et al. Multiparameter flow-cytometric quantitation of epidermal growth factor receptor and c-erbB-2 oncoprotein in normal and neoplastic tissues of the female genital tract. *Gynecol Oncol* 1991; **42**: 256–64.

133 Malejczyk J, Malejczyk M, Urbanski A, et al. Constitutive release of IL6 by human papillomavirus type 16 (HPV16)-harboring keratinocytes: a mechanism augmenting the NK-cell-mediated lysis of HPV-bearing neoplastic cells. *Cell Immunol* 1991; **136**: 155–64.

134 Eustace D, Han X, Gooding R, Rowbottom A, Riches P, Heyderman E. Interleukin-6 (IL-6) functions as an autocrine growth factor in cervical carcinomas *in vitro*. *Gynecol Oncol* 1993; **50**: 15–19.

135 Tartour E, Gey A, Sastre-Garau X, et al. Analysis of interleukin 6 gene expression in cervical neoplasia using a quantitative polymerase chain reaction assay: evidence for enhanced interleukin 6 gene expression in invasive carcinoma. *Cancer Res* 1994; **54**: 6243–8.

136 Bascom CC, Wolfshohl JR, Coffey Jr RJ, et al. Complex regulation of transforming growth factor beta 1, beta 2, and beta 3 mRNA expression in mouse fibroblasts and keratinocytes by transforming growth factors beta 1 and beta 2. *Mol Cell Biol* 1989; **9**: 5508–15.

137 Coffey Jr RJ, Bascom CC, Sipes NJ, Graves-Deal R, Weissman BE, Moses HL. Selective inhibition of growth-related gene expression in murine keratinocytes by transforming growth factor beta. *Mol Cell Biol* 1988; **8**: 3088–93.

138 Shipley GD, Pittelkow MR, Wille Jr JJ, Scott RE, Moses HL. Reversible inhibition of normal human prokeratinocyte proliferation by type beta transforming growth factor-growth inhibitor in serum-free medium. *Cancer Res* 1986; **46**: 2068–71.

139 Braun L, Durst M, Mikumo R, Crowley A, Robinson M. Regulation of growth and gene expression in human papillomavirus-transformed keratinocytes by transforming growth factor-beta: implications for the control of papillomavirus infection. *Mol Carcinog* 1992; **6**: 100–11.

140 Braun L, Durst M, Mikumo R, Gruppuso P. Differential response of nontumorigenic and tumorigenic human papillomavirus type 16-positive epithelial cells to transforming growth factor beta 1. *Cancer Res* 1990; **50**: 7324–32.

141 Comerci Jr JT, Runowicz CD, Flanders KC, et al. Altered expression of transforming growth factor-beta 1 in cervical neoplasia as an early biomarker in carcinogenesis of the uterine cervix. *Cancer* 1996; **77**: 1107–14.

142 Roberts AB, Sporn MB, Assoian RK, et al. Transforming growth factor type beta: rapid induction of fibrosis and angiogenesis *in vivo* and stimulation of collagen formation *in vitro*. *Proc Natl Acad Sci USA* 1986; **83**: 4167–71.

143 Hauser C, Dayer JM, Jaunin F, de Rochemonteix B, Saurat JH. Intracellular epidermal interleukin 1-like factors in the human epidermoid carcinoma cell line A431. *Cell Immunol* 1986; **100**: 89–96.

144 Martin P, Vass WC, Schiller JT, Lowy DR, Velu TJ. The bovine papillomavirus E5 transforming protein can stimulate the transforming activity of EGF and CSF-1 receptors. *Cell* 1989; **59**: 21–32.

145 Pim D, Collins M, Banks L. Human papillomavirus type 16 E5 gene stimulates the transforming activity of the epidermal growth factor receptor. *Oncogene* 1992; **7**: 27–32.

146 Straight SW, Hinkle PM, Jewers RJ, McCance DJ. The E5 oncoprotein of human papillomavirus type 16 transforms fibroblasts and effects the downregulation of the epidermal growth factor receptor in keratinocytes. *J Virol* 1993; **67**: 4521–32.

147 Hodivala KJ, Pei XF, Liu QY, et al. Integrin expression and function in HPV 16-immortalised human keratinocytes in the presence or absence of v-Ha-ras. Comparison with cervical intraepithelial neoplasia. *Oncogene* 1994; **9**: 943–8.

148 Hughes DE, Rebello G, al-Nafussi A. Integrin expression in squamous neoplasia of the cervix. *J Pathol* 1994; **173**: 97–104.

149 Cerri A, Favre A, Giunta M, Corte G, Grossi CE, Berti E. Immunohistochemical localization of a novel beta 1 integrin in normal and pathologic squamous epithelia. *J Invest Dermatol* 1994; **102**: 247–52.

150 Connor ME, Stern PL. Loss of MHC class-I expression in cervical carcinomas. *Int J Cancer* 1990; **46**: 1029–34.

151 Hilders CG, Houbiers JG, Krul EJ, Fleuren GJ. The expression of histocompatibility-related leukocyte antigens in the pathway to cervical carcinoma. *Am J Clin Pathol* 1994; **101**: 5–12.

152 Glew SS, Duggan-Keen M, Cabrera T, Stern PL. HLA class II antigen expression in human papillomavirus-associated cervical cancer. *Cancer Res* 1992; **52**: 4009–16.

153 Coleman N, Stanley MA. Analysis of HLA-DR expression on keratinocytes in cervical neoplasia. *Int J Cancer* 1994; **56**: 314–19.

154 Viac J, Guerin-Reverchon I, Chardonnet Y, Bremond A. Langerhans cells and epithelial cell modifications in cervical intraepithelial neoplasia: correlation with human papillomavirus infection. *Immunobiology* 1990; **180**: 328–38.

155 David AL, Taylor GM, Gokhale D, Aplin JD, Seif MW, Tindall VR. HLA-DQB1*03 and cervical intraepithelial neoplasia type III [letter] [see comments]. *Lancet* 1992; **340**: 52.

156 Wank R, Thomssen C. High risk of squamous cell carcinoma of the cervix for women with HLA- DQw3 [see comments]. *Nature* 1991; **352**: 723–5.

157 Zavada J, Zavadova Z, Pastorekova S, Ciampor F, Pastorek J, Zelnik V. Expression of MaTu-MN protein in human tumor cultures and in clinical specimens. *Int J Cancer* 1993; **54**: 268–74.

158 Liao SY, Brewer C, Zavada J, et al. Identification of the MN antigen as a diagnostic biomarker of cervical intraepithelial squamous and glandular neoplasia and cervical carcinomas. *Am J Pathol* 1994; **145**: 598–609.

159 Resnick M, Lester S, Tate JE, Sheets EE, Sparks C, Crum CP. Viral and histopathologic correlates of MN and MIB-1 expression in cervical intraepithelial neoplasia [see comments]. *Hum Pathol* 1996; **27**: 234–9.

160 Kato H, Torigoe T. Radioimmunoassay for tumor antigen of human cervical squamous cell carcinoma. *Cancer* 1977; **40**: 1621–8.

161 Bolli JA, Doering DL, Bosscher JR, et al. Squamous cell carcinoma antigen: clinical utility in squamous cell carcinoma of the uterine cervix. *Gynecol Oncol* 1994; **55**: 169–73.

162 Duk JM, de Bruijn HW, Groenier KH, et al. Cancer of the uterine cervix: sensitivity and specificity of serum squamous cell carcinoma antigen determinations. *Gynecol Oncol* 1990; **39**: 186–94.

163 Scheffner M, Munger K, Byrne JC, Howley PM. The state of the p53 and retinoblastoma genes in human cervical carcinoma cell lines. *Proc Natl Acad Sci USA* 1991; **88**: 5523–7.

164 Quade BJ, Park JJ, Crum CP, Sun D, Dutta A. *In vivo* cyclin E expression as a marker for early cervical neoplasia. *Mod Pathol* 1998; **11**: 1238–46.

165 Weaver EJ, Kovatich AJ, Bibbo M. Cyclin E expression and early cervical neoplasia in ThinPrep specimens. A feasibility study. *Acta Cytol* 2000; **44**: 301–4.

166 Lie AK, Skarsvag S, Skomedal H, Haugen OA, Holm R. Expression of p53, MDM2, and p21 proteins in high-grade cervical intraepithelial neoplasia and relationship to human papillomavirus infection. *Int J Gynecol Pathol* 1999; **18**: 5–11.

167 Skomedal H, Kristensen GB, Lie AK, Holm R. Aberrant expression of the cell cycle associated proteins TP53, MDM2, p21, p27, cdk4, cyclin D1, RB, and EGFR in cervical carcinomas. *Gynecol Oncol* 1999; **73**: 223–8.

10

Glandular lesions of the endocervix

BARBARA S DUCATMAN, LINDA L COOK

AN INCREASING PROBLEM

The diagnosis of endocervical glandular lesions is difficult. In particular, the differential diagnosis between reactive conditions, high-grade squamous lesions within glands and endocervical adenocarcinoma *in situ* has become a source of frustration to pathologists and gynecologists. In the last two decades this has been an increasing problem, most likely because of the increased frequency of detection of glandular lesions as a result of both better sampling devices and increased prevalence of endocervical adenocarcinoma. During this period, pathologists have re-examined the classification of glandular neoplasia and the pathogenesis of cervical adenocarcinoma, especially in view of molecular diagnostic testing.[1]

Initially the Ayre spatula was the instrument of choice for taking both endocervical and exocervical components of the Pap smear. Unfortunately, this device often did not go high enough into the cervical canal to sample either the transformation zone or endocervical glands. Recognizing this limitation, many clinicians switched to cotton-tipped swabs for sampling the endocervix. Although this was an improvement in that it reached higher, the cotton tip tended to entrap many of the cells that were of most interest.

In the 1980s, two new sampling devices were introduced. The first of these was the endocervical brush for sampling the endocervical canal. With this device, the Ayre spatula is still used for exocervical sampling. However, the other device – the cervical broom – does not have to be used with an Ayre spatula. Numerous studies have shown both the endocervical brush and the cervical broom to be more efficient (without significant differences) than the Ayre spatula or the Ayre spatula/cotton swab for sampling the endocervical canal.[2–5] These devices can be used with conventional and monolayer preparations.[6,7] The optimal collection device during pregnancy is more debatable, with most authors favoring the newer devices,[8–10] while others advocate the use of the Ayre spatula/swab.[11] Women who are sampled with the brush technique should be warned that spotting, although not clinically significant, is more likely to occur. Other devices such as the Cell Sweep, Unicum (a newer brush), the Papette, Szalay spatula, Papex spatula, WrGKK spatula and Exact touch have also been studied; again with improved collection compared with the Ayre spatula.[12–16]

At the same time, the frequency of adenocarcinoma has been increasing.[17–21] The incidence of endocervical adenocarcinoma in the USA doubled between the early 1970s and the mid-1980s.[22] The percentage of Pap smears with an endocervical component increased in one study, after the use of these devices from roughly half to three-quarters compared with previously.[23] The number of adenocarcinomas and adenocarcinoma *in situ* (AIS) increased as well, but was not statistically significant. Although the relative frequency of adenocarcinoma compared with squamous cancer has increased over the years because of better screening for cervical squamous precursors, there also appears to be an absolute increase in incidence. Interestingly, a recent study in Norway found this increase to be particularly significant for the endometrioid variant.[24]

The use of liquid-based cytological preparations may also increase the detection of glandular neoplasms. Ashfaq et al.[25] found a statistically significant decrease in non-glandular (squamous) lesions found on biopsy for cytological diagnosis of glandular neoplasia compared with conventional Pap smears. In addition, the number of false-negative cytologies on ThinPrep was decreased for biopsy-proven glandular lesions. Bai et al.[26] also reported better detection of glandular dysplasia/AIS and fewer non-specific cases on ThinPrep (see Chapter 3), with better correlation with histological findings. Thus, the use of liquid-based preparations seems to increase both sensitivity and specificity.

As in squamous carcinoma, the majority of adenocarcinomas contain human papillomavirus (HPV) DNA, in particular mucinous and adenosquamous carcinomas.[27] However, the associated HPV types appear limited to types 16, 18 and 31 (especially type 18 and, to a lesser degree, type 16). Human papillomavirus DNA is not found as frequently as it is in squamous carcinoma neither is it commonly associated with glandular dysplasias.[28–35] Duggan et al. found that HPV was more likely to be associated with endocervical adenocarcinomas arising after 1980, suggesting an increasing role for HPV in endocervical carcinogenesis.[29] In another study of adenocarcinomas, p53 mutations between exons 5 and 8 were more frequently associated with biologically aggressive tumors, whereas HPV type 16 or 18 infection appeared to be involved in less aggressive cases.[36]

Epidemiological studies have investigated numerous demographic factors including number of sexual partners, age at first intercourse, history of genital infections, obesity, smoking and the absence of Pap smears. Only oral contraceptive (OCP) use emerged as a potential risk factor; however this finding was not adjusted for HPV infection.[37,38] Other studies have noted a high frequency of OCP use in women with endocervical adenocarcinoma; these authors thought that it might be possibly associated with microglandular hyperplasia that is also seen with OCP use.[39] Other studies have noted an increased incidence of adenocarcinoma in women enrolled in family planning clinics on OCPs compared with intrauterine contraceptive device (IUDs).[40] Case-control studies have, in general, shown a roughly twofold increase in adenocarcinoma after OCP, with the greatest risk in recent and current users and after 12 years of oral contraceptive use.[22,37,41,42]

GLANDULAR DYSPLASIA: WHAT IS IT?

Most gynecologists and pathologists would agree that the finding of 'abnormal' glandular cells is increasing on Pap smears. Much of this relates to better sampling of both neoplastic glandular cells and benign variants of endocervical glandular cells, including sampling of the lower uterine segment, cervical endometriosis, tubal metaplasia of the endocervix, microglandular hyperplasia and reactive/reparative conditions (the differential diagnosis will be discussed later).

Although the prevalence of abnormal glandular cells on Pap smears seems to be increasing, the concept of 'glandular dysplasia' is still controversial. Zaino[1] suggested that glandular dysplasia should not be used as a diagnosis at this time because of limited knowledge about its reproducibility and biological significance. Lee et al.[43] tested a number of high- and low-grade glandular atypias for HPV and MIB-1 (the antibody clone for Ki-67, a marker for proliferation index) positivity and concluded that most AIS cases did not evolve from glandular atypias, although high-grade glandular atypias found in association with AIS might represent either subtle variants or precursors. Goldstein et al.[44] have agreed that no morphological evidence exists to support the existence of a spectrum of endocervical glandular changes that culminates in AIS. Therefore, many gynecology pathologists and cytopathologists do not render a diagnosis of 'glandular dysplasia' and only acknowledge the presence of AIS when the atypia is sufficient.

Despite the controversy, the term 'glandular dysplasia' has been used to denote potential precursor lesions of endocervical glandular epithelium (similar to those observed for squamous carcinoma), as separate from AIS. Other proposed terminology has included cervical intra-epithelial glandular neoplasia (CIGN) grade I, II and III,[45] atypical hyperplasia and low- and high-grade glandular intraepithelial lesion (GIL). These terms reflect the spectrum of neoplastic glandular atypia, the extreme of which is AIS, and link these to adenocarcinoma in a fashion analogous to squamous carcinomas. In one series, almost 10 per cent of all cervical adenocarcinomas were AIS.[46] As with squamous carcinoma, the mean age for presentation of AIS is 10 years younger than that of invasive adenocarcinoma and the majority of patients presented with abnormal bleeding.[46] The treatment of AIS is controversial, some authors recommend that diathermy loop excision (loop electrocautery excision procedure, LEEP) is adequate treatment if there is long-term careful follow-up,[47] whereas others believe that radical hysterectomy and pelvic lymph node evaluation be done.[46]

Proposed histological criteria for glandular dysplasia have included nuclear atypia, such as enlargement, hyperchromasia, pleomorphism and abnormal chromatin pattern, increased mitotic rate and an abnormal architectural pattern with mucin depletion, albeit with lesser degrees of severity than AIS.[45,48–50] Diagnostic reproducibility for these criteria have not been established, neither have serious attempts to grade these into high- and low-grade variants emerged over the years. The cytological criteria for glandular dysplasias, if these should indeed be diagnosed as a separate entity, are controversial.

In contrast, the cytological criteria for AIS are well established but variable, due in part to the inclusion of a spectrum of glandular neoplasia by most authors. Sheets, rosettes and 'picket fence' arrangements are seen, but the nuclei are more crowded than in normal endocervical glandular epithelium (Figs 10.1 and 10.2a).[51] Statistically significant predictors of AIS include three-dimensional groupings, hyperchromatic nuclei, altered nuclear polarity in most groups, increased nuclear to cytoplasmic ratio, feathering, apoptosis, and individual atypical cells (Figs 10.3a and 10.4a).[52]

On ThinPrep slides, AIS was described as showing dark groups and sheets with crowding and the traditional features of strips, feathering, rosettes and mitoses (Fig. 10.2b).[53] There was continuous depth of focus, variability of nuclear size and shape within groups, irregular nuclear membranes, uniformly stippled chromatin and at least occasional single atypical cells (Figs 10.3b and 10.4b).[53] Invasive lesions had many of the same features, with relatively more inflammation and lysed blood, particularly on conventional smears (Fig. 10.5a) Irregular nuclear membranes and the presence of nucleoli were more consistently identified than with conventional smears (Fig. 10.5b). Single cells were more common (Fig. 10.6).

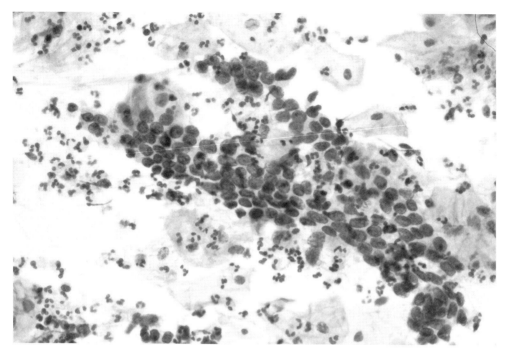

Figure 10.1 *Adenocarcinoma in situ. Note the honeycomb pattern and clean background. In contrast to normal endocervical cells, there is nuclear hyperchromasia with a coarsely granular chromatin pattern. The nucleus to cytoplasm ratio is markedly increased (conventional smear, original magnification ×40).*

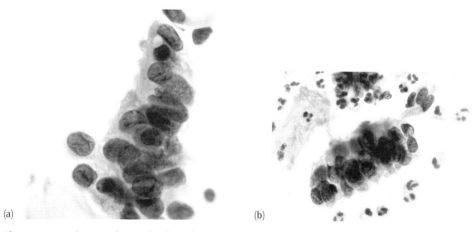

(a)   (b)

Figure 10.2 *Adenocarcinoma in situ with picket fence arrangement in the same patient. (a) Conventional. Nuclei are oval and stratified with nuclear enlargement and hyperchromasia. The chromatin pattern is coarsely granular (conventional smear, original magnification, ×100). (b) The cells are somewhat more overlapped compared with the conventional (ThinPrep, original magnification ×100).*

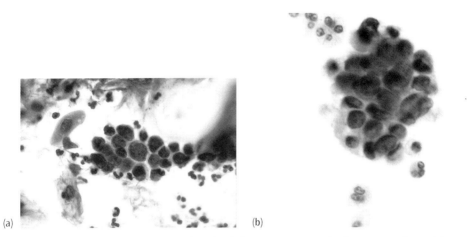

Figure 10.3 *Adenocarcinoma* in situ *with glandular arrangements in the same patient with two different preparatory techniques. Nuclei are dark and enlarged with an increased nucleus to cytoplasm ratio. (a) Conventional smear, original magnification* ×*100. (b) Note that there is more pronounced three-dimensionality (ThinPrep, original magnification* ×*100).*

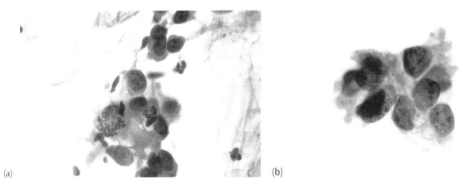

Figure 10.4 *Adenocarcinoma* in situ. *Scattered atypical single cells may be seen. (a) Note the mitotic figure (conventional smear, original magnification* ×*100). (b) ThinPrep, original magnification* ×*100.*

Although a 1986 study suggested that morphometric analysis might be able to distinguish micro-invasive endocervical adenocarcinoma from AIS,[54] the histological criteria for 'micro-invasive' adenocarcinoma is not well established[55] and this entity is probably not significant for cytology.

BENIGN MIMICS OF ENDOCERVICAL ADENOCARCINOMA AND AIS

Reactive and reparative conditions are a major diagnostic pitfall and are commonly included in the 'atypical glandular cells of undetermined significance' (AGUS) category. Reactive endocervical cells may be found singly, in sheets or small clusters. Small but prominent nucleoli are often found, and the chromatin pattern is even and vesicular to finely granular (Fig. 10.7).

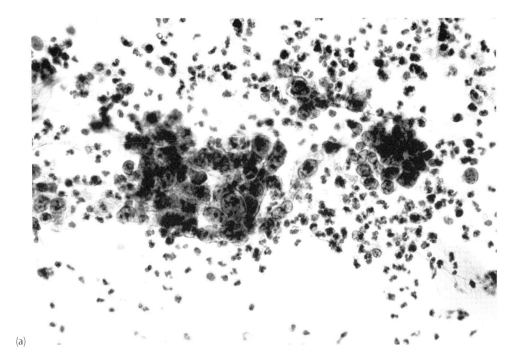

(a)

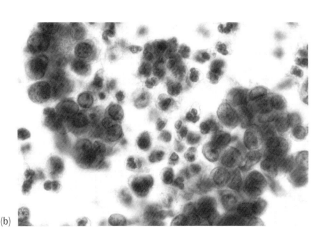

(b)

Figure 10.5 *Invasive endocervical adenocarcinoma (conventional smear). (a) Tumor diathesis of lysed blood and inflammatory cells (original magnification ×40). (b) Dyshesive cells with prominent nucleoli are noted in a dirty background (original magnification ×100).*

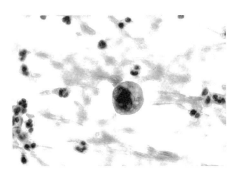

Figure 10.6 *Invasive endocervical adenocarcinoma. Single cells are usually easily found (conventional smear, original magnification ×100).*

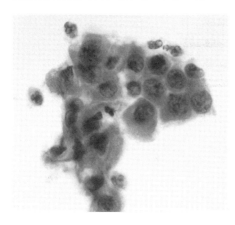

Figure 10.7 *Reactive. The cells are present singly. They resemble either endocervical or metaplastic cells with small but prominent nucleoli. However, there is no nuclear hyperchromasia or pleomorphism and the nuclear chromatin lacks granularity. Nuclear membranes are smooth, and there is no appreciable increase in the nucleus to cytoplasm ratio (ThinPrep, original magnification ×100).*

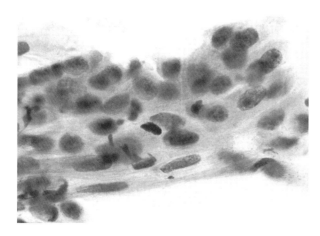

Figure 10.8 *Repair. Note the stretched out ('taffy-pull') appearance of the cells and nuclei. Cytoplasmic borders are distinct and nuclei are orderly arranged. Nucleoli may be prominent (conventional smear, original magnification ×100).*

Repair can be more troublesome. Such cases may have nuclei with a coarsely granular chromatin pattern, prominent nucleoli and frequent mitoses. The most important clues to the diagnosis are the presence of cells in a cohesive, stretched-out sheet ('taffy-pull') with prominent nucleoli (Fig. 10.8). These features are somewhat subtler on monolayer preparations.

Endometrial cells may be found because of sampling from the lower uterine segment or from endometriosis of the cervix.[56] The cells often appear different from the endometrial cells shed during menstruation. They are present during any time of the cycle and shed as large well-preserved sheets of cells with prominent nucleoli and scant cytoplasm. Endometrial cell 'whorls' and tubular structures, and stromal cells are seen in endometriosis (Fig. 10.9). In addition, absence of three-dimensional cell clusters, peripheral cell-sheet crowding, 'cell feathering' and pseudostratified cell strips aid in the distinction between cervical/vaginal endometriosis and adenocarcinoma.[57]

Lee[58] found that cervical smears from women with previous cone biopsies often contain crowded glandular cells that raised the possibility of AIS. However, the abnormal cells were less frequent and appeared as a continuum with benign cells, including endometrial cells. He postulated that some alteration of the endocervical histology following cone biopsy might be responsible. As with tubal metaplasia, this may present a dilemma in women that had cone biopsies for high-grade squamous intraepithelial lesion (HSIL) and are followed carefully.

Tubal metaplasia may pose a histological as well as a cytological problem. In a study of the prevalence of tubal metaplasia, we found it in 21 per cent of cone biopsy specimens and

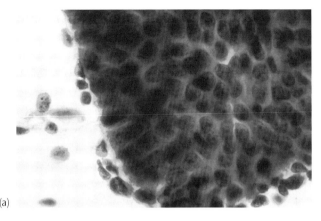

(a)

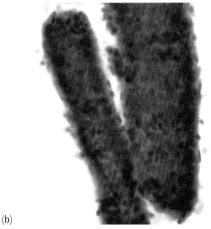

(b)

Figure 10.9 *Lower uterine segment. Stromal cells are attached to the outside of the cluster. These clusters are large and thick, but have an orderly arrangement. Individual nuclei are difficult to appreciate but are not enlarged or pleomorphic. (a) Conventional smear, original magnification ×100. (b) ThinPrep, original magnification ×40.*

62 per cent of hysterectomy specimens.[59] Tubal metaplasia is rarely observed in Pap smears. However, it may be a significant cause of false-positive smears for glandular neoplasia. When seen, it presents as flat sheets or cohesive clusters, and in palisade or mosaic patterns.[60] The nuclei may be hyperchromatic with granular cytoplasm. Ciliated cells can be appreciated only when they are viewed from the side (Fig. 10.10). They cannot be appreciated when they are 'en face.' Other features of tubal or tuboendometrioid metaplasia include a smaller cellular size, marked nuclear hyperchromasia with inconspicuous nucleoli, glandular structures without 'feathering' and lack of squamous dysplasia.[61]

Decidualized cells may rarely be seen in cervical cytology specimens from pregnant patients. These cells can be distinguished by their abundant granular cytoplasm. Although the nucleus is enlarged, the nuclear to cytoplasmic ratio is maintained (Fig. 10.11). A large but round nucleolus is usually seen. Decidualized cells are usually rare.

Selvaggi and Haefner[62] reviewed the smears and histological slides from three patients that showed microglandular endocervical hyperplasia. There were clusters of small to medium-sized cells with cytoplasmic vacuoles and engulfment of neutrophils, and nuclei containing coarse, granular chromatin and prominent nucleoli in two smears. The third smear had cells showing ample, vacuolated cytoplasm and vesicular nuclei with nucleoli. These findings were suggestive of endometrial adenocarcinoma in the former and endocervical adenocarcinoma in the latter. However, rare cases of AGUS with a microglandular-like pattern may actually represent endometrial adenocarcinoma.[63]

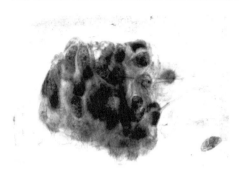

Figure 10.10 *Tubal metaplasia. Note the cells arranged in a picket fence arrangement. Nuclei may appear somewhat enlarged and hyperchromatic, but a coarsely granular chromatin pattern and nuclear pleomorphism are not seen. Note the cilia (conventional smear, original magnification ×100).*

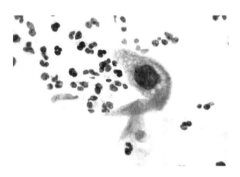

Figure 10.11 *Decidua. Rare single cells with enlarged nuclei with prominent nucleoli may be seen, but there is abundant granular cytoplasm and the nucleus to cytoplasm ratio is maintained (conventional smear, original magnification ×100).*

VARIANTS OF ENDOCERVICAL ADENOCARCINOMA

The majority of patients diagnosed with endocervical adenocarcinoma have the endocervical type. Other types include endometrioid, villoglandular papillary serous, minimal deviation adenocarcinoma and small-cell variants.

The endometrioid variant of AIS presents with a predominance of groups showing marked crowding, focal feathering, nuclear hyperchromatism with coarse chromatin and occasional mitotic figures. In contrast, sheets of cells, endometrial tubules and endometrial stroma favor a benign diagnosis.[64] Invasive endometrioid adenocarcinoma mimics endometrial adenocarcinoma and must be differentiated by fractional curettings or on hysterectomy.

Villoglandular carcinoma may not be recognized as malignant on Pap smears.[65] Cases of this malignancy have large cohesive and crowded groups and sheets of cells with loss of the normal honeycomb pattern, but nuclear changes are subtle and feathering is not observed. True papillary structures with stromal cores covered by columnar cells are found to be characteristic. Serous papillary carcinoma is similar to that found in the endometrium and ovary, with papillary clusters of cells with large vacuoles, highly atypical nuclei and often psammoma bodies.

Adenoma malignum or minimal deviation adenocarcinoma is a rare form of endocervical adenocarcinoma that closely mimics normal endocervical glands. As this tumor is usually not diagnosed until late in its course, the prognosis is dismal. It may be associated with Peutz–Jeghers syndrome. The most common presenting symptoms are menometrorrhagia, vaginal discharge, postmenopausal bleeding and abdominal swelling in decreasing order of frequency. The diagnosis is often established on the basis of the examination of a cervical biopsy specimen, endocervical curettage specimen or cone biopsy. The most important microscopic criteria for diagnosis are the presence of markedly abnormally and irregularly shaped glands, deeply invasive glands in a loose edematous or desmoplastic stromal response with foci that are less well-differentiated, vascular or perineurial invasion; and positive staining for carcinoembryonic antigen (CEA).[66] Histologically, adenoma malignum needs to be distinguished from benign endocervix and particularly from lobular endocervical glandular hyperplasia,[67] and cystic endocervical tunnel clusters.[68]

Cytological examination is usually not helpful as benign or only minimally atypical endocervical glands are noted. However, the smear of a biopsy-proven case has been described to show large sheets of columnar cells with focal acinar formation.[69] Irregularly packed, crowded nuclei are seen at the periphery of these sheets owing to turnover of the cell layers and their three-dimensional nature. Yellowish-orange staining of cytoplasmic mucins in these columnar cells by the Papanicolaou method has been touted as an important diagnostic clue aiding identification of mucinous adenoma malignum (in contrast to normal pinkish staining).[70] Immunostaining with HIK1083 (monoclonal antibody) may also be a useful tool in the diagnosis of these lesions by cytology as well as by histology.[69,70]

Small-cell carcinoma is sometimes considered a variant of adenocarcinoma. The cells are seen on Pap smears either arranged singly, or in loosely cohesive sheets, gland-like aggregates or files.[71,72] They have scanty cytoplasm, darkly staining nuclei with finely stippled chromatin and inconspicuous nucleoli. Tumor cells can have extremely pleomorphic, hyperchromatic and angulated nuclei with nuclear molding and smearing. Mitotic figures and karyorrhectic debris are also common.

OTHER NEOPLASMS

Endocervical adenocarcinoma may be confused with adenocarcinomas from other sites. Endometrial carcinoma will be thoroughly discussed in another chapter. Briefly, however, the most common differential diagnosis for malignant glandular cells on Pap smear is endocervical versus endometrial adenocarcinoma (Fig. 10.12). Although the use of combined immunohistochemical staining for vimentin and CEA is considered useful in this diagnosis on surgical pathology specimens,[73] this is not usually feasible on a conventional Pap smear. Papillary serous carcinomas present with hypercellular smears, a tumor diathesis, papillae, bare nuclei,

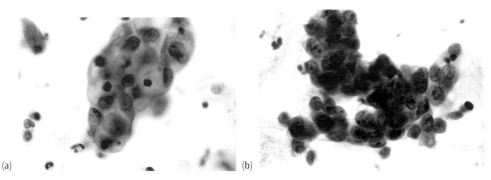

Figure 10.12 *Endometrial adenocarcinoma. Cells are more likely present in cell balls and nuclei are less hyperchromatic. However, the distinction between adenocarcinoma of endometrial and endocervical origins can be very difficult, if not impossible. The age of the patient and presenting symptoms can be helpful, but in such cases, a fractional D&C may be necessary. (a) Endometrial adenocarcinoma; note the cell ball with large cytoplasmic vacuoles (conventional smear, original magnification ×100). (b) Endometrial adenocarcinoma; although a cell ball is present, the cytoplasm is more granular in this case (ThinPrep, original magnification ×100).*

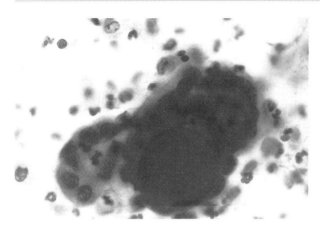

Figure 10.13 *Papillary serous carcinoma. Note the papillary structure with a central psammoma body (high power). Although the cell type can be accurately predicted by this pattern, the site of origin may be endocervix, endometrium or ovary (this case was ovarian). Extrauterine tumors are less likely to present with a tumor diathesis (conventional smear, original magnification ×100).*

and cells with large pleomorphic nuclei and bulky dense cytoplasm (Fig. 10.13).[74] These tumors may arise in ovary, endometrium or cervix, but when seen in cervical cytological specimens are most likely to originate from the endometrium. In that location they may be mixed with other variants (particularly typical endometrioid); however, the features of mixed tumors are similar to those of papillary serous carcinoma, suggesting preferential exfoliation.

Extrauterine carcinomas may also present on Pap smear. The conventional wisdom has held that a major diagnostic criterion for extrauterine carcinomas is a lack of tumor diathesis. However, a recent study found no statistically significant association of tumor diathesis with primary versus metastatic carcinoma and presence or absence of documented local involvement of the endometrium, cervix or vagina.[75]

The most common neoplastic lesion to present with glandular configurations is HSIL within glands. The presence of otherwise unequivocal HSIL in the smear and 'swirling' configuration within glandular structures is most helpful in predicting this lesion (Fig. 10.14).

AGUS: A PROBLEM DIAGNOSIS?

The diagnosis of AGUS appears to be increasing, in particular the 'favor premalignant/malignant category'.[76] In a review of 137 Pap smears initially classified as AGUS, approximately one-third were reclassified as negative, one-third remained AGUS, and the remainder were diagnosed as either atypical squamous cells of undetermined significance (ASCUS) or squamous intraepithelial lesions (SIL).[77] On colposcopic follow-up, approximately 14 per cent of these women had either HSIL or carcinoma, and the majority of these were identified by HPV testing. In another study, 41 per cent of cases with endocervical atypia had co-existing squamous dysplasia or atypia.[78]

Chin et al.[79] found a 0.29 per cent incidence of AGUS in 48 890 Pap smears from a community-based population. Although almost half of these women were not followed with colposcopy and biopsy, 61 per cent of those biopsied had positive findings, including five with cancer. The majority of positive biopsies were squamous neoplasia, but there were benign and malignant glandular lesions including AIS, endometrial hyperplasia, carcinoma and ovarian carcinoma. Postmenopausal women and women with vaginal bleeding were more likely to have a glandular lesion.

Similar results were found in a study of 44 217 Pap smears with a 0.24 per cent incidence of AGUS.[80] Tissue specimens were available for the majority and 37 per cent had significant

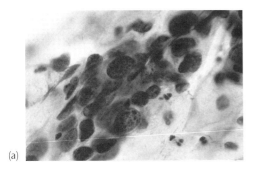

(a)

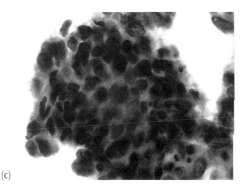

(c)

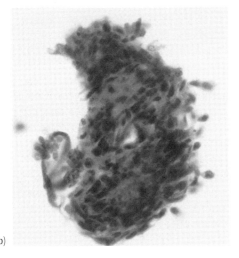

(b)

Figure 10.14 *High-grade squamous intraepithelial lesion in glands. This is the most common neoplasm found in conjunction with atypical glandular cells of undetermined significance (AGUS), favor neoplastic. The cells are found in glandular arrangements, but the nuclei are often more spindled and often appear to 'swirl' around the center. (a) Conventional smear, original magnification ×100. (b) Note the glandular acinus (ThinPrep, original magnification ×100). (c) ThinPrep, original magnification ×100.*

pathology; again squamous neoplasia was most frequent, especially in those with a previous history of this lesion. However, in older women and in those with AGUS 'favor neoplasia', endometrial hyperplasia and carcinoma were more likely. Obenson et al.[81] found that AGUS in postmenopausal women was highly predictive of endometrial pathology, although not necessarily malignancy.

Korn et al.[82] found a 0.27 per cent incidence of AGUS in 32 181 cervical smears. Approximately one-third had intraepithelial or invasive neoplasms with slightly more than half with LSIL or HSIL, and the remainder had glandular lesions of the endocervix or endometrium. Raab[83] considers AGUS to be misnamed, and it would be more appropriate to further subclassify most AGUS cases. Although cases diagnosed as AGUS may be AIS, the majority are squamous dysplasias. Even when the lesion is glandular, coexisting SIL was found in 50 per cent of the cases in one study.[84] Burja et al.[85] found that the majority of their AGUS cases had a clinically significant lesion, in particular, SIL. However, feathering, nuclear palisading and chromatin clearing could predict AIS/adenocarcinoma. Kim et al.[86] also found a significant percentage of women with AGUS on Pap smear (25 per cent) to have a clinically significant lesion and recommended good communication between pathologist and clinician, and immediate further diagnostic studies for this diagnosis. Atypical glandular cells of undetermined significance on Pap smears were correlated with significant findings in 45 per cent of patients (32 per cent with preinvasive or invasive lesions and 13 per cent with benign lesions) in another study from the University of Virginia.[87] Soofer and Sidawy[88] reviewed a total of 29 cases in which histological follow-up was available for AGUS (their AGUS rate was 0.11 per cent). AGUS was associated with clinically significant lesions, including HSIL, LSIL, endometrial lesions, AIS and invasive adenocarcinoma, in 25 per cent of patients. Most of the lesions were high grade and were detected histologically, although sometimes only after protracted follow-up.

Cenci et al.[89] showed that AGUS nuclei were more variable and had an intermediate value for area and shape between normal and neoplastic nuclei. In their study, the most useful cytological features in discriminating AGUS from neoplastic cells were normal endocervical cells singly or in sheets, and the absence of the following features: necrosis, bare atypical cells, papillary groups, anisonucleosis, irregular chromatin distribution and hyperchromasia. Another study of endocervical tissue and Pap smears concluded that reactive atypia of the endocervix could indeed be due to inflammatory–reparative changes, was possibly related to hormonal usage and could be separated from precursor lesions of endocervical adenocarcinoma.[90] These cells had large hyperchromatic nuclei, but they lacked the classic criteria for adenocarcinoma.

Roberts et al.[91] used the Australian modification of the Bethesda system that divides endocervical atypia into high-grade cases for predicting AIS, an inconclusive category that requires AIS be excluded and a low-grade category with minor changes. They concluded that this approach was better able to reflect the risk of underlying high-grade abnormalities and suggested that repeat cytology be the choice for low grade atypia (about 85 per cent of their cases) and cone biopsy for high-grade and inconclusive cases.[91]

Schindler et al.[92] similarly divided their AGUS smears into three categories. Most cases of AGUS-unqualified had mostly benign entities on follow-up with one-quarter of cases showing squamous neoplasia. Follow-up of AGUS-favor reactive also demonstrated mostly benign entities with a few cases of SIL. However, nearly half of the patients diagnosed with AGUS-favor neoplastic had pre-neoplastic or neoplastic lesions including AIS.

THE FUTURE: WHAT COULD HELP?

The overlap of cytological features between glandular benign and neoplastic lesions can make distinction of these lesions difficult. As previously described, the use of DNA HPV testing in liquid preparations may prove an important adjunct.[77] A number of other authors have studied the use of immunohistochemical stains as an adjunct in the detection of cervical neoplasia. Obviously, their use is difficult with conventional Pap smears. However, the increasing use of liquid-based preparations means that either additional slides for immunohistochemical studies or even possibly a cell block can be made from cellular samples. However the older, if not wiser, cytopathologist will remember a long history of adjunctive techniques that are just that – history.

For example, a combination of immunohistochemical stains including CEA and MIB-1 (both antibodies for immunostains) and p53 has been suggested to distinguish benign from malignant endocervical conditions on pathology examination.[93] Since increasing positivity of MIB-1 is seen with increasing degrees of both squamous and glandular neoplasia, this has the potential to become a useful adjunct.[94] Bcl-2 immunoreactivity is found in premalignant glandular but not squamous lesions of the cervix, suggesting a possible role for discriminating between these two.[95] (Bcl-2 is a monoclonal protein for an aberrant protein produced by gene translocation.)

The use of MN/CA9 antigen has also been thought to be useful in discriminating benign from dysplastic endocervical cells.[96,97] Liao and Stanbridge[96] studied the expression of MN/CA9 antigen, a tumor marker expressed in virtually all cervical carcinomas and cervical dysplasia, on cervical cytology specimens. Interestingly, this marker is expressed in normal endocervical cells, but only when there is coexisting dysplasia or carcinoma. Thus, MN/CA9 antigen might serve as an early biomarker of cervical neoplasia. The combination of detection via cytology and MN immunostaining discriminated between AGUS with corresponding squamous dysplasia or AIS and AGUS with reactive conditions.[96,97] It was postulated that MN/CA9 staining might be a useful adjunct for AGUS in cervical cytology.

In normal endocervical mucosa, immunoreactivity for CD44 and its splice variants was found to be absent or confined to only the basal portion of the glandular epithelium, whereas CD44 was diffusely expressed in 94 per cent of AIS and in 95 per cent of invasive adenocarcinomas with stronger expression.[98] In contrast to all other splice variants, CD44v9 demonstrated increased expression in nearly all *in situ* and invasive lesions compared with the normal tissue.[98]

Another study concluded that high iron diamine alcian blue and CEA might be useful in the diagnosis of endocervical adenocarcinoma.[99] Normal endocervical glands showed a predominance of sulfomucin, while adenocarcinoma predominantly showed sialomucin. CEA did not stain in normal or dysplastic endocervix, but was highly positive in adenocarcinoma. However, the use of high iron diamine alcian blue is not uniformly supported, as other authors have found no difference in the types of mucin in benign and malignant endocervical glands.[100,101] Although the use of special stains or immunostains is not practical with conventional Pap smears, this is possible with liquid-based techniques since multiple slides can be made.

REFERENCES

1 Zaino RJ. Glandular lesions of the uterine cervix. *Mod Pathol* 2000; **13**: 261–74.
2 Buntinx F, Brouwers M. Relation between sampling device and detection of abnormality in cervical smears: a meta-analysis of randomised and quasi-randomised studies [see comments]. *BMJ* 1996; **313**: 1285–90.
3 Luzzatto R, Boon ME. Contribution of the endocervical Cytobrush sample to the diagnosis of cervical lesions. *Acta Cytol* 1996; **40**: 1143–7.
4 Martin-Hirsch P, Jarvis G, Kitchener H, Lilford R. Collection devices for obtaining cervical cytology samples. *Cochrane Database Syst Rev* 2000; **2**.
5 Risberg B, Andersson A, Zetterberg C, Nordin B. Cervex-Brush vs. spatula and Cytobrush. A cytohistologic evaluation. *J Reprod Med* 1997; **42**: 405–8.
6 Selvaggi SM, Guidos BJ. Specimen adequacy and the ThinPrep Pap Test: the endocervical component. *Diagn Cytopathol* 2000; **23**: 23–6.
7 Spurrett B, Ayer B, Pacey NF. The inadequacies of instruments used for cervical screening. *Aust NZ J Obstet Gynaecol* 1989; **29**: 44–6.
8 Foster JC, Smith HL. Use of the Cytobrush for Papanicolaou smear screens in pregnant women. *J Nurse Midwifery* 1996; **41**: 211–17.
9 Paraiso MF, Brady K, Helmchen R, Roat TW. Evaluation of the endocervical Cytobrush and Cervex-Brush in pregnant women. *Obstet Gynecol* 1994; **84**: 539–43.
10 Stillson T, Knight AL, Elswick Jr RK. The effectiveness and safety of two cervical cytologic techniques during pregnancy. *J Fam Pract* 1997; **45**: 159–63.
11 Smith-Levitin M, Hernandez E, Anderson L, Heller P. Safety, efficacy and cost of three cervical cytology sampling devices in a prenatal clinic. *J Reprod Med* 1996; **41**: 749–53.
12 Broso PR, Buffetti G, Fabbrini T, Francone P, Orlassino R. The unicum and cytobrush plus spatula for cervical cytologic sampling: a comparison. *Acta Cytol* 1996; **40**: 222–5.
13 de Palo G, Stefanon B, Alasio L, Pilotti S. Exact Touch: a new device for cervical cytology. Comparison with Ayre spatula plus Cytobrush. *Cytopathology* 2000; **11**: 322–5.

14 Ferenczy A, Robitaille J, Guralnick M, Shatz R. Cervical cytology with the Papette sampler. *J Reprod Med* 1994; **39**: 304–10.

15 Kohlberger PD, Stani J, Gitsch G, Kieback DG, Breitenecker G. Comparative evaluation of seven cell collection devices for cervical smears. *Acta Cytol* 1999; **43**: 1023–6.

16 Tyau L, Hernandez E, Anderson L, Heller P, Edmonds P. The Cell-Sweep. A new cervical cytology sampling device. *J Reprod Med* 1994; **39**: 899–902.

17 Davis JR, Moon LB. Increased incidence of adenocarcinoma of uterine cervix. *Obstet Gynecol* 1975; **45**: 79–83.

18 Krishnamurthy S, Yecole BB, Jussawalla DJ. Uterine cervical adenocarcinomas and squamous carcinomas in Bombay: 1965–1990. *J Obstet Gynaecol Res* 1997; **23**: 521–7.

19 Peters RK, Chao A, Mack TM, Thomas D, Bernstein L, Henderson BE. Increased frequency of adenocarcinoma of the uterine cervix in young women in Los Angeles County. *J Natl Cancer Inst* 1986; **76**: 423–8.

20 Schwartz SM, Weiss NS. Increased incidence of adenocarcinoma of the cervix in young women in the United States. *Am J Epidemiol* 1986; **124**: 1045–7.

21 Vesterinen E, Forss M, Nieminen U. Increase of cervical adenocarcinoma: a report of 520 cases of cervical carcinoma including 112 tumors with glandular elements. *Gynecol Oncol* 1989; **33**: 49–53.

22 Ursin G, Peters RK, Henderson BE, d'Ablaing G, 3rd, Monroe KR, Pike MC. Oral contraceptive use and adenocarcinoma of cervix [see comments]. *Lancet* 1994; **344**: 1390–4.

23 Mitchell H, Medley G. Cytological reporting of cervical abnormalities according to endocervical status. *Br J Cancer* 1993; **67**: 585–8.

24 Alfsen GC, Thoresen SO, Kristensen GB, Skovlund E, Abeler VM. Histopathologic subtyping of cervical adenocarcinoma reveals increasing incidence rates of endometrioid tumors in all age groups: a population based study with review of all nonsquamous cervical carcinomas in Norway from 1966 to 1970, 1976 to 1980, and 1986 to 1990. *Cancer* 2000; **89**: 1291–9.

25 Ashfaq R, Gibbons D, Vela C, Saboorian MH, Iliya F. ThinPrep Pap Test. Accuracy for glandular disease. *Acta Cytol* 1999; **43**: 81–5.

26 Bai H, Sung CJ, Steinhoff MM. ThinPrep Pap Test promotes detection of glandular lesions of the endocervix. *Diagn Cytopathol* 2000; **23**: 19–22.

27 Pirog EC, Kleter B, Olgac S, et al. Prevalence of human papillomavirus DNA in different histological subtypes of cervical adenocarcinoma. *Am J Pathol* 2000; **157**: 1055–62.

28 Duggan MA, Benoit JL, McGregor SE, Inoue M, Nation JG, Stuart GC. Adenocarcinoma *in situ* of the endocervix: human papillomavirus determination by dot blot hybridization and polymerase chain reaction amplification. *Int J Gynecol Pathol* 1994; **13**: 143–9.

29 Duggan MA, McGregor SE, Benoit JL, Inoue M, Nation JG, Stuart GC. The human papillomavirus status of invasive cervical adenocarcinoma: a clinicopathological and outcome analysis. *Hum Pathol* 1995; **26**: 319–25.

30 Milde-Langosch K, Schreiber C, Becker G, Loning T, Stegner HE. Human papillomavirus detection in cervical adenocarcinoma by polymerase chain reaction. *Hum Pathol* 1993; **24**: 590–4.

31 Okagaki T, Tase T, Twiggs LB, Carson LF. Histogenesis of cervical adenocarcinoma with reference to human Papillomavirus-18 as a carcinogen. *J Reprod Med* 1989; **34**: 639–44.

32 O'Leary JJ, Landers RJ, Crowley M, et al. Genotypic mapping of HPV and assessment of EBV prevalence in endocervical lesions. *J Clin Pathol* 1997; **50**: 904–10.

33 Tase T, Okagaki T, Clark BA, Twiggs LB, Ostrow RS, Faras AJ. Human papillomavirus DNA in adenocarcinoma *in situ*, microinvasive adenocarcinoma of the uterine cervix, and coexisting cervical squamous intraepithelial neoplasia. *Int J Gynecol Pathol* 1989; **8**: 8–17.

34 Tase T, Okagaki T, Clark BA, Twiggs LB, Ostrow RS, Faras AJ. Human papillomavirus DNA in glandular dysplasia and microglandular hyperplasia: presumed precursors of adenocarcinoma of the uterine cervix. *Obstet Gynecol* 1989; **73**: 1005–8.

35 Yamakawa Y, Forslund O, Teshima H, Hasumi K, Kitagawa T, Hansson BG. Human papillomavirus DNA in adenocarcinoma and adenosquamous carcinoma of the uterine cervix detected by polymerase chain reaction (PCR). *Gynecol Oncol* 1994; **53**: 190–5.

36 Jiko K, Tsuda H, Sato S, Hirohashi S. Pathogenetic significance of p53 and c-Ki-ras gene mutations and human papillomavirus DNA integration in adenocarcinoma of the uterine cervix and uterine isthmus. *Int J Cancer* 1994; **59**: 601–6.

37 Brinton LA, Huggins GR, Lehman HF, et al. Long-term use of oral contraceptives and risk of invasive cervical cancer. *Int J Cancer* 1986; **38**: 399–44.

38 Brinton LA, Tashima KT, Lehman HF, et al. Epidemiology of cervical cancer by cell type. *Cancer Res* 1987; **47**: 1706–11.

39 Dallenbach-Hellweg G. On the origin and histological structure of adenocarcinoma of the endocervix in women under 50 years of age. *Pathol Res Pract* 1984; **179**: 38–50.

40 Vessey MP, Lawless M, McPherson K, Yeates D. Neoplasia of the cervix uteri and contraception: a possible adverse effect of the pill. *Lancet* 1983; **ii**: 930–4.

41 Parazzini F, la Vecchia C, Negri E, Maggi R. Oral contraceptive use and invasive cervical cancer. *Int J Epidemiol* 1990; **19**: 259–63.

42 Thomas DB, Ray RM. Oral contraceptives and invasive adenocarcinomas and adenosquamous carcinomas of the uterine cervix. The World Health Organization Collaborative Study of Neoplasia and Steroid Contraceptives. *Am J Epidemiol* 1996; **144**: 281–9.

43 Lee KR, Sun D, Crum CP. Endocervical intraepithelial glandular atypia (dysplasia): a histopathologic, human papillomavirus, and MIB-1 analysis of 25 cases. *Hum Pathol* 2000; **31**: 656–64.

44 Goldstein NS, Ahmad E, Hussain M, Hankin RC, Perez-Reyes N. Endocervical glandular atypia: does a preneoplastic lesion of adenocarcinoma *in situ* exist? *Am J Clin Pathol* 1998; **110**: 200–9.

45 Gloor E, Hurlimann J. Cervical intraepithelial glandular neoplasia (adenocarcinoma *in situ* and glandular dysplasia). A correlative study of 23 cases with histologic grading, histochemical analysis of mucins, and immunohistochemical determination of the affinity for four lectins. *Cancer* 1986; **58**: 1272–80.

46 Hopkins MP, Roberts JA, Schmidt RW. Cervical adenocarcinoma in situ. *Obstet Gynecol* 1988; **71**: 842–4.

47 Houghton SJ, Shafi MI, Rollason TP, Luesley DM. Is loop excision adequate primary management of adenocarcinoma *in situ* of the cervix? *Br J Obstet Gynaecol* 1997; **104**: 325–9.

48 Brown LJ, Wells M. Cervical glandular atypia associated with squamous intraepithelial neoplasia: a premalignant lesion? *J Clin Pathol* 1986; **39**: 22–8.

49 Casper GR, Ostor AG, Quinn MA. A clinicopathologic study of glandular dysplasia of the cervix. *Gynecol Oncol* 1997; **64**: 166–70.

50 Jaworski RC. Endocervical glandular dysplasia, adenocarcinoma *in situ*, and early invasive (microinvasive) adenocarcinoma of the uterine cervix. *Semin Diagn Pathol* 1990; **7**: 190–204.

51 Bousfield L, Pacey F, Young Q, Krumins I, Osborn R. Expanded cytologic criteria for the diagnosis of adenocarcinoma *in situ* of the cervix and related lesions. *Acta Cytol* 1980; **24**: 283–96.

52 Biscotti CV, Gero MA, Toddy SM, Fischler DF, Easley KA. Endocervical adenocarcinoma *in situ*: an analysis of cellular features. *Diagn Cytopathol* 1997; **17**: 326–32.

53 Johnson JE, Rahemtulla A. Endocervical glandular neoplasia and its mimics in ThinPrep Pap tests. A descriptive study. *Acta Cytol* 1999; **43**: 369–75.

54 Clark AH, Betsill Jr WL. Early endocervical glandular neoplasia. II. Morphometric analysis of the cells. *Acta Cytol* 1986; **30**: 127–34.

55 Yeh IT, LiVolsi VA, Noumoff JS. Endocervical carcinoma. *Pathol Res Pract* 1991; **187**: 129–44.

56 Hanau CA, Begley N, Bibbo M. Cervical endometriosis: a potential pitfall in the evaluation of glandular cells in cervical smears. *Diagn Cytopathol* 1997; **16**: 274–80.

57 Mulvany NJ, Surtees V. Cervical/vaginal endometriosis with atypia: A cytohistopathologic study. *Diagn Cytopathol* 1999; **21**: 188–93.

58 Lee KR. Atypical glandular cells in cervical smears from women who have undergone cone biopsy. A potential diagnostic pitfall. *Acta Cytol* 1993; **37**: 705–9.

59 Jonasson JG, Wang HH, Antonioli DA, Ducatman BS. Tubal metaplasia of the uterine cervix: a prevalence study in patients with gynecologic pathologic findings. *Int J Gynecol Pathol* 1992; **11**: 89–95.

60 Ducatman BS, Wang HH, Jonasson JG, Hogan CL, Antonioli DA. Tubal metaplasia: a cytologic study with comparison to other neoplastic and non-neoplastic conditions of the endocervix. *Diagn Cytopathol* 1993; **9**: 98–103.

61 Hirschowitz L, Eckford SD, Phillpotts B, Midwinter A. Cytological changes associated with tubo-endometrioid metaplasia of the uterine cervix [see comments]. *Cytopathology* 1994; **5**: 1–8.

62 Selvaggi SM, Haefner HK. Microglandular endocervical hyperplasia and tubal metaplasia: pitfalls in the diagnosis of adenocarcinoma on cervical smears. *Diagn Cytopathol* 1997; **16**: 168–73.

63 Shidham VB, Dayer AM, Basir Z, Kajdacsy-Balla A. Cervical cytology and immunohistochemical features in endometrial adenocarcinoma simulating microglandular hyperplasia. A case report. *Acta Cytol* 2000; **44**: 661–6.

64 Lee KR, Genest DR, Minter LJ, Granter SR, Cibas ES. Adenocarcinoma *in situ* in cervical smears with a small cell (endometrioid) pattern: distinction from cells directly sampled from the upper endocervical canal or lower segment of the endometrium [see comments]. *Am J Clin Pathol* 1998; **109**: 738–42.

65 Chang WC, Matisic JP, Zhou C, Thomson T, Clement PB, Hayes MM. Cytologic features of villoglandular adenocarcinoma of the uterine cervix: comparison with typical endocervical adenocarcinoma with a villoglandular component and papillary serous carcinoma. *Cancer* 1999; **87**: 5–11.

66 Gilks CB, Young RH, Aguirre P, DeLellis RA, Scully RE. Adenoma malignum (minimal deviation adenocarcinoma) of the uterine cervix. A clinicopathological and immunohistochemical analysis of 26 cases. *Am J Surg Pathol* 1989; **13**: 717–29.

67 Nucci MR, Clement PB, Young RH. Lobular endocervical glandular hyperplasia, not otherwise specified: a clinicopathologic analysis of thirteen cases of a distinctive pseudoneoplastic lesion and comparison with fourteen cases of adenoma malignum [see comments]. *Am J Surg Pathol* 1999; **23**: 886–91.

68 Segal GH, Hart WR. Cystic endocervical tunnel clusters. A clinicopathologic study of 29 cases of so-called adenomatous hyperplasia. *Am J Surg Pathol* 1990; **14**: 895–903.

69 Sato S, Ito K, Konno R, Okamoto S, Yajima A. Adenoma malignum. Report of a case with cytologic and colposcopic findings and immunohistochemical staining with antimucin monoclonal antibody HIK-1083. *Acta Cytol* 2000; **44**: 389–92.

70 Ishii K, Katsuyama T, Ota H, et al. Cytologic and cytochemical features of adenoma malignum of the uterine cervix [published erratum appears in *Cancer* 1999; **87**: 395]. *Cancer* 1999; **87**: 245–53.

71 Proca D, Keyhani-Rofagha S, Copeland LJ, Hameed A. Exfoliative cytology of neuroendocrine small cell carcinoma of the endometrium. A report of two cases. *Acta Cytol* 1998; **42**: 978–82.

72 Zhou C, Hayes MM, Clement PB, Thomson TA. Small cell carcinoma of the uterine cervix: cytologic findings in 13 cases. *Cancer* 1998; **84**: 281–8.

73 Dabbs DJ, Sturtz K, Zaino RJ. The immunohistochemical discrimination of endometrioid adenocarcinomas. *Hum Pathol* 1996; **27**: 172–7.

74 Wright CA, Leiman G, Burgess SM. The cytomorphology of papillary serous carcinoma of the endometrium in cervical smears. *Cancer* 1999; **87**: 12–18.

75 Gupta D, Balsara G. Extrauterine malignancies. Role of Pap smears in diagnosis and management. *Acta Cytol* 1999; **43**: 806–13.

76 Eddy GL, Ural SH, Strumpf KB, Wojtowycz MA, Piraino PS, Mazur MT. Incidence of atypical glandular cells of uncertain significance in cervical cytology following introduction of the Bethesda System. *Gynecol Oncol* 1997; **67**: 51–5.

77 Ronnett BM, Manos MM, Ransley JE, et al. Atypical glandular cells of undetermined significance (AGUS): cytopathologic features, histopathologic results, and human papillomavirus DNA detection. *Hum Pathol* 1999; **30**: 816–25.

78 Goff BA, Atanasoff P, Brown E, Muntz HG, Bell DA, Rice LW. Endocervical glandular atypia in Papanicolaou smears. *Obstet Gynecol* 1992; **79**: 101–4.

79 Chin AB, Bristow RE, Korst LM, Walts A, Lagasse LD. The significance of atypical glandular cells on routine cervical cytologic testing in a community-based population. *Am J Obstet Gynecol* 2000; **182**: 1278–82.

80 Cheng RF, Hernandez E, Anderson LL, Heller PB, Shank R. Clinical significance of a cytologic diagnosis of atypical glandular cells of undetermined significance. *J Reprod Med* 1999; **44**: 922–8.

81 Obenson K, Abreo F, Grafton WD. Cytohistologic correlation between AGUS and biopsy-detected lesions in postmenopausal women. *Acta Cytol* 2000; **44**: 41–5.

82 Korn AP, Judson PL, Zaloudek CJ. Importance of atypical glandular cells of uncertain significance in cervical cytologic smears. *J Reprod Med* 1998; **43**: 774–8.

83 Raab SS. Can glandular lesions be diagnosed in Pap smear cytology? *Diagn Cytopathol* 2000; **23**: 127–33.

84 Siziopikou KP, Wang HH, Abu-Jawdeh G. Cytologic features of neoplastic lesions in endocervical glands. *Diagn Cytopathol* 1997; **17**: 1–7.

85 Burja IT, Thompson SK, Sawyer Jr WL, Shurbaji MS. Atypical glandular cells of undetermined significance on cervical smears. A study with cytohistologic correlation. *Acta Cytol* 1999; **43**: 351–6.

86 Kim TJ, Kim HS, Park CT, et al. Clinical evaluation of follow-up methods and results of atypical glandular cells of undetermined significance (AGUS) detected on cervicovaginal Pap smears. *Gynecol Oncol* 1999; **73**: 292–8.

87 Veljovich DS, Stoler MH, Andersen WA, Covell JL, Rice LW. Atypical glandular cells of undetermined significance: a five-year retrospective histopathologic study. *Am J Obstet Gynecol* 1998; **179**: 382–90.

88 Soofer SB, Sidawy MK. Atypical glandular cells of undetermined significance: clinically significant lesions and means of patient follow-up. *Cancer* 2000; **90**: 207–14.

89 Cenci M, Mancini R, Nofroni I, Vecchione A. Endocervical atypical glandular cells of undetermined significance. I. Morphometric and cytologic characterization of cases that 'cannot rule out adenocarcinoma in situ'. *Acta Cytol* 2000; **44**: 319–26.

90 Ghorab Z, Mahmood S, Schinella R. Endocervical reactive atypia: a histologic–cytologic study. *Diagn Cytopathol* 2000; **22**: 342–6.

91 Roberts JM, Thurloe JK, Bowditch RC, Laverty CR. Subdividing atypical glandular cells of undetermined significance according to the Australian modified Bethesda system: analysis of outcomes. *Cancer* 2000; **90**: 87–95.

92 Schindler S, Pooley Jr RJ, De Frias DV, Yu GH, Bedrossian CW. Follow-up of atypical glandular cells in cervical-endocervical smears. *Ann Diagn Pathol* 1998; **2**: 312–17.

93 Cina SJ, Richardson MS, Austin RM, Kurman RJ. Immunohistochemical staining for Ki-67 antigen, carcinoembryonic antigen, and p53 in the differential diagnosis of glandular lesions of the cervix. *Mod Pathol* 1997; **10**: 176–80.

94 Mittal K. Utility of proliferation-associated marker MIB-1 in evaluating lesions of the uterine cervix. *Adv Anat Pathol* 1999; **6**: 177–85.

95 Nakamura T, Nomura S, Sakai T, Nariya S. Expression of *bcl-2* oncoprotein in gastrointestinal and uterine carcinomas and their premalignant lesions. *Hum Pathol* 1997; **28**: 309–15.

96 Liao SY, Stanbridge EJ. Expression of the MN antigen in cervical Papanicolaou smears is an early diagnostic biomarker of cervical dysplasia. *Cancer Epidemiol Biomarkers Prev* 1996; **5**: 549–57.

97 Liao SY, Stanbridge EJ. Expression of MN/CA9 protein in Papanicolaou smears containing atypical glandular cells of undetermined significance is a diagnostic biomarker of cervical dysplasia and neoplasia. *Cancer* 2000; **88**: 1108–21.

98 Lu D, Tawfik O, Pantazis C, Hobart W, Chapman J, Iczkowski K. Altered expression of CD44 and variant isoforms in human adenocarcinoma of the endocervix during progression. *Gynecol Oncol* 1999; **75**: 84–90.

99 Kase H, Kodama S, Tanaka K. Observations of high iron diamine-alcian blue stain in uterine cervical glandular lesions. *Gynecol Obstet Invest* 1999; **48**: 56–60.

100 Lapertosa G, Baracchini P, Fulcheri E, Tanzi R. Patterns of mucous secretion in normal and pathological conditions of the endocervix. *Eur J Gynaecol Oncol* 1986; **7**: 113–19.

101 Maes G, Fleuren GJ, Bara J, Nap M. The distribution of mucins, carcinoembryonic antigen, and mucus-associated antigens in endocervical and endometrial adenocarcinomas. *Int J Gynecol Pathol* 1988; **7**: 112–22.

11

Endometrial cells and extrauterine carcinoma

DAVID R GENEST

HISTORICAL OVERVIEW OF ENDOMETRIAL CELLS ON PAP SMEAR

As early as 1962, Koss and Durfee reported on the significance of endometrial cells on vaginal cytological smears.[1] This important early paper used a composite definition for the term of 'abnormal endometrial cells' which included the following: (1) cytologically atypical endometrial cells; (2) normal-looking endometrial cells in postmenopausal patients; (3) endometrial cells after day 10 of the cycle; (4) numerous histiocytes; (5) abundant blood; and (6) an elevated maturation index in postmenopausal women. (Note that criteria 1 and 2 are analogous to the criteria currently used by the Bethesda System, as further discussed in Chapter 9.) Using the foregoing composite definition of 'abnormal endometrial cells' on vaginal cytology, Koss and Durfee reported that 65 per cent of 80 patients with symptomatic endometrial adenocarcinoma had abnormal endometrial cells present. Furthermore, 63 per cent of 85 asymptomatic patients with abnormal endometrial cells on vaginal cytology had significant endometrial pathology on follow-up, such as cancer (26 per cent), hyperplasia (27 per cent), polyps (8 per cent) and endometritis (2 per cent).

A number of questions concerning abnormal endometrial cells on vaginal cytology raised by the important early study of Koss and Durfee have been more fully addressed by subsequent studies over the subsequent 35 years. These questions and their answers in the subsequent medical literature are summarized in the remainder of this section.

Endometrial cells on premenopausal Pap smear

The first question raised was: is the shedding of endometrial cells on Pap smears from premenopausal women influenced by the menstrual cycle and method of contraception? Several investigators have demonstrated that approximately 20–40 per cent of Pap smears taken during the menstrual or early proliferative phase (days 1–10) contain endometrial cells that appear benign.[2,3] In contrast, only 2 per cent of Pap smears taken from day 11 through menses have endometrial cells present.[2] It has also been demonstrated that rates of endometrial cell exfoliation on Pap smear are strongly influenced by the contraceptive method: endometrial exfoliation rates are doubled by the intrauterine device and halved by oral contraceptives.[3]

Cytologically benign endometrial cells in premenopausal versus postmenopausal patients

PREMENOPAUSAL

Several studies have shown that 'normal' endometrial cells on Pap smears of premenopausal women (especially those under the age of 40 years) are rarely, if ever, associated with malignancy. Ng et al.[4] and Gondos and King[5] found no adenocarcinomas among women who were less than 40 years of age and had benign-appearing endometrial cells on Pap smear.

POSTMENOPAUSAL

Among older women, the rates of cancer associated with endometrial cells on Pap smears in the two foregoing studies were 2 per cent at ages 40–49 years, 4 per cent at ages 50–59 years and 13 per cent at ages above 59 years.[4,5] Furthermore, Cherkis et al.[6] found endometrial cancer in 21 per cent of women above the age of 59 years who had 'normal' endometrial cells on pap smear. These findings indicate that a woman's age and/or menopausal status strongly influence the significance of endometrial cells on Pap smear, and that in postmenopausal women benign endometrial cells should be reported as an abnormality that needs further investigation.

It is possible that the presence of postmenopausal bleeding and the use of hormone replacement therapy may modify the risk of cancer associated with benign endometrial cells on Pap smear in postmenopausal women. A recent study (which did not control for bleeding or exogenous hormones) found that 15 per cent of postmenopausal patients with benign endometrial cells on Pap smear had endometrial carcinoma.[7] However, another study of benign-appearing endometrial cells in postmenopausal women found that abnormal bleeding was the significant factor.[8] The prevalence of hyperplasia/carcinoma was 10 per cent with postmenopausal bleeding versus 0 per cent with no bleeding in the presence of endometrial cells on Pap smears.[8] The preliminary results of a recent study of women undergoing hormone replacement therapy showed that women receiving hormones are 41 per cent more likely to shed benign endometrial cells on Pap smear (1.4 per cent with hormones versus 0.99 per cent without hormones), but much less likely to have endometrial carcinoma when endometrial cells were present on the Pap smears (1.3 per cent with hormones versus 3.4 per cent without hormones).[9]

Utility of vaginal pool sample in the detection of endometrial carcinoma on Pap smear

Although Koss and Durfee initially made this suggestion in 1962,[1] no subsequent study has directly compared the sensitivities of specimens from these two anatomical sites (vaginal pool versus cervix) for the detection of endometrial carcinoma. However, several large studies using Pap smears from either the vaginal pool or the cervix in the general ('low-risk') populations have found comparable sensitivities for the detection of endometrial cancer. For example, Mitchell et al.[10] and Koss et al.,[11] studying cervical samples and cervico-vaginal samples, respectively, reported a sensitivity of 28 per cent. Such low sensitivities strongly support the proposition by

Burk et al.[12] that Pap smears should not be viewed as a method to routinely screen the general population for endometrial adenocarcinoma.

Histiocytes and an elevated maturation index

Despite the early suggestion by Koss and Durfee,[1] subsequent cytological studies have failed to substantiate any significant independent associations between either histiocytes or an elevated maturation index and endometrial cancer.[13–15] Blumenfeld et al.[13] compared the sensitivity and specificity of endometrial cells alone on Pap smear with those of endometrial cells with histiocytes on Pap smear for detecting endometrial cancer in postmenopausal women. The addition of 'histiocytes' to 'endometrial cells' as criteria for further evaluation increased the sensitivity from 61 per cent to 82 per cent, but decreased the specificity from 99 per cent to 67 per cent.[13] The latter result led to 33-times more 'false-positives' (i.e. an increase in false-positive rate from 1 per cent to 33 per cent). Zucker et al. further assessed this issue in a study of postmenopausal Pap smears.[15] Regression analysis was used to determine the individual influences of histiocytes, maturation index and endometrial cells on the cytological identification of endometrial cancers. They demonstrated that neither histiocytes nor maturation index was independently associated with endometrial cancer; however, endometrial cells on Pap smear were strongly associated with endometrial cancer ($P = 0.0001$).[15] In addition, they found that the degree of atypia of endometrial cells is very closely linked to the likelihood of endometrial cancer (see next paragraph). A recent post-Bethesda study of histiocytes on Pap smears confirmed their lack of independently predictive value for endometrial cancer.[14]

Atypical endometrial cells

Zucker et al., in their study of postmenopausal Pap smears, graded the degree of cytological atypia of endometrial cells as absent, atypical, suspicious or positive.[15] The rates of endometrial cancer were 0 per cent, 33 per cent, 66 per cent and 100 per cent for these categories, respectively. Cherkis et al.[6] graded endometrial cytological atypia as type I (nuclear enlargement and increased nucleus-to-cytoplasm ratio), type II (type I characteristics plus hyperchromasia or altered chromatin), or type III (type II characteristics plus prominent nucleoli). With this schema, they found endometrial cancer rates to be 0 per cent, 13 per cent and 41 per cent among women with endometrial cells showing type I, II and III atypia, respectively.[6] Yancey et al.[16] classified endometrial cells as typical, atypical (nuclear enlargement, overlapping, molding, and hyperchromasia) or suspicious (three-dimensional molded groups, nucleoli, and extensive chromatin clumping). Based on this grading system, endometrial cancer rates in premenopausal women were 0 per cent, 0 per cent and 100 per cent, and in postmenopausal women were 0 per cent, 23 per cent and 61 per cent, for typical, atypical and suspicious categories, respectively.

Collectively, the foregoing results strongly suggest that endometrial cytological atypia warrants histological evaluation, regardless of the patient's age or menopausal status. Several post-Bethesda studies of atypical glandular cells of undetermined significance (AGUS) have found that 40–80 per cent of patients with Pap smears diagnosed as 'AGUS, favor endometrial neoplasia' had carcinoma on follow-up.[17–19] Furthermore, even when the diagnosis of AGUS is not further qualified as suggesting an endometrial origin, several studies have found a substantial risk for endometrial cancer (up to 10 per cent).[18–20] This suggests that in postmenopausal women with AGUS, it is prudent to evaluate both the cervix and the endometrium by tissue sampling.

Factors that influence the detectability of endometrial carcinoma

Do tumor-related factors, such as grade, stage, and histological type, influence the detectability of endometrial cancer on Pap smear? This question has been addressed by several studies. As expected, high-grade tumors, high-stage tumors and tumors with non-endometrioid histology are more readily detected cytologically. Kim and Underwood[21] found that the percentage of endometrioid tumors with positive or suspicious cytology depended upon histological architectural grade (grade 1 = 25 per cent ; grade 2 = 44 per cent, and grade 3 = 50 per cent). Schneider et al.[22] demonstrated that an increasing histological architectural grade or an increasing histological nuclear grade rendered a higher proportion of suspicious or positive Pap smears (architectural grade 1 = 55 per cent, architectural grade 2 = 53 per cent and architectural grade 3 = 75 per cent; nuclear grade 1 = 63 per cent ; nuclear grade 2 = 80 per cent and nuclear grade 3 = 86 per cent). Conversely, Costa et al.[23] showed strong associations between 'false' negative Pap smears and the following features: endometrioid histology ($P < 0.005$), grade 1–2 tumors ($P < 0.005$), stage 1 tumors ($P < 0.005$) and 'small' tumor size ($P < 0.05$).

Collectively, these results suggest an explanation for the low sensitivity (approximately 25 per cent) of endometrial cancer detection by Pap smear: at the time of initial presentation the majority of endometrial cancers are tumors with a low stage, a low grade, and an endometrioid histology (all of which compromise the cytopathologist's best efforts).

CURRENT STATUS OF ENDOMETRIAL CELLS ON PAP SMEAR

The 1988 Bethesda System for reporting cervical/vaginal cytological diagnoses[24,25] recommended that endometrial cells be reported as 'epithelial cell abnormalities' if they fall into one of the three categories: cytologically benign endometrial cells (glandular or stromal) in a postmenopausal woman; atypical endometrial glandular cells of undetermined significance; endometrial adenocarcinoma. These categories are discussed below.

Cytologically benign endometrial cells (glandular or stromal) in a postmenopausal woman

According to the Bethesda System, cytologically benign endometrial cells need not be reported in premenopausal women.

As shown in the first section of this chapter (Historical Overview), endometrial cells are often found on Pap smears in premenopausal women but rarely, if ever, associated with cancer. The explanatory notes on the endometrial cells section in the Bethesda System imply that benign appearing endometrial cells in postmenopausal women on hormonal therapy may not be as significant as in women not using hormones.[25] Preliminary data from a recent study supported this assumption.[9] Olmstead et al. reported that two (1.3 per cent) of 154 women who were on hormone replacement therapy and had benign appearing endometrial cells on Pap smear were found on follow-up to have endometrial cancer compared with eight (3.4 per cent) of 232 women who were not on hormones and had benign appearing endometrial cells on Pap smear.[9] Both of the women who were on hormone replacement therapy and found to have carcinoma on follow-up for endometrial cells on Pap smear had abnormal vaginal bleeding.[9]

Criteria in the Bethesda System for categorizing endometrial cells have been fully described and well illustrated in the 1994 monograph by Kurman and Solomon.[25] Cytologically benign endometrial cells may appear as single cells or more commonly cell clusters (Fig. 11.1).

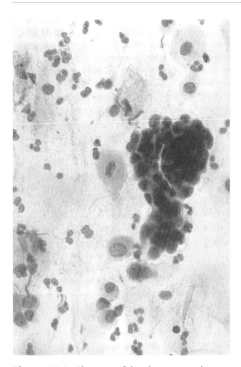

Figure 11.1 *Clusters of benign-appearing endometrial cells in a premenopausal woman (day 7 of menstrual cycle). The nuclear size of endometrial cells is similar to that of adjacent intermediate squamous cells. The nuclei are relatively regular but slightly crowded and without nucleoli; the cytoplasm is scant and inconspicuous (conventional smear, original magnification ×100).*

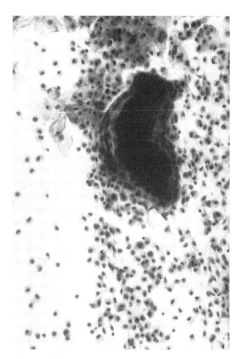

Figure 11.2 *Exodus body (endometrial cells spontaneously exfoliated from menstrual endometrium); day 8 of menstrual cycle. There is a central hyperchromatic core of tightly compacted stromal cells and a peripheral collar of endometrial epithelium. The background contains numerous small, individual stromal cells and histiocytes (conventional smear, original magnification ×40).*

With menses and other causes of stromal breakdown, endometrial cells often appear as 'blue balls' (Fig. 11.2), which are double-contoured masses with central stromal cells and peripheral epithelial cells. Endometrial epithelial nuclei are approximately the size of intermediate squamous nuclei with small, inconspicuous nucleoli; there is scant, basophilic cytoplasm. Endometrial stromal cells are spindled, with small, oval nuclei, and scant cytoplasm (Fig. 11.3).

The differential diagnosis of spontaneously exfoliated endometrial cells on Pap smears includes the following entities: (1) lower uterine segment direct endometrial sampling (Fig. 11.4), characterized by relatively well-preserved large tissue sheets of stroma surrounding tubular glands with occasional mitoses;[26] (2) lymphocytes as seen in follicular cervicitis and usually associated with tingible body; (3) histiocytes, which may closely resemble endometrial stromal cells (Fig. 11.3); (4) cervical endometriosis; (5) endocervical tubal metaplasia (cilia are a characteristic feature, although they may be difficult to spot); (6) high-grade (syncytial) squamous intraepithelial lesion; (7) endocervical glandular neoplasia; and (8) small cell carcinoma, which may closely resemble clusters of stromal breakdown, however, numerous mitoses may be present.

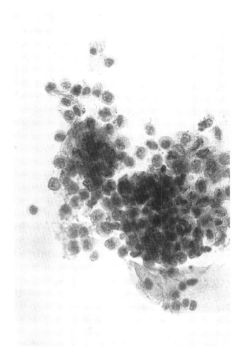 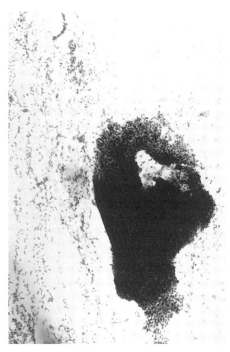

Figure 11.3 *Endometrial stromal cells (day 8 of menstrual cycle). These cells have round to oval nuclei and slightly spindled cytoplasm; many cells closely resemble histiocytes (conventional smear, original magnification ×100).*

Figure 11.4 *Directly sampled endometrial cells from lower uterine segment. Several large sheets of endometrial glandular and stromal cells were identified. Although this finding was mentioned in the cytological diagnosis (endometrial cells consistent with direct lower uterine sampling), it was not reported as a significant abnormality (conventional smear, original magnification ×20).*

Atypical endometrial glandular cells of undetermined significance

Cytologically atypical endometrial cells of undetermined significance are characterized by slight nuclear enlargement and hyperchromasia, small nucleoli and occasionally vacuolated cytoplasm (Figs 11.5–11.7); they usually occur in small groups of 5 to 10 cells. According to the Bethesda definition, atypical endometrial cells of undetermined significance imply a borderline category, exhibiting nuclear atypia exceeding obviously benign reactive/reparative changes, but lacking unequivocal features of invasive adenocarcinoma. The clinical significance of such atypical endometrial cells has not been determined. The significance of varying degree of atypia in endometrial cells on Pap smear as defined by different investigators was reviewed in the previous section.

Endometrial adenocarcinoma

Cells from endometrial adenocarcinoma are characterized by variations in nuclear size and polarity, hyperchromasia, irregular chromatin distribution, parachromatin clearing,

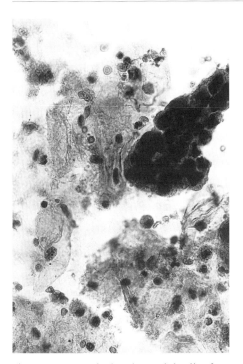

Figure 11.5 *Atypical endometrial cells of undetermined significance in a postmenopausal woman; a subsequent endometrial curettage demonstrated an endometrial polyp. There is slight nuclear enlargement, hyperchromasia and irregularity (conventional smear, original magnification ×100).*

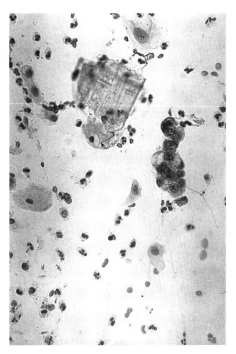

Figure 11.6 *Atypical endometrial cells of undetermined significance; these were found in a 40-year-old woman with an intrauterine device. Several small clusters of endometrial cells were present; in the endometrial cluster illustrated, there is vacuolated cytoplasm and slight nuclear enlargement (conventional smear, original magnification ×40).*

prominent nucleoli and cytoplasmic vacuolization (Figs 11.8 and 11.9). Single cells and small, loose clusters are found. A watery, finely granular tumor diathesis is sometimes seen in the background.

FUTURE DIRECTIONS OF ENDOMETRIAL CELLS ON PAP SMEAR

Computer technology

Will computer technology improve the sensitivity of the Pap smear for the detection of endometrial cancer? Preliminary reports suggest that the use of the PAPNET (see Chapter 3) cytological screening system for quality control of cervical smears may not alter the low sensitivity for endometrial cancer.[27] One recent PAPNET study stated that retrospective PAPNET screening correctly identified 15 out of 16 neoplastic smears; however, these were all cervical tumors. The one missed tumor in this study was an endometrial carcinoma with a single cluster of vacuolated cancer cells.[27]

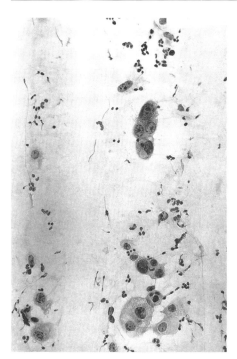

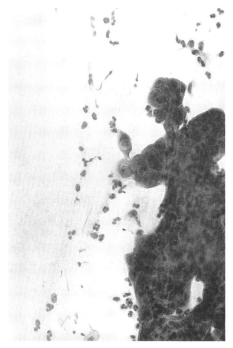

Figure 11.7 *Atypical endometrial cells of undetermined significance in a postmenopausal woman; well-differentiated mucinous adenocarcinoma of the endometrium was found. Small clusters of vacuolated endometrial cells with moderate nuclear atypia were present (conventional smear, original magnification ×40).*

Figure 11.8 *Adenocarcinoma of the endometrium, characterized by numerous crowded sheets of atypical endometrial cells in a postmenopausal patient; this was diagnosed as 'suspicious' for endometrial carcinoma. Well-differentiated endometrial adenocarcinoma was found at hysterectomy (conventional smear, original magnification ×40).*

Preoperative cervicovaginal smear in patients with endometrial cancer

Several recent reports have suggested that the presence of malignant endometrial cells in preoperative cervical cytology is strongly associated with high-grade endometrial tumors or with deep myometrial invasion, cervical involvement, or extrauterine spread to pelvic and para-aortic lymph nodes.[28–31] Another report suggested that the cervical smear may be superior to endocervical curettage for identifying cervical involvement by endometrial cancer.[32] Two patterns of malignant endometrial cells were noted on Pap smear in this study: (1) a 'sloughing' pattern, indicative of insignificant tumor exfoliation (characterized by rounded, three-dimensional cell balls); and (2) an 'abraded' pattern, indicative of direct sampling of cervical metastatic tumor (characterized by loosely cohesive sheet-like cell groups displaying 'natural cellular configurations' with frayed edges). This observation needs to be confirmed in other studies before they can be applied for clinical purposes.

Postoperative vaginal smear in patients with endometrial carcinoma

A recent study by Shumsky et al.[33] showed that routine vaginal cytological follow-up may have little use in the identification of recurrences following surgery for endometrial cancer. Although

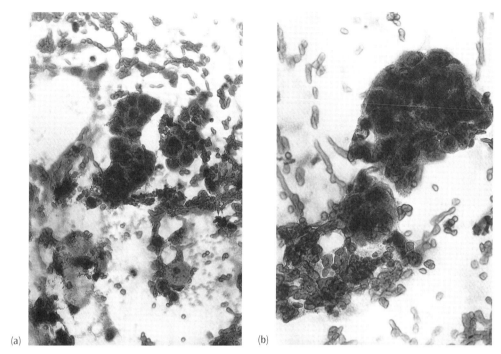

(a) (b)

Figure 11.9 *Adenocarcinoma of the endometrium. Premenopausal woman with irregular bleeding; Pap smear showed abundant blood, and numerous clusters of highly atypical endometrial cells, with nuclear crowding, chromatin clumping and prominent nucleoli. This was diagnosed as positive for adenocarcinoma, consistent with endometrial primary; a poorly differentiated endometrial carcinoma was found at hysterectomy. Conventional smear, original magnification ×40 in (a) and ×100 in (b).*

clinical follow-up identified 53 vaginal recurrences among 317 patients treated by hysterectomy for endometrial carcinoma, none of these were 'occult' recurrences identified initially by positive cytology alone.[33]

Directly sampled endometrial cytology and cancer surveillance

In the 1980s and 1990s, numerous studies have investigated the cytology of the directly sampled endometrium. Although reports suggest that the sensitivity of this technique for the identification of endometrial cancer may be very high (90–97 per cent), this method has not gained wide acceptance.[11,34,35] One reason could be resistance among gynecologists, who consider tissue sampling the gold standard for evaluation of the endometrium. Even advocates of direct endometrial sampling concede that symptomatic (bleeding) patients should be evaluated by endometrial biopsy rather than by directly sampled cytology.[36] Thus, the unresolved question is whether direct endometrial cytology is useful for the evaluation of asymptomatic women.

The direct endometrial sample is obtained by aspiration with a cannula, or scraping with an Endocyte or Endopap sampler or brushing with a cytobrush. In earlier reports, the sampling tool was immediately smeared onto two or three slides before ethanol fixation.[11] More recently, brush samples have been liquid-fixed then centrifuged, yielding four to six slides per case.[37] In addition, any grossly identifiable tissue fragments are removed and processed histologically as cellblocks or mini-biopsies (as discussed below, this is very important for identifying malignant cases).

In the early report by Koss et al.[11] about 1 per cent of endometrial samples in asymptomatic women was positive or suspicious, and approximately 5 per cent were atypical. Among 2586 samples, 11 were positive (follow-up: nine cancers and two negatives), 16 were suspicious (follow-up: seven cancers, four hyperplasias, and five negatives), 125 were atypical (follow-up: one cancer, 17 hyperplasias, and 107 negatives), and 2434 were negative (with four cancers subsequently detected).[11] In this study, the sensitivity and specificity of abnormal cytology (atypical, suspicious or positive) for an abnormal endometrium (hyperplasia or cancer) were 90 per cent and 96 per cent, respectively.

In a more recent study by van Hoeven et al.,[36] only four out of 1983 (about 0.2 per cent) of samples were positive or suspicious (all four had cancer on follow-up); in addition, 21 out of 1983 (1 per cent) were atypical (one had cancer on follow-up). The sensitivity and specificity of abnormal cytology for endometrial cancer in this study were 83 per cent and 99 per cent, respectively.

In directly sampled endometrial specimens, cytological features of endometrial hyperplasia and low-grade carcinoma may overlap.[37] High-grade carcinomas are generally readily diagnosed owing to considerable nuclear atypia, loss of polarity, hypercellularity, solid cell aggregates, tumor diathesis and absence of stroma. At the other end of the malignancy spectrum, however, low-grade carcinomas and atypical hyperplasias may be indistinguishable: both have moderate nuclear atypia, some retention of polarity, and a paucity of stroma. In this setting, marked cellularity and a tumor diathesis would favor carcinoma.

Most reports concerning directly sampled endometrial cytology state that the histological evaluation of tissue fragments (cellblock or mini-biopsy) is very important in cases with malignancy. In one recent study, the diagnostic accuracy for directly sampled endometrial cytology alone versus directly sampled endometrial cytology combined with cell block or mini-biopsy was 56 per cent (cytology alone) versus 100 per cent (cytology and histology) for atypical hyperplasia, 67 per cent (cytology alone) versus 100 per cent (cytology and histology) for low grade carcinoma, and 85 per cent (cytology alone) versus 100 per cent (cytology and histology) for high grade carcinoma.[37]

EXTRAUTERINE CARCINOMA ON PAP SMEAR

Occasionally, extrauterine cancer cells are present on Pap smear. This most commonly occurs with advanced-stage adenocarcinoma of the ovary, gastrointestinal tract or breast; other metastatic tumors such as melanoma, lymphoma, sarcoma or squamous cell carcinoma are extremely rare.[38–40] In comparison with cervical or endometrial adenocarcinomas, the malignant cells from extrauterine adenocarcinomas are often found in a clean background, without tumor diathesis or blood. Psammoma bodies may be seen with ovarian or fallopian tubal primary cancers (as well as with endometrial papillary serous tumors, ovarian borderline tumors, peritoneal adenocarcinomas, pancreatic carcinoma, intrauterine devices and various benign conditions). Malignant cells will be present on Pap smears in approximately 20–30 per cent of ovarian and tubal cancers; they tend to be large, frankly malignant cells (larger than endometrial adenocarcinoma cells), present in papillary clusters or as single cells, with prominent nucleoli, occasionally with psammoma bodies, in a clean background (Fig. 11.10). Mucinous ovarian tumors may have a prominently vacuolated cytoplasm. Borderline serous neoplasia tends to have more psammoma bodies, and less pronounced cytological atypia. A recent study of extrauterine malignancies diagnosed by Pap smear[38] reported that the

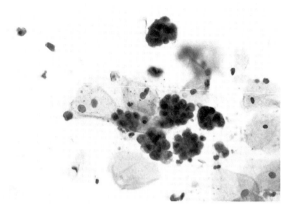

Figure 11.10 *Papillary serous carcinoma of the ovary. Previously healthy premenopausal woman with increasing abdominal girth for 2 weeks; Pap smear showed many papillary clusters of atypical epithelial cells with nuclear molding and overlapping in a clean background. Occasional psammoma bodies were also found. This was diagnosed as positive for papillary serous carcinoma consistent with an ovarian primary tumor. Cytology of the peritoneal and pleural fluids a few days later showed similar cell clusters; the patient expired 3 weeks later without surgery or autopsy (conventional smear, original magnification ×40).*

majority of tumors originated in the ovary (49 per cent), gastrointestinal tract (18 per cent) or breast (18 per cent), and that in the great majority of cases (85 per cent) there was a known history of a primary tumor at the time of the positive Pap smear.

REFERENCES

1 Koss LG, Durfee GR. Cytologic diagnosis of endometrial adenocarcioma. Result of ten years of experience. *Acta Cytol* 1962; **6**: 519–31.
2 Liu W, Barrow MJ, Spitler MF, Kochis AF. Normal exfoliation of endometrial cells in premenopausal women. *Acta Cytol* 1963; **7**: 211–14.
3 Vooijs GP, van der Graaf Y, Vooijs MA. The presence of endometrial cells in cervical smears in relation to the day of the menstrual cycle and the method of contraception. *Acta Cytol* 1987; **31**: 427–33.
4 Ng AB, Reagan JW, Hawliczek S, Wentz BW. Significance of endometrial cells in the detection of endometrial carcinoma and its precursors. *Acta Cytol* 1974; **18**: 356–61.
5 Gondos B, King EB. Significance of endometrial cells in cervicovaginal smears. *Ann Clin Lab Sci* 1977; **7**: 486–90.
6 Cherkis RC, Patten Jr SF, Dickinson JC, Dekanich AS. Significance of atypical endometrial cells detected by cervical cytology. *Obstet Gynecol* 1987; **69**: 786–9.
7 Wu HH-J, Schuetz MJ, Cramer HM. Benign endometrial cells in postmenopausal women: a study of 61 cases with histologic follow-up (Abstr). *Acta Cytol* 1999; **43**: 912.
8 Gomez-Fernandez CR, Ganjei-Azar P, Capote-Dishaw J, Averette HE, Nadji M. Reporting normal endometrial cells in Pap smears: an outcome appraisal. *Gynecol Oncol* 1999; **74**: 381–4.
9 Olmstead J, Mount S, Drejet A. Benign endometrial cells on the Papanicolaou smear in women over the age of 50 taking hormone replacement therapy (Abstr). *Acta Cytol* 1999; **43**: 913.
10 Mitchell H, Giles G, Medley G. Accuracy and survival benefit of cytological prediction of endometrial carcinoma on routine cervical smears. *Int J Gynecol Pathol* 1993; **12**: 34–40.

11 Koss LG, Schreiber K, Oberlander SG, Moussouris HF, Lesser M. Detection of endometrial carcinoma and hyperplasia in asymptomatic women. *Obstet Gynecol* 1984; **64**: 1–11.

12 Burk JR, Lehman HF, Wolf FS. Inadequacy of papanicolaou smears in the detection of endometrial cancer. *N Engl J Med* 1974; **291**: 191–2.

13 Blumenfeld W, Holly EA, Mansur DL, King EB. Histiocytes and the detection of endometrial adenocarcinoma. *Acta Cytol* 1985; **29**: 317–22.

14 Nguyen TN, Bourdeau JL, Ferenczy A, Franco EL. Clinical significance of histiocytes in the detection of endometrial adenocarcinoma and hyperplasia. *Diagn Cytopathol* 1998; **19**: 89–93.

15 Zucker PK, Kasdon EJ, Feldstein ML. The validity of Pap smear parameters as predictors of endometrial pathology in menopausal women. *Cancer* 1985; **56**: 2256–63.

16 Yancey M, Magelssen D, Demaurez A, Lee RB. Classification of endometrial cells on cervical cytology. *Obstet Gynecol* 1990; **76**: 1000–5.

17 Duska LR, Flynn CF, Chen A, Whall-Strojwas D, Goodman A. Clinical evaluation of atypical glandular cells of undetermined significance on cervical cytology. *Obstet Gynecol* 1998; **91**: 278–82.

18 Eddy GL, Strumpf KB, Wojtowycz MA, Piraino PS, Mazur MT. Biopsy findings in five hundred thirty-one patients with atypical glandular cells of uncertain significance as defined by the Bethesda system. *Am J Obstet Gynecol* 1997; **177**: 1188–95.

19 Eddy GL, Wojtowycz MA, Piraino PS, Mazur MT. Papanicolaou smears by the Bethesda system in endometrial malignancy: utility and prognostic importance. *Obstet Gynecol* 1997; **90**: 999–1003.

20 Veljovich DS, Stoler MH, Andersen WA, Covell JL, Rice LW. Atypical glandular cells of undetermined significance: a five-year retrospective histopathologic study. *Am J Obstet Gynecol* 1998; **179**: 382–90.

21 Kim HS, Underwood D. Adenocarcinomas in the cervicovaginal Papanicolaou smear: analysis of a 12-year experience. *Diagn Cytopathol* 1991; **7**: 119–24.

22 Schneider ML, Wortmann M, Weigel A. Influence of the histologic and cytologic grade and the clinical and postsurgical stage on the rate of endometrial carcinoma detection by cervical cytology. *Acta Cytol* 1986; **30**: 616–22.

23 Costa MJ, Kenny MB, Naib ZM. Cervicovaginal cytology in uterine adenocarcinoma and adenosquamous carcinoma. Comparison of cytologic and histologic findings. *Acta Cytol* 1991; **35**: 127–34.

24 The 1988 Bethesda System for reporting cervical/vaginal cytologic diagnoses: developed and approved at the National Cancer Institute Workshop in Bethesda, Maryland, December 12–13, 1988. *Hum Pathol* 1990; **21**: 704–8.

25 Kurman RJ, Soloman D. *The Bethesda system for reporting cervical/vaginal cytologic diagnosis: Definitions, criteria and explanatory notes for terminology and specimen adequacy.* New York: Springer-Verlag, 1994.

26 de Peralta-Venturino MN, Purslow MJ, Kini SR. Endometrial cells of the 'lower uterine segment' (LUS) in cervical smears obtained by endocervical brushings: a source of potential diagnostic pitfall. *Diagn Cytopathol* 1995; **12**: 263–8; discussion 8–71.

27 Koss LG, Lin E, Schreiber K, Elgert P, Mango L. Evaluation of the PAPNET cytologic screening system for quality control of cervical smears. *Am J Clin Pathol* 1994; **101**: 220–9.

28 Demirkiran F, Arvas M, Erkun E, et al. The prognostic significance of cervico-vaginal cytology in endometrial cancer. *Eur J Gynaecol Oncol* 1995; **16**: 403–9.

29 DuBeshter B. Endometrial cancer: predictive value of cervical cytology [editorial; comment]. *Gynecol Oncol* 1999; **72**: 271–2.

30 DuBeshter B, Warshal DP, Angel C, Dvoretsky PM, Lin JY, Raubertas RF. Endometrial carcinoma: the relevance of cervical cytology. *Obstet Gynecol* 1991; **77**: 458–62.

31 Larson DM, Johnson KK, Reyes Jr CN, Broste SK. Prognostic significance of malignant cervical cytology in patients with endometrial cancer. *Obstet Gynecol* 1994; **84**: 399–403.

32 Zuna RE, Erroll M. Utility of the cervical cytologic smear in assessing endocervical involvement by endometrial carcinoma. *Acta Cytol* 1996; **40**: 878–84.

33 Shumsky AG, Stuart GC, Brasher PM, Nation JG, Robertson DI, Sangkarat S. An evaluation of routine follow-up of patients treated for endometrial carcinoma. *Gynecol Oncol* 1994; **55**: 229–33.

34 Bistoletti P, Hjerpe A, Mollerstrom G. Cytological diagnosis of endometrial cancer and preinvasive endometrial lesions. A comparison of the Endo-Pap sampler with fractional curettage. *Acta Obstet Gynecol Scand* 1988; **67**: 343–5.

35 LaPolla JP, Nicosia S, McCurdy C, et al. Experience with the EndoPap device for the cytologic detection of uterine cancer and its precursors: a comparison of the EndoPap with fractional curettage or hysterectomy. *Am J Obstet Gynecol* 1990; **163**: 1055–9; discussion 9–60.

36 van Hoeven KH, Zaman SS, Deger RB, Artymyshyn RL. Efficacy of the Endo-pap sampler in detecting endometrial lesions. *Acta Cytol* 1996; **40**: 900–6.

37 Maksem JA, Knesel E. Liquid fixation of endometrial brush cytology ensures a well-preserved, representative cell sample with frequent tissue correlation. *Diagn Cytopathol* 1996; **14**: 367–73.

38 Gupta D, Balsara G. Extrauterine malignancies. Role of Pap smears in diagnosis and management. *Acta Cytol* 1999; **43**: 806–13.

39 Ng AB, Teeple D, Lindner EA, Reagan JW. The cellular manifestations of extrauterine cancer. *Acta Cytol* 1974; **18**: 108–17.

40 Takashina T, Ono M, Kanda Y, Sagae S, Hayakawa O, Ito E. Cervicovaginal and endometrial cytology in ovarian cancer. *Acta Cytol* 1988; **32**: 159–62.

Index